ENDORSEMENT

"This book offers the most comprehensive and up-to-date resource for yoga therapists and mental health professionals in the field of mental health that I have seen. It is a needed text in the field and will be valuable to all who want not just an overview but an in-depth exploration of the connections between yoga and mental health and the possibilities for its application. The contributors to the book are all knowledgeable and respected members of their respective communities. Heather Mason and Kelly Birch have achieved the seemingly impossible to gather together such a remarkable collection of knowledge, wisdom, and practice in one very thoroughly researched and organized volume. The references alone are impressive, comprehensive, and helpful, and each chapter is packed with value.

The opening chapter provides a thorough overview of the history and evolution of yoga. Then follows a look at how the connection between yoga and the field of mental health has unfolded through to the present day. Comprehensive chapters on various conditions where yoga might play a role are very well informed and researched and offer practices and scope of practice guidelines for the reader. Here the yoga therapist can very quickly get a thorough primer into working with clients experiencing such conditions as depression, anxiety, or trauma and several others. Working with children has its own chapter and the book also offers a useful perspective on what the future holds in the bridging of yoga and traditional therapy.

I have no hesitation in highly recommending this book, and I have no doubt it will become required reading in many yoga therapy training programs going forward."

— **Michael Lee,** MA, Dip.Soc.Sci., ERYT-500, C-IAYT, international conference presenter and founder of Phoenix Rising Yoga Therapy

"My heart is full of joy in reading Heather Mason and Kelly Birch's beautifully edited and in-depth book on the integration of yoga and mental health. From the start, in my training as a psychologist and practitioner of yoga in the 1970s, I was fortunate to learn these as complementary approaches and how each informs and strengthens the other. When combined, each catalyzes the healing effects of the other. Yoga is educational as well as therapeutic, as indeed are Western approaches to mental health. This is their strength. Both provide tools and interventions to the student-client-practitioner that build a strong foundation of mental health. They both offer us interventions for nourishing wellbeing, resilience, and a sense of harmony within ourselves and in our relationship with the world around us. I am enriched by, and grateful for, the depth of insight, knowledge, and wisdom that comes forth in every page and chapter of Mason and Birch's book. I therefore offer a deep bow of gratitude to them, and each author, for making this seminal book available. I will be recommending *Yoga for Mental Health* to all my students who yearn for guidance, as they traverse their path to health, healing, and wholeness."

— **Richard Miller,** PhD, co-founder of the International Association of Yoga Therapists, founding editor of the *International Journal of Yoga Therapy*, and founding director of the Integrative Restoration Institute

"Mason and Birch have curated the most comprehensive explication of the science of yoga by expert scientists and scholars yet. With much confusion in the current literature and a plethora of styles in yoga studios around the globe, the contributors to the book have been able to illustrate with great clarity the essential components of yoga practices as they may apply in contemporary yoga teaching and in a therapeutic context, while being careful to not unwittingly ignore or dismiss the deepest and most subtle features of such practices. This book is a treasured resource for any integrative mental health provider interested in using yoga therapeutically in the most informed capacity."

— **David Vago**, PhD, Research Director,
  Osher Center for Integrative Medicine,
  Vanderbilt University Medical Center

"The management of mental health conditions is one of the most challenging aspects of modern healthcare, and this book provides a comprehensive, theoretically grounded, and practically applicable guide to how yoga-based practices can be used for this scope. It spans a broad range of mental health conditions, and the individual chapters written by world experts in the field beautifully outline both their commonalities and unique characteristics when it comes to therapeutic needs. It is a most significant contribution to the field of mental health and integrative healthcare, and an invaluable resource for yoga therapists, instructors and practitioners, and mental health providers alike."

— **Laura Schmalzl**, PhD, Associate Professor, Southern California University of Health Sciences (SCU) Editor in Chief, *International Journal of Yoga Therapy*

"The mind remains a mystery, but advances in neuroscience are fast overturning the idea that it's all in the brain. As psychology and psychotherapy rediscover the body as the source of emotion, the question arises as to how the flows of feeling that arise there, and that so profoundly shape how we view ourselves and the world, can be regulated. Millions of people have experienced the contribution yoga can make, but until now, health professionals wanting to understand yoga's potential as a mental health intervention had nowhere to turn. This book meets the need of those

of us who want not only to see the research evidence, but also to hear the rich experience of colleagues who have used yoga in the clinic and the classroom."

— Professor **David Peters**
  Director, Westminster Centre for Resilience
  University Polyclinic
  University of Westminster

"*Yoga for Mental Health* is a groundbreaking book for mental health professionals and yoga practitioners. It introduces mental health professionals to the power of the yoga in healing and it gives yoga practitioners the science and knowledge they need to integrate into the field of mental health. This book functions as the bridge between psychology and yoga, creating a paradigm shift and consequently transforming both fields of study. Every mental health professional should read this book if they would like to have a glimpse into the next generation of training in the field of mental health. Yoga teachers and yoga therapists can use this comprehensive guide to mental health with the goal of improved teaching and keeping their students safe."

— **Amy Wheeler**, PhD, President of the Board,
  International Association of Yoga Therapists

"Heather Mason and Kelly Birch have put together an incisive collection of chapters on the most current uses of yoga techniques in the field of mental health. This is a beautifully written and edited book that will prove invaluable for clinicians who want to be up-to-date on the latest—and very effective—uses of yoga with a wide spectrum of patients. Clinicians of all sorts will be thrilled to have this new resource."

— **Stephen Cope**, Senior Scholar in Residence, Kripalu Center for Yoga and Health, and bestselling author of *Yoga and the Quest for the True Self*

YOGA FOR MENTAL HEALTH

YOGA FOR MENTAL HEALTH

Editors
Heather Mason and Kelly Birch

Forewords
B. N. Gangadhar MD
Timothy McCall MD

Contributors

Lucy Arnsby-Wilson

Samantha Bottrill

Catherine Cook-Cottone

Holger Cramer

Laura Douglass

Michelle Fury

Patricia Gerbarg

Lana Jackson

Lisa Kaley-Isley

Sat Bir Singh Khalsa

Daniel J. Libby

Dana Moore

Lisa Sanfilippo

Shivarama Varambally

Elizabeth Visceglia

Amy Weintraub

Janice White

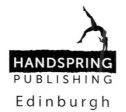

HANDSPRING
PUBLISHING
Edinburgh

HANDSPRING PUBLISHING LIMITED
The Old Manse, Fountainhall,
Pencaitland, East Lothian
EH34 5EY, Scotland
Tel: +44 1875 341 859
Website: www.handspringpublishing.com

First published 2018 in the United Kingdom by Handspring Publishing

Reprinted 2019

ISBN 978-1-909141-35-3
ISBN Kindle eBook 978-1-912085-26-2

British Library Cataloguing in Publication Data
A catalogue record for this book is available from the British Library

Library of Congress Cataloguing in Publication Data
A catalog record for this book is available from the Library of Congress

Notice
Neither the Publisher nor the Authors assume any responsibility for any loss or injury and/or damage to persons or property arising out of or relating to any use of the material contained in this book. It is the responsibility of the treating practitioner, relying on independent expertise and knowledge of the patient, to determine the best treatment and method of application for the patient.

All reasonable efforts have been made to obtain copyright clearance for illustrations in the book for which the authors or publishers do not own the rights. If you believe that one of your illustrations has been used without such clearance please contact the publishers and we will ensure that appropriate credit is given in the next reprint.

Commissioning Editor Sarena Wolfaard
Project Manager Morven Dean
Copy editor Dylan Hamilton
Chapter opening artwork Sophie Birch-Bridges
Cover artwork Brigitte McReynolds (www.brigittemcreynolds.com)
Designer Bruce Hogarth
Indexer Aptara, India
Typesetter DiTech Process Solutions, India
Printer Bell and Bain Ltd, Glasgow

The Publisher's policy is to use paper manufactured from sustainable forests

The
Publisher's
policy is to use
paper manufactured
from sustainable forests

CONTENTS

Read. 1, 2, 6

ACKNOWLEDGMENTS

I would like to thank Handspring and, in particular, Sarena Wolfaard, for believing in the vision of this book. My deep appreciation goes to my brilliant co-editor, Kelly Birch—without you none of this would have come to light—you are a gifted editor and a dear friend. To the many authors who contributed to this book, your knowledge has taught me so much about my own field—it was an honor to work with you.

I would also like to thank all my teachers whose wisdom and dedication taught me how yoga could change my life. My professional work is an organic emergence of insights that I gained in my own process of self-healing. In particular, I would like to thank Jeff Oliver and Marcus Sorenson, who have helped me to become who I am today.

Dr. Robin Monro of the Yoga Biomedical Trust, thank you for believing in me and for allowing me to teach my first course on yoga therapy for depression and anxiety all those years ago. I offer sincere thanks to Patricia Gerbarg, MD, and Sat Bir Singh Khalsa, PhD, who have helped shape my academic and professional career through their sage advice.

To my family, thank you for listening, and for providing endless feedback on my writing at the expense of your busy schedules, and to Courtenay Howe, who helped with all the little details that put everything in place.

Finally, I would like to thank Elsie, the most wonderful dog I have ever known. Her sweet and ever-loving nature is a constant reminder of how to create bliss and community. She is a true yogi.

Heather Mason

Thank you, Sarena Wolfaard, for your support and guidance, and to all the amazing team at Handspring Publishing for their various talents, and especially to Morven Dean. Thank you, Heather, my co-editor and dear friend, for having the vision to start this book and for inviting me on this extraordinary journey with you; and for your expertise, your pioneering spirit, and your moxie.

My deep gratitude goes to all of the contributors to this book—it has been my honor to work with such an outstanding collection of people, I've learned so much from you. Thank you for making this book possible.

To all the researchers and yoga practitioners for their contributions to the wealth of knowledge on yoga and mental health.

To my extended family, thank you for all your encouragement and love. Special thanks to my daughter, Sophie, for creating the drawings at the start of each chapter while busy at university. Endless gratitude to my partner, Michael, who continues to be there for me in all of the ways that matter in life.

Profound thanks to all my teachers in all their forms past and present.

Kelly Birch

PREFACE

This book is intended as a professional resource for (1) mental health professionals interested in the potential for yoga interventions that facilitate the therapeutic process, and who want to learn ways in which yoga can catalyze and deepen this process across a broad spectrum of mental health approaches; (2) yoga professionals with a focus on mental health and wellbeing who want to expand their understanding of how yoga relates to mental health approaches and their knowledge of best practices; and (3) yoga practitioners and other interested parties who want to know more about this rapidly evolving integrative approach to yoga and mental health.

Yoga is a comprehensive mind-body practice that is particularly effective for self-regulation, mood management, fostering resilience, and promotion of wellbeing. Inherently, yoga is a system for improving mental health and alleviating suffering at the deepest levels. Readers may be struck by the congruence of yogic philosophical ideas and those of modern psychology and neuroscience. Consequently, yoga's potential as a key component of integrative and complementary mental health is now being recognized internationally.

In 2012, Heather, along with Jane Ryan of Confer, co-organized a conference entitled Yoga, the Brain and Mental Health. Leading yoga researchers gave keynote speeches to hundreds of yoga teachers, yoga therapists, and mental health providers. It was there that we met for the first time and discovered our mutual love for yoga and mindfulness and their implications for mental healthcare. It was there, too, that Heather met Sarena Wolfaard from Handspring, who proposed this book as a way to share the message of yoga's efficacy in mental health with those around the world. Heather assembled an outstanding group of experts in the fields of research, mental health, and yoga who agreed to contribute their expertise, two authors collaborating on each chapter to present cutting-edge information and treatments featuring yoga and mental health conditions with a focus on wellbeing. In 2013, Heather invited Kelly to become co-editor.

About the editors

We both come from a background of extensive experience and training in the contemplative practices of yoga and mindfulness. We know first-hand the depth and breadth of the practices described in this book in the application of mental health in our own lives and the profound impact they have had, and we have seen them transform the lives of students and clients over the years.

Approach to mental health

Chapters are organized around the classifications found in the fifth edition of the *Diagnostic and Statistical Manual of Mental Disorders* (commonly referred to as the DSM-5), published by the American Psychiatric Association. This manual, the result of collaboration between several hundred contributors, is widely used by clinicians to diagnose mental health disorders and provides a common language for describing clusters of symptoms that are recognized in mental healthcare and frequently used in research. Our approach in this book is holistic: mental health conditions are considered to arise from multifactorial biological, psychological, spiritual, social, and environmental factors.

Organization

The format of the book is designed for consistency and ease of reading. Chapter 1 introduces the reader to the yogic viewpoint of mental health and wellbeing, and the psychological and neurological rationale for yoga's usage in mental health conditions. Each subsequent chapter is organized into a clinical overview of mental health conditions, followed by sections on current research and the rationale for incorporating yoga into the treatment of the condition, recommended yoga practices, and future directions.

Terms used in the book

In Chapter 1 you will find a description of how we distinguish between yoga teaching and yoga therapy. In each chapter, the terms yoga teacher and yoga therapist refer to guidelines specifically for those professional designations, and the terms yoga teacher/therapist or yoga professional refers to guidelines that apply to both. The terms mental health provider, mental health professional, clinician, and psychologist are used variously by different authors and refer to any provider in the field of mental health with recognized credentials for working independently with clients/patients. Generally, the words client and patient refer to recipients of individual yoga therapy or mental health, and student refers to an attendee of a yoga class. The term yoga is used broadly to refer to the comprehensive system described in Chapter 1 (except where specified by authors). We use the gender-neutral term they in the singular form rather than he or she.

Bridging yoga and mental healthcare

We anticipate that in future years there will be a growing integration of mental healthcare and yoga. It is our sincere hope that this book contributes to bridging these complementary disciplines and provides growing awareness of how yoga may help reduce the global burden of mental health challenges.

FOREWORD *by B. N. Gangadhar*

Yoga comes from the root word *yuj*, which means "merging," or "union." At a spiritual level, it refers to the joining of one's personal consciousness and the cosmic consciousness. In the journey toward transcendence, yoga results in several health benefits, both physical and psychological. These measurable effects are increasingly recognized by the medical world, engendering a new perspective, whereby yoga is now used to treat individuals with a variety of disease conditions.

All traditional texts on yoga allude to its effects on the mind. For example, the very second aphorism of the Patanjali *Yoga Sutras* is "*Yogah chitta vritti nirodhah*" (yoga is subduing the modifications of mind). Hence, it is not surprising that the preponderance of the applications of yoga are for mental health–related reasons. In recent years, yoga has been the focus of attention as therapy in psychiatry practice, both as a primary treatment and as an adjunct. A substantial body of literature has accumulated that can guide clinical practice with reference to applying yoga as a treatment in clinical situations. This book, *Yoga for Mental Health*, edited by Heather Mason and Kelly Birch, has chapters that are exhaustive and insightful reviews on the use of yoga in several psychiatric conditions, informing this emerging field and driving it forward. As a significant and unprecedented reference, *Yoga for Mental Health* is a unique voice guiding both mental health professionals and yoga experts on how to safely and comprehensively bring yoga into mental healthcare.

In their navigation of this topic, the editors have covered most of the common psychiatric conditions that are known to benefit from yoga (anxiety, depression, psychoses, ADHD and other childhood conditions, insomnia, trauma-related conditions, and eating disorders). Accordingly, this book makes a compelling case for including a yoga professional as a member of the mental healthcare team. Each chapter, in exploring a mental health condition from a modern perspective, followed by an analysis of the yoga perspective of this condition, research supporting yoga's efficacy, and recommendations for the use of yoga and yoga therapy in the treatment of the condition, provides a thorough foundation for the marrying of the yogic and mental healthcare worlds in a mode that best informs professionals and will lead to great benefit for patients.

In the final chapter, Future Directions, the authors have discussed the specific needs for further yoga research in mental health. This chapter is an in-depth study of the topic, offering novel insights, and deserves special appreciation. All yoga-promoters should diligently pay attention to this tenth chapter, which delineates several issues relating to yoga research in clinical populations. Each of these also merit attention by yoga researchers. As a researcher myself, I am familiar with many of these challenges and feel they must be addressed for the field to grow. The standardization of the intervention and matching yoga procedures to specific symptoms or specific mental health conditions are major issues. Importantly, yoga philosophy and practice did not evolve as a medical practice to cure diseases. Yoga scholars have described certain benefits of yoga that clinicians approximate to treat mental health. This too deserves validation and standardization. Future efforts should hence consider the challenges to match yoga research with modern mental health interventions.

In summary, yoga is lifestyle for harnessing the immense potential of the mind to heal the ailments afflicting the mind. The editors should be credited for their efforts to collate such an extensive and thought-provoking text. Without a doubt, this book serves as a ready reference for all psychiatric hospitals, clinics, and yoga therapy centers.

B. N. Gangadhar, MD, DSc
Senior Professor of Psychiatry and Program Director
NIMHANS Integrated Center for Yoga
National Institute of Mental Health and Neurosciences
Bengaluru, India
August 2018

FOREWORD *by Timothy McCall*

We are at a crisis point in mental health. Rates of clinical depression, anxiety disorders, attention-deficit diagnoses, among others, are soaring. Meanwhile, resources are stretched thin and the number of therapists inadequate to fully meet the need. Yoga is inexpensive, when skillfully applied safe, and, as the research summarized in this book demonstrates, backed by growing evidence that suggests it can help many patients on the road to improved psychological well-being. There are many ways to understand the mission of yoga. One that I favor is that we are trying to identify and help change habit patterns—of thought, word, or deed—that do not serve our clients. These could be anything from slumping posture, to rough, erratic breathing, to a tendency to judge themselves harshly. Such habits, which the yoga texts call *samskaras*, are said to deepen over time like ruts in a muddy road.

The idea is to craft a therapeutic yoga practice that facilitates the development of new counter-habits. Such a practice might consist of yoga poses, relaxation techniques, visualizations, meditation, breathing exercises, or some combination of these, depending on the situation and the client's preferences. When that practice is repeated regularly, eventually the new habits become sufficiently strong that they may start to out-compete the old ones. How long that takes depends in part on how deeply etched the old habits are in the nervous system.

Patanjali, the great codifier of yoga philosophy and practices, laid out in his second-century CE *Yoga Sutras* a formula for success in yoga: regular practice without interruption over a long period of time. Although he could not have been aware of neuroplasticity, his prescription takes advantage of it. This is why yoga teachers stress that a daily practice—even if done for a few minutes—is the best way to foster improvements in health and well-being. Longer yoga sessions if done only once or twice a week seem less effective at bringing lasting change.

Even if a new *samskara* is successfully developed, seeds of the old behavior continue to exist, yoga teaches, and this is consistent with modern neuroscience. Neural networks may attenuate with lack of use, but are prone to be reactivated if old habits recur. This is why a man who quit smoking decades ago can find out he has lost his job, stop at a bar on the way home, bum a cigarette and be up to a pack a day by morning. No one without a prior smoking *samskara* will do this. When the students of an Indian yoga therapist I interviewed ask how long they need to keep up their practice, he replies, "How long do you need to keep brushing your teeth?"

As *Yoga for Mental Health* thoroughly demonstrates, mental health disorders are often associated with dysregulation of the autonomic nervous system (ANS). Some people with anxiety disorders, for example, have an ANS that is exquisitely reactive to stress. They may find themselves responding to even seemingly minor events as if they are life-threatening. But the level of ANS reactivity, yoga teaches, can also be viewed as a *samskara*. Some people with a history of early life trauma, for example, become progressively more sensitized over time. With each new stress, the groove gets a little deeper.

Because the breath is the one autonomic function that can be controlled voluntarily, it plays a crucial role in therapeutic yoga. When the breath changes, it affects every other component of the ANS, as well as the organs it innervates. When I work with people with such disorders as insomnia or panic attacks, I consider it good news if I detect a breathing dysfunction. That is because experience has taught me that if we can re-pattern how the person breathes, it can lead to major improvements in symptoms, sometimes in short order.

Contrary to what non-practitioners might expect, not all yoga practices are relaxing. Some, like strong back-bending postures or repeated sun salutations, can be powerful stimuli of the sympathetic nervous system. When yoga students perform these challenging practices with non-judgmental awareness and slow, smooth breathing, they are learning to modulate their ANS response. What begins on a yoga mat can spread to other areas of their lives.

That is a big claim, and one that so far here I am only basing on anecdotal evidence. As persuasive as such experiences may be to the yoga therapist and client, they are not going to convince physicians, insurance companies, or scientifically minded members of the general public. For that we need research.

It is a testament to the tremendous growth in the scientific investigation of yoga that it is now possible to publish a professional-level textbook on the use of the ancient practice as well as modern adaptations of it for psychological disorders. In cataloging—and critically evaluating—the wealth of scientific data now accumulating, proposing credible mechanisms of actions for yoga's effects, and offering practical implementation guidelines for each condition covered, *Yoga for Mental Health* provides an invaluable service. Editors Heather Mason and Kelly Birch brings years of experience in both the science and the practice of yoga for psychological health and healing, and have assembled leading figures in the field to contribute individual chapters. This book will be welcomed by psychologists, psychiatrists, nurses, social workers, and the many other mental healthcare professionals who are curious about how the tools of yoga might help them do what they do better. It should also help pave the way for the increasing acceptance of this generally safe, inexpensive, and potentially life-enhancing practice by the medical profession, governmental agencies, and healthcare systems. That's a *samskara* that could make the world a calmer, healthier, and happier place.

Timothy McCall, MD
August 2018

Timothy McCall, MD, is a board-certified internist, *Yoga Journal*'s medical editor since 2002, and the author of the bestselling *Yoga as Medicine: The Yogic Prescription for Health and Healing* (Bantam Books). He co-edited and contributed to the 2016 textbook *The Principles and Practice of Yoga in Health Care* (Handspring Publishing). Dr McCall's articles have appeared in dozens of publications, including the *New England Journal of Medicine, JAMA*, and the *Los Angeles Times*, and he serves on the editorial board of the *International Journal of Yoga Therapy*. His latest book is *Saving My Neck: A Doctor's East/West Journey through Cancer* (Whole World Publishing). Timothy lives in Burlington, Vermont, and lectures and teaches yoga therapy seminars worldwide. For more information, see www.DrMcCall.com

EDITORS

Heather Mason is the founder and director of The Minded Institute, an organization that trains professionals and develops, implements, and researches innovative methods for mental health treatment based on the fusion of yoga therapy, mindfulness techniques, neuroscience, physiology, and psychotherapy. She is also the founder of the Yoga Health Care Alliance, which integrates yoga into healthcare.

Heather (RYT 500) has MAs in Psychotherapy and Buddhist Studies and an MSc in Medical Physiology; she has also completed extensive academic training in neuroscience. She is a yoga therapist and a Mindfulness-Based Cognitive Therapy facilitator. Committed to the integration of yoga into healthcare, Heather created and taught an elective at the Boston University School of Medicine for first- and second-year medical students, focusing on the neural correlates and clinical applications of yoga. She has also lectured in Harvard's Mind-Body Medicine Class alongside global leaders in mind-body medicine research. She continues to lecture at various universities on this topic.

Previously, Heather lectured on the neurobiology of PTSD, and on the neurological mechanisms of yoga and mindfulness as relevant interventions, at the world-renowned Boston Trauma Center. In 2008, she developed a program for patients with PTSD at Maudsley Hospital in London, one of the UK's leading psychiatric hospitals. As part of her mission to incorporate yoga into society, she co-organized national yoga therapy conferences in the UK. She is also a yoga researcher, and her main area of interest is how pranayama effects the central nervous system.

Heather, and other leaders within the yoga world, including researchers, NHS staff, and parliamentarians, have been meeting at the House of Lords since 2016 to work toward promoting the long-term beneficial effects of yoga on physical and mental health. In 2018, a group was formed specifically for this purpose, and Heather was nominated as the secretariat representative for the All-Party Parliamentary Group on Yoga in Society.

Kelly Birch has an MS in Clinical Mental Health Counseling and is a board-certified counselor with an integrative psychotherapy practice. She has extensive training in yoga (E-RYT 500) and yoga therapy and is certified as a yoga therapist (C-IAYT) by the International Association of Yoga Therapists (IAYT). Since 2004, Kelly has taught yoga to diverse populations including community classes and veterans, as well as to private yoga therapy clients. She has also trained in teaching mindfulness, including Mindfulness-Based Stress Reduction.

From 2010 to 2017, Kelly was the editor in chief of *Yoga Therapy Today*, the professional membership magazine published by the IAYT. She was the founding editor of the *Journal of Yoga Service*, a peer-reviewed publication of the Yoga Service Council, which she edited for two years. Kelly was copyeditor and text developer on the *Principles and Practice of Yoga in Health Care* (published by Handspring in 2016) and is currently a freelance book editor. She is also adjunct faculty at Endicott College in Massachusetts, and is a frequent guest lecturer on mindfulness and yoga at Southern Oregon University in Ashland, Oregon.

With a BA in biology, Kelly worked in scientific research in the San Francisco Bay Area for several years, as a molecular biology technologist at Stanford Health Center, a research assistant at a biotech company, and as a laboratory coordinator on a large molecular epidemiology project with Children's Hospital Oakland Research Institute and University of California, Berkeley.

CONTRIBUTORS

Lucy Arnsby-Wilson, MSc, DClinPsych
Clinical Psychologist, Yoga Therapist and Teacher Trainer
Director and founder of The Maya Project cic
www.themayaproject.org.uk, Stroud, Gloucestershire, UK

Samantha Bottrill, DClinPsy
Senior Clinical Psychologist, The Maudsley Child and
Adolescent Eating Disorder Service, London, UK, Yoga
Therapist, Senior supervisor and lecturer, The Minded
Institute London, UK

Catherine Cook-Cottone, Associate Professor, Licensed
Psychologist, Registered Yoga Instructor
Co-Editor in Chief, *Eating Disorders: Journal of Treatment and
Prevention*
Founder and President of Yogis in Service
Recent books:
*Mindfulness and Yoga in Schools: A Guide for Teachers and
Practitioners*
*Mindfulness and Yoga for Self-Regulation: A Primer for Mental
Health Professionals*
*Mindfulness for Anxious Kids: A Workbook to Help Children Cope
with Anxiety, Stress, and Worry*

Holger Cramer, PhD
Research Director at the Department of Internal and
Integrative Medicine, Kliniken Essen-Mitte, Faculty of
Medicine, University of Duisburg-Essen, Essen, Germany

Laura Lee Douglass, PhD
Dean of Professional Studies, Assistant Faculty Endicott
College, Beverly, MA, USA

Michelle J. Fury, LPC, C-IAYT
Colorado School of Medicine Faculty, Yoga Therapist,
Denver, CO, USA
Author of *Using Yoga Therapy to Promote Mental Health in
Children and Adolescents* (Handspring Publishing)

Patricia Gerbarg, MD
Assistant Clinical Professor in Psychiatry, New York Medical
College, Integrative Psychiatrist and Co-Founder of Breath-
Body-Mind, Kingston, NY, USA

Lana Jackson, BSc Hons, DClinPsych
Senior Clinical Psychologist and Yoga Therapist for Mental
Health, Sussex Partnership NHS Trust and Private Practice
Brighton, UK

Lisa Kaley-Isley, PhD, E-RYT-500, C-IAYT
Yogacampus Yoga Therapy Diploma Course, board
member, supervisor, and lecturer
The Yoga Therapy Clinic at The Life Centre, Islington,
Clinical Director
International Association of Yoga Therapists, Accreditation
committee and Advisory Council member
Life Tree Yoga with Lisa
Yoga Therapist, Yoga Therapy Educator, and Yoga Teacher

Sat Bir Singh Khalsa, PhD
Assistant Professor of Medicine, Harvard Medical School
Director of Research, Kundalini Research Institute Director
of Research, Yoga Alliance, Editor in Chief, *International
Journal of Yoga Therapy,* Boston, MA, USA
Co-editor of *Principles and Practice of Yoga in Health Care*
(Handspring Publishing)

Daniel J. Libby, PhD
Clinical Psychologist and Founder of Veterans Yoga Project
Alameda, CA, USA

Dana Moore, MAR, MA, OSB Oblate
Santa Fe, NM, USA

Lisa Sanfilippo, BSc, MSc
Yoga Therapist, Senior Yoga Teacher, Member IAYT, Teacher
Trainer, Triyoga UK and Yoga Therapy Trainer, Yogacampus
UK, Founder, Super Sleep Yoga (TM) and Sleep Recovery
Yoga (TM)

Shivarama Varambally, MD
Professor of Psychiatry and Officer-in-Charge, NIMHANS
Integrated Center for Yoga, National Institute of Mental
Health and Neurosciences, Bengaluru, India

Elizabeth Visceglia, MD, CIAYT
Assistant Clinical Professor of Psychiatry, Mount Sinai
School of Medicine, New York City, NY, USA

Amy Weintraub, MA, C-IAYT, YACEP, ERYT-500
Founder of LifeForce Yoga Healing Institute, Author of
Yoga for Depression (Broadway Books) and *Yoga Skills for
Therapists* (W.W.Norton)

Janice White MA (Traditions of Yoga & Meditation)
Yoga Therapist C-IAYT, London, UK

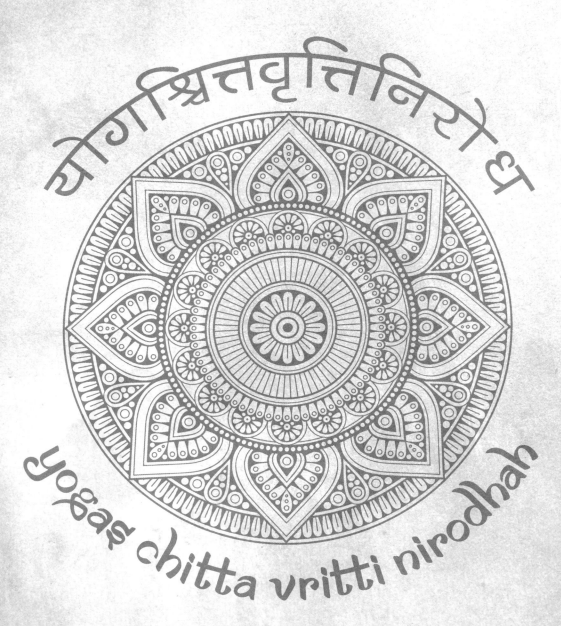

योगश्चित्तवृत्तिनिरोध

yogaş chitta vritti nirodhah

Yoga Sutra II.2 ~ Patanjali

Introduction
Heather Mason and Janice White

The growth in yoga practice

On December 11, 2014, Narendra Modi, the Prime Minister of India, appealed to the General Assembly of the United Nations (UN) to mark June 21 each year as *International Yoga Day*, declaring that yoga "embodies unity of mind and body; thought and action; restraint and fulfilment; harmony between man and nature; a holistic approach to health and well-being" (Government of India, 2015). In response, 177 UN member states sponsored the proposal and it was passed without the need for a vote, reflecting a global interest in the practice of yoga. Since then, annual celebrations have been held worldwide with support from international governments and the World Health Organization (WHO). Yoga is now globally recognized as having the potential to improve wellbeing.

There were 20.4 million people practicing yoga in the United States in 2012 and 36 million in 2016.

The number of people practicing yoga has been steadily growing, and it has increased exponentially in recent years. According to a survey by the American magazine *Yoga Journal* and the Yoga Alliance there were 20.4 million people practicing yoga in the United States in 2012 and 36 million in 2016, representing an increase of 75% in just four years (Yoga Alliance, 2016).

The number of people practicing yoga in order to derive some form of therapeutic benefit for a health condition has also risen. As reported by Barnes, Bloom, and Nahin (2008), survey data from the Centers for Disease Control and Prevention's National Center for Health Statistics revealed that in 2007, four out of ten Americans had used complementary and alternative medicine (CAM) over the last twelve months to manage a health complaint, with 6.1% practicing yoga for this purpose. Another report showed that by 2015 this figure had risen to 9.5% (Clarke, Black, Stussman, Barnes, & Nahin, 2015). Both these surveys and others consistently reveal that a sizable proportion of individuals who practice yoga do so for stress relief and/or to manage a mental health condition (Cramer et al., 2016; Penman, Stevens, Cohen, & Jackson, 2012).

Alongside an expansion in the practice of yoga for health management, there has been a simultaneous rise in research and professional development related to the therapeutic application of yoga in mental healthcare. A bibliometric analysis of research trends from 1967 to 2013 found a three-fold increase in yoga research from 2004 to 2013, with the greatest preponderance of studies dedicated to yoga's influence on mental health (Jeter, Slutsky, Singh, & Khalsa, 2015). Although research is still in the incipient phase and requires more rigor, reviews investigating the evidence for yoga's efficacy in mental health are encouraging (Balasubramaniam, Telles, & Doraiswamy, 2013; Büssing, Michalsen, Khalsa, Telles, & Sherman, 2012; Hendriks, de Jong, & Cramer, 2017).

In 2003, only five schools were registered with the International Association of Yoga Therapists (IAYT), a professional membership organization that supports education and research in yoga and whose mission is to establish yoga as a recognized and respected therapy. To date, 185 member schools have joined the IAYT; there are 28 IAYT-accredited yoga therapy programs, with a further 21 pending (The International Association of Yoga Therapists, 2017). It is a minimum requirement of IAYT accreditation that all yoga therapy training programs incorporate a mental health component within their curriculum, resulting in a rise in the number of yoga therapists trained at an entry level to apply yoga to mental health populations. In addition, shorter specialist programs—some available to both yoga teachers and mental health professionals—that focus on the application of yoga to specific mental health conditions are also on the increase. The Big UK Yoga Survey conducted in 2016 found that 3.7% of yoga teachers were already offering classes for depression and anxiety, and specialist classes addressing all aspects of mental health including trauma, depression, anxiety, eating disorders, insomnia, addictions, and child and adolescent mental health, can now be found.

> Mental health professionals are working in tandem with yoga teachers/therapists in prescribing yoga to their clients, along with bringing its practice into their clinical work to provide better support for patients' recoveries.

Recent academic commentary in research journals suggests that yoga is now firmly established in the domain of clinical practice within the mental healthcare sector (Nyer, Nauphal, Roberg, & Streeter, 2018; Reddy & Vijay, 2016; Uebelacker & Broughton, 2018; Varambally & Gangadhar, 2016). Mental health professionals are working in tandem with yoga teachers/therapists in prescribing yoga to their clients, along with bringing its practice into their clinical work to provide better support for patients' recoveries. There has been a notable rise in the use of yoga in inpatient settings for acute mental health conditions such as schizophrenia (Machleidt & Ziegenbein, 2008; Rao, Varambally, & Gangadhar, 2013). Similarly, the American Psychological Association (APA), the United Kingdom's National Health Service (NHS), and The Indian Ministry of AYUSH (Ayurveda, Yoga, Unani, Siddha, and Homeopathy) all refer to the potential of yoga as a complementary treatment in mental healthcare.

In many ways this may seem an innovation, and of course it is. On the other hand, one of the primary goals of yoga has always been psychological development, albeit (in the early tradition) for spiritual aspirations. Contemporary psychological interest in yoga may have a new and specific flavor, but in the field of psychology, interest in yoga dates back to Karl Jung, who spoke extensively about the connections between yogic philosophy and psychological concepts in his seminar to the Psychological Club of Zurich (Jung, 1932).

Yogic perception of the mind

How the mind operates and how it can be controlled is a central aspect of the yoga tradition. Although this tradition has its origins in ancient India, there isn't one unbroken linear thread of philosophy and practice that connects it to the present day. Contemporary yoga, its theory and practice, is the result of a confluence of various influences, both from within and without the Indian tradition.

Notably, in his highly influential book, *Yoga Body: The Origins of Modern Posture Practice*, Mark Singleton (2010) describes how the development during the twentieth century of the physical systems of postural practice (which have become designated as "yoga") owes as much of a debt to "harmonial gymnastics," bodybuilding, muscular Christianity, and other systems of western physical exercise as to the description of postures and exercises found in the haṭha yoga texts.

The *Vedas*, the oldest sacred texts of the Indian tradition (c. 1500 BCE), are primarily concerned with ritual practice. Although the word *yoga* does appear in the *Vedas*, it does not refer to the complex of mind-body practices or the goal of those practices. The *Vedas* describe the concept of *prana* as a vitalizing lifeforce (Atharvaveda 6.12) (Chand, 1982), and the *Rg Vedic* hymn to the long-haired sage (10.136) suggests the potential of an early ascetic tradition similar to later yogic practices (Mallinson & Singleton, 2017).

However, it isn't until the *Katha Upanishad* in the third century BCE that we encounter the first references to yoga as a technique to control the mind:

When the five perceptions are stilled,
Together with the mind,
And not even reason bestirs itself;
They call it the highest state.
When senses are firmly reined in,
That is Yoga, so people think.
From distractions a man is then free,
For Yoga is the coming-into-being,
As well as the ceasing-to-be.

(KU: 6.10-11) (Olivelle, 1996)

The *Upanishads* explore a range of philosophical questions such as the nature of reality, the origins of the universe, and the nature of the individual self. Two terms come to the fore in the Upanishadic literature: *brahman*, referring to the absolute universal reality, and *atman*, the self, the essential nature of the individual (although it is also used in the texts to refer to the physical body). The attainment of knowledge about these two aspects, and their relationship to each other, is a central motif of the *Upanishads*.

Achieving this knowledge leads to self-realization and spiritual enlightenment. In the framework of the *Upanishads*, this meant liberation from the cycle of birth, death, and rebirth, and mental concentration is the first step to achieving salvation. The practitioner is exhorted to calm the mind by taking control of the senses and withdrawing from external phenomena.

> The unruffled mind is likened to a lamp in a spot sheltered from wind that does not flicker.

The *Bhagavad Gita*, a section of the Indian epic the *Mahabharata* (500–200 BCE), draws heavily on ideas from the *Upanishads*: the mind is described as restless, turbulent, strong, and stubborn, "as difficult to control as wind" (6.34). The *Bhagavad Gita* advocates the attainment of *sthithaprajna* (the state of steadiness of mind), *samatvam* (mental evenness), and *shanti* (mental peace). The unruffled mind is likened to a lamp in a spot sheltered from wind that does not flicker (6.18), or is compared to a tortoise with its limbs drawn in (2.58).

In the *Bhagavad Gita*, the disturbed mind is said to be in thrall to negative emotional states such as anger, jealousy, greed, and fear. The consequences of allowing these states to go unchecked leads to further mental imbalance; for example, anger leads to delusion, delusion leads to confused memory, and confused memory leads to the destruction of reason (2.63).

However, it is perhaps in the Yoga Sutras (YS) (Feuerstein, 1989) ascribed to Patanjali that we find the most detailed exposition of the mind, in both its settled and disturbed states. The YS consists of 196 verses and commentary believed to date from 325–425 CE, although they were most likely compiled from older sources (Mallinson & Singleton, 2017, p. xvi). Although the YS has achieved a central position in the canon of yoga literature, it has little to say about physical practice but much to say about working with the mind. In the yogic tradition, because mental refinement is necessary for spiritual transformation, the yogic path is geared toward development of the mind. This is clearly expressed in the second sutra of Patanjali's work as "*Yogas citta vritti nirodhah*" ("Yoga is the restriction of the fluctuations of consciousness") (Feuerstein, 1989).

Citta, meaning consciousness or awareness, is presented in the YS as consisting of the desiring or lower mind (*manas*), egoity (*ahamkara*), and intellect or discriminating faculty (*buddhi*.) The *vrittis* (literally meaning "whirls") are the fluctuations of mind that lead to a state of mental agitation and confusion, often described by use of the metaphor of ripples disturbing the surface of a lake. The techniques of yoga enable the practitioner to achieve the stilling or restriction (*nirodhah*) of these fluctuations, leading to equanimity of mind and ultimately to *samadhi*, a state of deep meditative absorption. The YS describes several stages of *samadhi*, the ultimate being unknowable and indescribable, because it transcends what we are able to apprehend with the mind.

Patanjali also speaks of five mental afflictions (*kleshas*) that prevent us from realizing our true nature as the unchanging self. The five afflictions are

- ignorance or nescience (*avidya*);

- egoism (*asmita*);

- attachment to pleasure (*raga*);

- aversion (*dvesha*); and

- clinging to physical life (*abhinivesa*).

Each of these *kleshas* produces *samskaras,* subliminal dispositions or mental imprints; in other words, all behavior leaves traces in our consciousness. These traces are like grooves in the mind, where the memories of all behaviors are laid down. It is similar to the grooves of a vinyl record: each time the record is played, the grooves determine the sound that is heard. Therefore, the *samskaras* function as memory traces that cause us to repeat past behaviors, in a potentially destructive pattern.

In Patanjali's system, the goal of yoga is the gradual suppression or restriction (*nirodhah*) of the activities and processes (*vrittis*) occurring in the mind complex (*citta*) as a result of the *samskaras*. The route to dealing with these fluctuations of mind is a two-step process of *abhyasa* (practice), which Patanjali defines in YS 1.3 as specific effort applied to the maintenance of mental calm and stability, along with the cultivation of an attitude of *vairagya* (dispassion). Wisdom comes to the person who practices the eight limbs of yoga (*ash-tangayoga*), a series of auxiliary methods (Mallinson & Singleton, 2017, p. 7) to attain the goal of yoga.

Patanjali outlines a number of options for the focus of concentration during this mental effort that include

- our attitudes toward all beings and circumstances. Four types of attitude are advocated: friendliness or lovingness, compassion or support, happiness or goodwill, and neutrality or acceptance (1.33);

- cultivating a specific object of focus (1.32): specific suggestions are given, including breath practice, awareness of sensations or sensory input, inner luminosity, contemplation of a stable mind free from attachments, and focusing on the flow of consciousness achieved in the sleep or dream state (1.34–1.38);

- meditation on whatever the practitioner finds pleasing and useful (1.39).

Therefore, mental equilibrium is achieved through actively cultivating certain states of mind and not others.

History of yoga as a therapeutic intervention

Improved physical and mental health was not the original goal of yoga, although the YS (1.30–32) does describe ill health as one of the barriers to practice, a barrier that is further compounded by mental and physical pain. It is not until the hatha yoga literature from the thirteenth to fifteenth centuries that we find any reference to the therapeutic benefits of practices; for example, the *Hatha Yoga Pradipika* (Akers, 2002) claims that the practice of asana leads to "steadiness, health and lightness of body" (2.13). In the early literature, the word *asana* simply referred to a way of sitting (Mallinson & Singleton, 2017, p. 86); only later did it acquire its modern meaning of a physical posture.

In the hatha yoga literature, certain postures and breath practices are said to have specific physiological benefits; for example, *paschimottanasana* (seated forward bend) is said to stimulate digestion (2.25), *suryabheda* ("vitalizing") breath to cure intestinal worms (2.50), and *ujjayi* ("victorious") breath to deal with phlegmatic problems (2.52). However, despite praising these associated physiological benefits, the ultimate aim of these practices remained spiritual.

Although many of the techniques and practices described in the hatha yoga literature will be familiar to contemporary yoga practitioners, it was not until the late nineteenth and early twentieth century that we come across the systematization of physical postures and breathing exercises as a blueprint for health and wellbeing.

Swami Vivekananda (born Narendranath Datta), through his speech at the first World's Parliament of Religions in 1893 and subsequent lectures, was a key figure in introducing the West to many aspects of Hinduism and yoga. However, it was in the 1920s, through the work of Swami Kuvalayananda (born Jagannath G. Gune) and Shri Yogendra (born Manibhai Haribhai Desai) that yoga therapy, defined as the adaptation and application of yoga practices to treat specific physical and mental health conditions, emerged as a discipline (Alter, 2004, p. 87).

Kuvalayananda and Yogendra were the first to fully take the study of yoga into the realm of scientific experiment. In 1921, Kuvalayananda established the Kaivalyadhama Yoga Institute in Lonavla, India; the institute is committed to scientific investigation into the physiological effects of haṭha yoga techniques, and the efficacy of those practices as a therapeutic approach to treat disease. Experiments at Kaivalyadhama investigated the effects of yoga practices on heart rate, blood pressure, and other physical measures, then published the results in its house journal, *Yoga Mimamsa*. Kaivalyadhama

was open to the public, and Kuvalayananda's aim was to encourage people to practice yoga as a way of maintaining health (Alter, 2004, p. 85). Similarly, Yogendra opened a research center, the Yoga Institute at Santa Cruz in Mumbai (formerly Bombay); he later traveled to the United States to set up an institute.

The idea of yoga as a practice with benefits for health and wellbeing in addition to its spiritual aims was propagated in the West by a number of influential Indian teachers. These included T. Krishnamacharya, whose son T. K. V. Desikachar developed Viniyoga, a form of yoga therapy tailored to the individual. Krishnamacharya's other students included K. Pattabhi Jois, the founder of the Ashtanga yoga style (distinct from Patanjali's *ashtangayoga* system); B. K. S. Iyengar, who placed particular emphasis on postural alignment and the use of props; and Indra Devi, a Russian woman who was instrumental in bringing yoga to the West. While Pattabhi Jois and Iyengar advocated systems of yoga practice for general health, Desikachar championed an individualized approach tailored to each person's unique needs and capabilities, delivered one-on-one by a yoga therapist.

Another influential teacher was Swami Sivananda of Rishikesh, founder of the Divine Life Society (DLS). The teachings of Sivananda, a former medical doctor, spread globally, both through the widespread dissemination of low-cost yoga manuals printed by the DLS, and through the work of his students, the Swamis Vishnudevananda and Satyananda. The former established Sivananda Vedanta Yoga Centers worldwide, extolling the mental and physical benefits of the five points of yoga: proper exercise, proper breathing, proper relaxation, proper diet, and positive thinking and meditation. Satyananda went on to establish the Bihar School of Yoga, whose many publications on yoga have an emphasis on the benefits of yoga practices for physical and mental health, often supporting their claims with references to research studies.

Defining yoga in contemporary research

Contemporary medical and scientific research into yoga is still an evolving field, and the rigor and quality of its methodology and results are often questioned (Elwy et al., 2014), in particular those of the older Indian studies (Alter, 2004, p. 34). The myriad of practices that are categorized as yoga have made it challenging to make definitive statements about the totality of yoga as a therapeutic intervention.

Patanjali's *ashtangayoga* system has frequently been used as the model for a working definition of yoga in contemporary research studies (Khalsa, 2016). The techniques and practices used must fit under one or more of the headings of the eight limbs described in the YS. This allows researchers to differentiate between yoga and practices that might bear some relation to it, for example, stretching as part of a physical exercise regime as opposed to asana, or slow breathing as opposed to *ujjayi*, a controlled form of breathing that reduces airflow by a slight contraction of the glottis (Mason et al., 2013).

> The myriad of practices that are categorized as yoga have made it challenging to make definitive statements about the totality of yoga as a therapeutic intervention.

Laura Schmalzl, co-editor in chief of the *International Journal of Yoga Therapy* (*IJYT*) and an associate professor of health sciences at Southern California University, has argued for a more rigorous and secularized approach to an operational definition of what she describes as yoga-based practices (YBP) (Schmalzl, Powers, & Henje Blom, 2015). She defines YBP as "modern psychophysiological therapeutic practices that employ a series of movement, breath, and attention-based techniques inspired by a variety of yogic traditions" (Schmalzl et al., 2015, p. 2).

This marks a shift from the work of the early researchers who, although interested in the therapeutic benefits of yoga for specific conditions, were originally motivated by exploring the efficacy of the practices to improve general health (Alter, 2004). For example, it was only after the death of Kuvalayananda in 1966 that research into tailored interventions for specific conditions began in earnest at Kaivalyadhama (Alter, 2004).

Indeed, this marks the difference between the generalized approach of yoga as a practice to improve overall mental and physical wellbeing and yoga therapy, which is tailored to the alleviation of specific physical and mental health challenges as well as increasing resilience and overall wellbeing in the client. For this reason, the training of a yoga therapist is more in-depth than that of a yoga teacher and requires the therapist to be familiar with a range of physical and mental health conditions, to possess the ability to read and understand a medical diagnosis, and to have a clear sense of how to prescribe yoga practices relevant to a diagnosis (although the yoga therapist does not actually diagnose physical or mental health conditions).

Although both yoga and yoga therapy can be delivered either in group sessions or one-on-one, the difference is that a yoga therapist will undertake a detailed interview with an assessment of the client prior to embarking on the practice (see Appendix for an example of an intake form), and an individualized treatment plan will be drawn up that is modified periodically according to the client's response to treatment. Particularly, but not exclusively, in the field of yoga therapy for mental health, the therapeutic alliance—the relationship of trust that the client forms with their therapist—is critical to achieving positive outcomes.

In the field of modern mental healthcare, the comprehensive model of Patanjali's eight limbs, alongside the *kosha* model (see later in this chapter), offers supplementary approaches to treat those suffering from mental health conditions. The holistic view of the individual inherent in the *kosha* system is in alignment with practices and techniques already embraced by many professionals working in mental healthcare. This aspect, along with yoga's current popularity as a method for improving general wellbeing, goes some way toward explaining its attractiveness as a therapeutic intervention in the field of mental healthcare.

The eight limbs of yoga

The multi-tiered framework known as the eight limbs of yoga (*ashtangayoga*) found in Patanjali's YS is a system that displays a remarkable congruence with the principles of modern mental healthcare.

The first two limbs of this eightfold path are the *yamas* and *niyamas*. The *yamas* are self-regulating behaviors related to how we interact with others and the world around us, advocating *ahimsa* (nonviolence), *satya* (truthfulness), and *aparigraha* (not grasping or seeking to possess), among others. The *niyamas* are internal personal practices that include *santosha* (contentment) and *tapas* (self-discipline). Collectively, the *yamas* and *niyamas* promote positive perceptions and actions that lead to wellbeing. The next two limbs are pranayama (breath practice) and asana (postures, in the modern usage) that promote self-regulation by balancing the autonomic nervous system (ANS); asana also helps to keep the body supple and strong. The appreciation of the role of exercise in mental wellbeing is growing rapidly, and asana can be seen as a form of it (see also the earlier section covering the history of yoga as a therapeutic intervention).

The fifth limb is *pratyahara*, withdrawal of the senses from external stimuli, aimed at providing a mental space to perceive the mind with greater clarity. The sixth limb, *dharana*, is focused concentration. In most mental health conditions the mind is unruly, and learning to maintain flexible attention rather than having a scattered focus is a vital component of developing mental quietude. A mind that is unable to self-sooth does not have the ability to apply sustained concentration, so development of this skill is critical to working with mental health issues.

The last two limbs, *dhyana*, a deep level of meditative concentration, and *samadhi*, an indescribable state of deep meditative absorption, in which the practitioner achieves oneness with the universal, are beyond the scope of mental healthcare. However, a felt sense of present moment awareness can foster a sense of connection, whether to self or others, and is a vital aspect of emotional wellbeing.

The *kosha* model

There are other models of physical, psychological, and spiritual wellbeing from the yoga tradition that find parity with, and may even enhance, paradigms of modern mental healthcare, including the biopsychosocial model. The *kosha* system is perhaps the most widely used in contemporary schools of yoga therapy as an assessment and diagnostic tool. The concept of the *koshas* as a way of understanding a person's physical, mental, and energetic constitution first appears in the *Taittiriya Upanishad*, a pre-Buddhist text dating from around the middle of the first millennium BCE. It was expanded upon by later yogic philosophers such as Sankara in the eighth or ninth century CE. The *kosha* model conceives of a person as consisting of five bodies, or sheaths—that is, layers or aspects of the whole person that interconnect with each other so that something impacting one sheath has a corresponding effect on the others. To achieve a state of wellbeing, each aspect must be in balance. The *koshas* are described here from the densest (only the *annamaya kosha* consists of matter) to the subtlest:

1. *Annamaya kosha*, the "food body," or the physical body. What a person eats, how one sleeps, moves, and holds posture all influence this

sheath. It is also called the food body because at death it will become food for other creatures.

2. *Pranamaya kosha*, the "energy body," consists of *prana*, the vital lifeforce. The breath can have a profound influence on this sheath and also on physical and mental health.

3. *Manomaya kosha*, the sheath of "mind-stuff," or the mental and emotional sheath, is where thought, will, and desire reside. This *kosha* also includes the motor and sensory organs. *Manomaya kosha* supports action in the world based on input it receives from the senses. However, if desire overtakes wisdom, then actions may give rise to suffering.

4. *Vijnanamaya kosha*, is composed of the intellect and the wisdom faculty. When strong, this *kosha* supports the others, through insight and awareness, to engage in practices that foster wellbeing.

5. *Anandamaya kosha*, the body of bliss or joy, the deepest aspect of the individual self. A modern iteration of *anandamaya kosha* is that which gives us a sense of connection or purpose within the world. This is conceived of as the finest veil separating the individual from connecting with the divine, or higher self, in which the individual experiences a sense of wholeness or integration. It also relates to a person's sense of connection with the universal or their higher purpose in the world.

> A yoga therapist might suggest ways that the client can connect to other people, or to nature, to inspire a sense of greater meaning and purpose.

In many yoga therapy trainings and therapeutic applications, the *kosha* model is the lens through which the therapist views a person's health complaint. Therefore, the primary complaint is believed to arise from a confluence of different factors, and the therapeutic plan will take into consideration treatment that will positively impact all the *koshas*. For a mental health condition, this might include yoga postures that will give the mind a point of focus, reduce tension, and impart a feeling of inner strength. Lifestyle suggestions and sleep stewardship recommendations might also be included. Breath practices are likely to be taught, and a therapist might help a client to highlight thoughts that create emotional pain, then advise how to shift attention and ingrained patterns of thought through yoga practices. Finally, a yoga therapist might suggest ways that the client can connect to other people, or to nature, to inspire a sense of greater meaning and purpose.

This comprehensive approach to mental health treatment using the *kosha* model dovetails with advances in psychiatric medicine, psychology, and counseling that view the symptoms of mental health conditions from a multifactorial viewpoint and their treatment as requiring a holistic approach.

Efficacy of yoga in mental health

There are a number of reasons why yoga may be an attractive intervention for individuals with mental health issues. Uebelacker summarizes the rationale for yoga's efficacy in mental health in a meta-analysis on yoga for depression: "First, current strategies for treating depression are not sufficient for many individuals. Second, many patients have concerns about existing treatments. Yoga may be an attractive alternative or a good adjunctive strategy. Third, aspects of yoga—including mindfulness promotion and exercise—are thought to be 'active ingredients' of other successful treatments for depression. Fourth, there are plausible biological, psychological, and behavioral mechanisms by which yoga may have an impact on depression" (Uebelacker et al., 2010, p. 25).

In addition, certain philosophical tenets espoused by the yoga tradition have an appeal to many mental healthcare practitioners. The philosophy of the higher self as pure consciousness or sheer awareness (*cit*), unchanging and unaffected by the fluctuations of the lower mind (*manas*), provides a contrast to the tendency of many modern psychological interventions to focus on the diagnosis and fixing of pathology. In the yogic view, mental health issues arise when the *vrittis* hold sway over an individual's attention so that the state of pure consciousness is obscured; the level of this obscuration correlates to the level of mental suffering experienced by the individual. Based on this view, the mind cannot be inherently tarnished, nor can someone be defined by their mental health complaint. At the deepest level, there is nothing to be fixed—a viewpoint that supports radical acceptance of self. As the psychologist Carl Rogers, founder of the humanistic approach to psychotherapy, famously stated, "The curious paradox is that when I accept myself just as I am, then I can change." Rogers eloquently describes a major tenet underpinning the value of yoga in mental health as described in this book. This philosophical standpoint is also important in reducing the stigma associated with mental health conditions, which leads to better outcomes, partly because individuals are more likely to seek treatment when they feel less shame about what is troubling them but also because negative perceptions about their mental health condition add an additional layer of stress (Sirey, 2008).

Social connection

As well as challenges with personal fragmentation, mental health problems include difficulties in effectively connecting with other people. The Sanskrit word *yoga* originates from the root *yuj*, meaning to attach or to join together. The use of the word in certain contexts implies "a state of conjunction or union" (Mallinson & Singleton, 2017, p. 4), so that yoga can be perceived as a practice that fosters connection.

Psychophysiological evidence (see later in this chapter) suggests that yoga practices themselves facilitate personal and interpersonal integration. The yoga community and the sense of belonging it can create may further enrich the experience of connectedness. Group classes support the emergence of *sangha*; the term *sangha*, borrowed from the Buddhist tradition, traditionally refers to an organized assembly of beings who communally aspire for enlightenment by cultivating wisdom and compassion. A *sangha* potentially offers a place of refuge where individuals can trust in the goodwill of its members and find safety within. Although much less formal, within the context of the yoga community, the notion of kind beings collaboratively practicing toward betterment engenders an environment where connection and communication may feel safer than in other aspects of their lives.

> A *sangha* potentially offers a place of refuge where individuals can trust in the goodwill of its members and find safety within.

Given that social isolation increases both the risk of developing and the severity of presentation in many mental health issues (Cornwell & Waite, 2009), yoga's ability to bring individuals together in a safe and nurturing environment is an important part of its value. Research has found that reduced social isolation is correlated with improved health behaviors commensurate with better mental health (Kawachi, 2001). Social support may also trigger a physiological cascade, such as a reduction in stress hormones, which organically improves mental wellbeing (Umberson & Karas Montez, 2010). Recognizing the significance of social networks in health, the NHS in the UK has developed social prescribing, whereby a patient is referred to an activity group commissioned by the NHS to improve health outcomes.

Research into yoga interventions has found a correlation between practice, mental health, and positive health behaviors (Ross, Bevans, Friedmann, Williams, & Thomas, 2013; Ross, Friedmann, Bevans, & Thomas, 2012). In this self-perpetuating triad it may be that practice supports social connection, fueling improved health behaviors, which combine to improve mental health.

Psychophysiology

Although there is heterogeneity, all mental health issues present with dysregulation in the nervous system correlated with a common cluster of subjective symptoms. Discussions of aberrant activity in these various systems are threaded throughout this book, and here we provide an overview to present clarity regarding how they interact. Imbalances may present in the autonomic nervous system, altered levels of certain neurotransmitters and biochemicals, and increased activity in fear networks with decreased activity in brain regions that support inhibition, regulation, and reappraisal. Many of these shared threads are positively impacted by yoga practice and will each now be explored in turn.

The *Bhagavad Gita* defines three qualities of energy, or fundamental forces, called the *gunas* (literally, strands or fibers), whose interplay creates the ever-changing universe of *prakriti* (matter). *Rajas* is the quality of action or change, *tamas* is stillness and density, and *sattva* is purity and balance. This ancient system provides a basic construct for considering the classification of modern psychological concepts whereby individuals have either too much *rajas* and are therefore anxious and lack the ability to inhibit responses, or they are lethargic and somewhat immobilized, unable to garner the strength to move and change. A disorder may be defined by a tendency toward one of these, or it could be characterized by an oscillation between both states, as is often seen in trauma or bipolar disorders. Healing involves finding a balance between these qualities, with *sattva* as the primary state.

The autonomic nervous system

The autonomic nervous system (ANS), a branch of the peripheral nervous system, is composed of the sympathetic nervous system (SNS) and the parasympathetic nervous system (PNS). These two systems are coordinated to help people respond to constantly changing internal and external environments. The SNS mobilizes energy for action, and it is instrumental in orchestrating the stress response: stimulating the release of the hormones epinephrine and norepinephrine, sympathetic activity increases heart and respiratory rate, effectively increasing blood flow to muscles and the brain, readying them for fight or flight. During heightened activity, nonessential physiological processes are downregulated so that energy can be directed toward survival. In contrast, PNS activity is associated with a sense of safety and ease, colloquially referred to as the "rest and digest system." Parasympathetic activity is associated with reduced heart and breath rate, healthy blood flow throughout the entire body, and the building of immune cells. There are many sympathetic nerves that exit the spine that stimulate various organs; the vagus is the main parasympathetic nerve, exiting the brain stem and stimulating many different organs including the heart, lungs, and stomach, and is therefore responsible for a substantial share of the peripheral activity of the ANS.

> During heightened activity, nonessential physiological processes are downregulated so that energy can be directed toward survival.

A majority of people with mental health issues present with overactivity of the SNS and underactivity of the PNS (Chalmers, Quintana, Abbott, & Kemp, 2014). Dysregulation in the ANS co-arises with reduced flexibility between these two systems, leading to consistent stress and reducing the capacity for coping with daily life. Flexibility with the ANS is generally inferred from heart rate variability

(HRV). HRV is the measure of beat-by-beat variation in heart rate over time as influenced by sympathetic nerve fibers and the vagus nerve. The sympathetic fibers release norepinephrine, increasing heart rate, while the vagus releases acetylcholine, reducing heart rate. Flexibility between these aspects of the ANS is determined by the level of variation in the heart rate. A person with high flexibility can manage a stressful situation by effectively mobilizing resources and can relax once the situation has passed. Intriguingly, but perhaps not surprisingly, there is a link between HRV, autonomic flexibility, and cognitive flexibility. Hence, physiological flexibility is matched by the ability to change one's perspective and to see things from various angles, both signs of mental wellbeing. The idea that ANS elasticity and fluid neurological responses are interdependent is known as neurovisceral integration (Thayer, Hansen, Saus-Rose, & Johnsen, 2009). Herein, the mutual flexibility in the central and peripheral nervous systems engenders the subjective experience of integration. Therefore, increasing HRV is an important target for affecting the multifactorial psychophysiological symptoms of mental ill health.

Although HRV indicates the health of both the SNS and the PNS, the vagus nerve can exert more control over levels of HRV than the sympathetic fibers because the rate of vagal firing can significantly exceed the sympathetic output to the heart. When measuring HRV, high frequency output is assigned to vagal activity, while low (and in particular very low) frequencies are assigned to sympathetic output. The rate of vagal firing is often referred to as vagal tone. Consequently, HRV measurements are also an indicator of vagal tone (Shaffer & Ginsberg, 2017).

Stephen Porges, a pioneer in psychophysiology, is internationally recognized for his polyvagal theory, which elaborates on the classical descriptions of the SNS and the PNS and specifically focuses on the two branches of the vagus nerve, the ventral and the dorsal, each of which has a distinct function. Linking evolutionary biology to neuroscience and mental health, Porges expounds on the hierarchy of three different possible responses governed by the ANS, all of which support survival. These responses include social communication, which is mediated by the ventral branch of the vagus; mobilization, modulated by the SNS; and immobilization, controlled by the dorsal vagus. If social communication can be used to promote survival, then this is the first choice of the ANS; mobilization, or action, will be the next choice; and immobilization is the last resort. The level of threat combined with the inherent flexibility of the ANS will determine which response is used (Figure 1.1).

> Freezing offers the evolutionary benefits of retaining physiological resources by immobilizing the mammal and also by preventing further aggression when confronted by an attacker too powerful to fight or flee from.

The phylogenetically newest branch of the vagus nerve, unique to mammals, is the ventral vagus complex (VVC), and the dorsal vagus complex (DVC) is the oldest. The DVC initiates the last-resort "freeze" response when the nervous system perceives it is under insurmountable threat. Unlike the VVC, the DVC is unmyelinated, meaning that the nerve is not surrounded by a fatty sheath that expedites signaling transmission. However, it can rapidly reduce heart rate, which leads to behavioral shutdown, such as the fainting or numbing that can occur in times of overwhelming threat. Freezing offers the evolutionary benefits of retaining physiological resources by immobilizing the mammal and also by preventing further aggression when confronted by an attacker too powerful to fight or flee from. A maladaptive freeze response is often found in individuals with a trauma history, for example, in cases of emotional numbing.

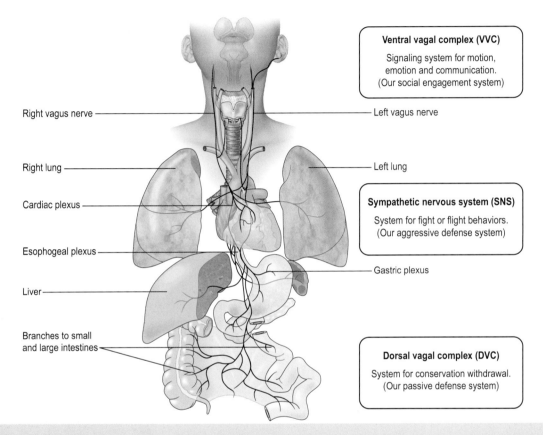

Ventral vagal complex (VVC)

Signaling system for motion, emotion and communication. (Our social engagement system)

Right vagus nerve ——————— ——————— Left vagus nerve

Right lung ———————— ———————— Left lung

Cardiac plexus ————————

Esophogeal plexus ————————

Liver ————————

Branches to small and large intestines ————————

———————— Gastric plexus

Sympathetic nervous system (SNS)

System for fight or flight behaviors. (Our aggressive defense system)

Dorsal vagal complex (DVC)

System for conservation withdrawal. (Our passive defense system)

Figure 1.1
Polyvagal theory. The ventral vagal pathway, the sympathetic nerves, and the dorsal vagal pathway

The VVC promotes survival through bonding and cooperation with other mammals (tend and befriend). Vagal activity downregulates sympathetic drive, reducing heart rate and curbing activity of the hypothalamic-pituitary-adrenal (HPA) axis. Therefore, VVC activity is also linked to a sense of personal and mental flexibility. The VVC has myelinated fibers, enabling it to send fast signals, hence its capacity to override sympathetic responses. This branch of the vagus innervates the throat, permitting voice modulation, and the face, facilitating expressions that forge connections with others. When an individual is relaxed, the VVC is active and provides fluency in interpersonal connections via changes in voice, expression, and a sense of relaxation. The ability to access this mode of being, which Porges calls the social engagement network, is based on a level of perceived safety; it also requires that the SNS is not overreactive. Accordingly, those with mental health issues often struggle with ventral vagal activity and are unable to access its benefits, instead living primarily in fight or flight mode (Porges, 2009, 2011). This leaves them feeling internally fragmented, attached to habitual ways of thinking, disconnected from others, and often socially isolated.

How yoga works on the autonomic nervous system

One of the most notable physiological effects of yoga is its ability to increase HRV and theoretically to increase ventral vagal tone, which in turn may support better internal integration and connectedness with others. Researchers believe that yoga's impact on HRV is primarily derived primarily from asana and pranayama and potentially the result of their combined effects (Cohen & Tyagi, 2016). There may also be additional influences from other yoga practices such as chanting, which may stimulate the vagus. It is well established that exercise generally increases HRV, through sympathetic activation and reverse reflex mechanisms that downregulate SNS activity post-exertion (Routledge, Campbell, McFetridge-Durdle, & Bacon, 2010) to return the body to homeostasis. This effect may be found in yoga, for example, strong asana practice can be categorized as exercise and may produce a similar effect of SNS stimulation; the practice of *savasana* (a resting pose) may downregulate post-asana. Similarly, stretching, a component of most asana practice, may also support greater HRV by increasing PNS activity. Although the mechanism remains unclear, research indicates that PNS drive increases during passive stretching (Inami, 2014). By contrast, in active static stretching, SNS drive increases and PNS activity post-stretching is greater than before. Whether practicing intense asana with rigorous flow, gentle postures, or strong long holds stretches, it is likely that parasympathetic activity will increase either during or after practice, thereby promoting greater HRV.

Respiratory science as well as research on pranayama indicates that variations in breathing can have marked effects on vagal tone and HRV. During inhalation there is a dampening of VVC output activity and increased sympathetic output to the heart, while during exhalation vagal output to the heart is upregulated (Lehrer & Gervirtz, 2014; Porges, 2011; Steffen, Austin, DeBarros, & Brown, 2017). Long slow breathing, as taught during many yoga classes, increases the activity of both systems, enhancing HRV. Likewise, another common practice of making the exhalation longer than the inhalation also enhances HRV, and it may support vagal tone by consistently increasing its activity (Brown & Gerbarg, 2012).

In addition to sending signals from the brain and evoking parasympathetic responses throughout the body, the vagus nerves send signals from the body to the brain, effectively promoting parasympathetic responses from the bottom up. Indeed, 80% of vagal fibers are afferent, traveling from the body to the brain, in contrast to efferent fibers, which travel from the brain to the body (Janig, 2006). Researchers hypothesize that during yoga practice information is sent from the body via the vagus nerve to the brain, engendering neurological changes that result in relaxation, and which may over time promote lasting mental wellbeing. The discrete mechanism through which asana may give rise to such effects is not clear, although respiratory mechanisms have been mapped: the vagus is threaded throughout the respiratory tract and easily stimulated by slow controlled breathing (Brown & Gerbarg, 2005, 2012).

Continual vagal stimulation through asana and slow controlled breathing may enhance vagal tone (Cohen & Tyagi, 2016). Consequently, it can be argued that by reducing the reactivity of the SNS through yoga, an individual will find it easier to activate the social engagement network, thereby enhancing an experience of connection—a theory supported by qualitative and anecdotal evidence. In a small interpretive phenomenological study investigating the effects of yoga on women with major depressive disorder, participants reported reductions in depression and cited feelings of connectedness as a major mediating factor (Kinser, Bourguignon, Taylor, & Steeves, 2013). A qualitative study examining the effect of yoga on interpersonal relationships found that it increased social interaction, personal transformation, and supported better interpersonal connection. These comingling factors culminated in an experience of spiritual transcendence and connection to something greater than the self (Ross, Friedmann, Bevans, & Thomas, 2014).

Yoga and GABA

Chris Streeter devised a comprehensive hypothesis of how yoga might positively influence mental health, drawing on theories of yoga's influence on the vagally-mediated parasympathetic response as well as her previous research, which asserted that yoga practice is correlated with increased gamma aminobutyric acid (GABA), the major inhibitory neurotransmitter in the brain. GABA is counterbalanced by glutamate, the primary excitatory neurotransmitter in the brain. GABA directly represses fear-based pathways and supports higher brain structures by inhibiting signals and activity of fear networks. In 2007, Streeter discovered that yoga increased GABA post-practice, and in 2010 her research revealed that yoga increased GABA levels more than metabolically matched exercise. In 2012, Streeter hypothesized that vagal stimulation via yoga triggered the release of GABA throughout the central nervous system (CNS), and that this marked increase in GABA induced both short- and long-term effects. In her view, the short-term effect is relaxation post-yoga practice. The long-term effect of increased GABA could be alterations in the neural pathways necessary for inhibiting fear responses, with the consequence of also enhancing cognitive reappraisal and reframing, as well as interoception (awareness of internal body states)—all vital components of mental health (Streeter, Gerbarg, Saper, Ciraulo, & Brown, 2012; Streeter et al., 2007, 2010).

If accurate, Streeter's hypothesis helps to further elucidate the efficacy of yoga in mental health issues (Figure 1.2). Across the spectrum of disorders, neuroscientists find increased amygdala activity and volume coupled with attenuation, and reduced activity in the prefrontal cortex (PFC) in comparison to age-matched controls (Drevets, Price, & Furey, 2008; Etkin & Wager, 2007). A limbic structure, the amygdala is instrumental in triggering the fear response (among other functions) through both sympathetic pathways and the HPA axis, which releases cortisol. The PFC, a higher brain structure, is known for its role in executive functioning, that is, the ability to receive multiple inputs and to determine appropriate responses. Accordingly, the PFC has both inhibitory and excitatory projections to and from other regions of the brain, and attempts to manage competing goals based on previous experience and current input (Jadhav, Rothschild, Roumis, & Frank, 2016). Mental health necessitates that the PFC can adequately inhibit amygdala activity. This permits flexible responses as opposed to those merely geared toward survival. In individuals with mental health issues the amygdala possesses greater connectivity to other brain structures, creating the potential to perceive a host of innocuous inputs as threatening. Without proper inhibition from the PFC, a person is not able to easily downgrade fear and/or reappraise inputs as nonthreatening, and may in turn cause the PFC to generate negative cognitions and activate fear networks (Arnsten, 2009).

Streeter's hypothesis suggests that GABA may inhibit amygdala activity, while also influencing PFC activity suppressing the amygdala.

The effects of mindfulness

In addition to the influence of afferent input on neurological processes, the mindful attention cultivated via

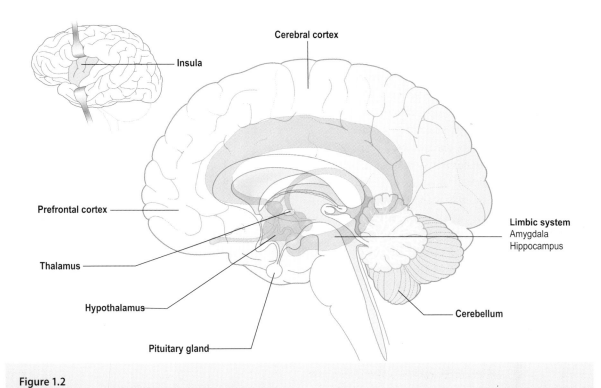

Cerebral cortex

Insula

Prefrontal cortex

Thalamus

Hypothalamus

Pituitary gland

Limbic system
Amygdala
Hippocampus

Cerebellum

Figure 1.2
Areas of the brain commonly implicated in mental health

yoga practice may promote cortical activity and support greater mental wellbeing. Mindfulness is a quality of mind that involves nonjudgmental awareness of present-moment mind-body experience. Mindfulness meditation involves several practices such as seated and walking meditation, designed to help a person notice sensations and thoughts as they arise without reacting to them. Through this bare attention, the difference between projected and actual experience is gleaned, catalyzing self-insight and promoting freedom from habitual responses. Mindfulness is often distinguished from other types of meditation that encourage atten-

tion on one point of focus with the purpose of developing concentration with the goal of self-realization.

> Mindfulness is a quality of mind that involves nonjudgmental awareness of present-moment mind-body experience.

Unlike the afferent, bottom-up mechanisms already described, mindfulness is a top-down strategy relying on self-monitoring and direct response inhibition to alter the relationship to experience (Guendelman, Medeiros, & Rampes, 2017). Research asserts that mindfulness recruits frontal lobe structures, exerting top-down effects that move from cortex through to viscera. Brain scans reveal various functional and anatomical changes associated with mindfulness. Notably, mindfulness practice is correlated with increases in prefrontal cortex (PFC) volume and activity, reduced amygdala activity, increased anterior cingulate cortical activity and volume (related to attentional control), and volume and normalizing activity in the insula (a structure implicated in body awareness and, relatedly, self-awareness). Mindfulness, especially in novices, recruits PFC and anterior cingulate activity, enabling a person to attend to but not react to thoughts or sensory input. This garners inhibition of habitual responses, bolstering concentration, reappraisal, innovative thinking, and executive functioning—all mental faculties that are compromised in mental health disorders (Guendelman et al., 2017; Hölzel et al., 2011; Lutz, Brühl, Scheerer, Jäncke, & Herwig, 2016).

Although a distinction is usually made between mindfulness practice and yoga, yoga practice is often conducted with the purpose of additional mindful intention, while asana practice naturally directs the mind to sensation, and so mindfulness is inherent in the practice. Therefore, mindfulness is often understood as intrinsic to yoga practice. Given the modern focus on the body-based aspects of yoga, the link between mindfulness of the body and sensations and yoga practice is most readily evident. Theory and evidence provide a rationale for yoga's role in increasing body awareness, a vital component of mental well-being. A highly complex phenomenon, body awareness includes proprioception, awareness of the body in space, and interoception, awareness of the inner workings of the body.

Proprioception

Proprioception, the sense of the position of our body parts, helps in sensory integration and may also help us be aware of self-boundaries and identity (Nasrallah,

2012); proprioceptive awareness is compromised in many mental health conditions (Arnfred, Raballo, Morup, & Parnas, 2015; Izawa et al., 2012; Zucker et al., 2013), partly because high levels of rumination may inhibit afferent signaling regarding the body position. However, during the act of both moving and stretching, sensory bodies on the skin, in the muscles, and the tendons are consistently signaling to the brain, offering interoceptive and proprioceptive cues (ScienceDirect, 2018). Therefore, the practice of asana is perfectly suited for increasing proprioception, and research on elderly participants has indicated that yoga practice enhances proprioception (Wooten, Signorile, Desai, Paine, & Mooney, 2018).

Interoception

Interoception is a combination of actual sensory input and our perception of it, providing an embodied experience of how we feel, thereby contributing to our overall sense of self (Craig, 2009). Together, interoception and proprioception mediate the relationship between the inner state and the outer world.

Interoception is a bidirectional process between the body and the brain. Interoceptive awareness melds raw sensory input from the body provided through thalamic subcortical pathways with the higher cortical structures responsible for encoding salience and meaning (Paulus & Stein, 2010). Together, cortical and subcortical thalamic networks work in tandem to provide a landscape of what we feel and information on how to respond. Interoceptive accuracy (IA) is a term that refers to the ability to accurately perceive sensations from the body. High levels of IA imply that pre-existing expectations about sensations are not transposed onto present-moment feelings. High IA is associated with better mental health outcomes, because individuals who clearly sense messages from the body have a greater potential to respond in appropriate and adaptive ways (Farb & Mehling, 2016).

Compromised IA is common in mental health disorders and speaks to the disconnect between the body and the mind (Decety & Moriguchi, 2007; Downar, Blumberger, & Daskalakis, 2016; Manoliu et al., 2013). High levels of rumination, associated with hyperactivity in the medial PFC (mPFC), are associated with inhibition of sensory input to cortical regions (Farb & Mehling, 2016; Kerr, Sacchet, Lazar, Moore, & Jones, 2013). Accordingly, individuals struggle to care appropriately for their needs because body signals are dampened or seen as alarming. For example, if a person is tired but does not clearly perceive signs of fatigue and does not stop to rest when necessary, this can augment negative emotions, which in turn may be interpreted as depression. Similarly, an anxious person may misconstrue the elevated heart rate that accompanies exercise as a sign of distress and will therefore avoid exercise, something that could be helpful in anxiety management. All of these may indicate impaired brain functions related to interoception.

> If a person is tired but does not clearly perceive signs of fatigue and does not stop to rest when necessary, this can augment negative emotions.

Possibly the clearest understanding of how mental health issues influence interoception comes from the world-renowned neuroanatomist A. D. Craig, who has developed groundbreaking theories regarding the insula. He hypothesizes that the insula possesses a perceptual map of bodily states, which is why it is sometimes referred to as the interoceptive cortex. The main site of interoception, the insula communicates with the mPFC, which appraises the meaning of sensation (Craig, 2009). Aberrant activity within the insula and between the insula and the mPFC are seen across the spectrum of mental health issues, and jointly create a distorted experience of the body, its input, and the sense of self.

Research reveals that the practice of mindfulness creates connections within the insula and between the insula and other brain regions, providing greater IA. Simply noticing a sensation, with the specific cue not to react, appears to recruit inhibitory mPFC circuits, thereby downregulating fear responses and allowing for clear perception (Farb, Segal & Anderson, 2013; Kerr et al., 2013).

In the case of mental health problems, individuals may struggle with mindfulness. Teasdale, one of three pioneers of Mindfulness-Based Cognitive Therapy (MBCT)—a mindfulness intervention for preventing relapse of depressive episodes—states that "…factors such as difficulty in concentrating and the intensity of negative thinking may preclude acquisition of the attentional control skills central to the programme" (Teasdale et al., 2000, p. 60). Likewise, fear around sensory input may prevent a person from staying present with what is felt.

Mindfulness through physical yoga practices

For many people, the practice of yoga asana is an easier way to develop awareness of the body than seated and walking meditation or body scanning. To begin with, yoga (in particular asana) naturally engenders mindfulness as attention is pinned to the present moment, in part due to the intensity of sensation (Schmalzl, 2015), augmented by intentional inward focus. In addition, asana is often practiced with slow controlled breathing, generating a parasympathetic response, thereby fostering the relaxation needed to remain with the experience while simultaneously inhibiting negative cognitions (Gard, Noggle, Park, Vago, & Wilson, 2014). This confluence of factors helps a practitioner to stay present with sensations and thoughts, even unpleasant ones, without overreacting or escaping. The asanas can create a safe microcosm where a person may experiment with sensory experience, knowing that distress can be relieved by simply exiting the posture. Practitioners may begin to understand that some challenging sensations lead to pleasant experiences and that one need not flee from them. For instance, staying in a challenging posture might build strength in the body and this feels good. Evidence for the connection between yoga practice, interoception, and tolerance of sensations comes from a study that investigated pain tolerance in practitioners in comparison to yoga-naïve controls: practitioners exhibited more gray matter in the insula, anterior cingulate, and the mPFC, and were able to tolerate pain for twice as long as the controls; when interviewed, the yoga practitioners reported using strategies that evoked parasympathetic responses, such as slow breathing in cooperation with nonjudgmental awareness (Villemure, Ceko, Cotton, & Bushnell, 2014).

Increased body awareness and tolerance of sensations may also support cognitive reappraisal of thought. In other words, mindfulness of the body facilitates mindfulness of mental processes. For example, while performing asana, a person may begin to inquire into, rather than blindly believe in, negative cognitions. The thought "I will never be good enough to do this posture" is revealed as untrue after discovering that the pose is in fact achievable. This may engender the insight that if this idea is not true, perhaps other self-limiting beliefs are also inaccurate. Progression of such cognitive reappraisal allows a practitioner to distil projections from actual experience, reducing distress and promoting novel ways of perceiving experiences rather than simply defaulting to habitual negative beliefs. This, in turn, may increase the sense of self-efficacy in a practitioner.

In summary, asana and pranayama may provide a structure for the development of mindfulness through body awareness, buttressing positive neuroplasticity in higher brain structures, which then support better emotion regulation through mindfulness of thought.

Embodiment, movement, and mental flexibility

As a mindful movement practice, yoga may also enhance higher brain processing through other pathways. The research psychiatrist Adele Diamond is interested in the overlap between motor and cognitive development, especially how the cerebellum, generally thought to relate only to motor control, is also instrumental in cognitive pathways. She suggests that when planning a new movement, the cerebellic prefrontal cortex pathway is recruited, and that this coactivation enhances functionality of both structures (Diamond, 2000). Because yoga asana involves a wide variety of movements, it follows that it may enhance PFC activity, particularly for those individuals who would otherwise struggle with engagement of the higher brain processes. Gard et al. (2015) published research reporting that the greatest difference between practitioners of mindfulness and yoga and non-practitioners was connectivity between the caudate and higher cortical structures such as the PFC. The caudate is part of a larger structure known as the basal ganglia, which is essentially a group of subcortical nuclei. The basal ganglia and the caudate are involved in initiation and inhibition of movement; previously thought to only play a role in controlling movement, it is now known that the caudate is also connected to the PFC and plays a role in learning acquisition and cognitive flexibility. Commenting on Gard's research, Schmalzl hypothesized that when practicing yoga, the process of moving into and out of one pose after another requires planning, inhibition, and learning, thus recruiting frontal cortical circuits and strengthening the connections between the caudate and cortical regions. Remarkably, greater connectivity between the caudate and PFC not only furthers initiation and inhibition of movement, but affords the same mental skills; in other words the ability to inhibit thinking, to shift thinking, and choosing to engage in specific (and often helpful) types of thinking (Schmalzl et al.,

2015). For someone with mental health issues who struggles with cognitive flexibility, the development of the kind of mental flexibility that naturally emerges through controlled mindful movement, as practiced in yoga, may represent a much easier path.

> To begin with, yoga (in particular asana) naturally engenders mindfulness as attention is pinned to the present moment, in part due to the intensity of sensation (Schmalzl, 2015), augmented by intentional inward focus.

Additional biochemical changes

The stress response in the body is orchestrated by the SNS and the HPA axis. The HPA axis stimulates the release of cortisol, the body's major stress hormone. Mental health problems often present with dysregulation of the HPA axis, primarily with elevated cortisol secretion (Heinze, Lin, Reniers, & Wood, 2016; Vreeberg et al., 2010). Exceptions are found in posttraumatic stress disorder (PTSD), where there may be a blunted cortisol response, but this is the exception rather than the rule in mental health disorders (Morris, Rao, & Garber, 2012). An array of trials investigating yoga's efficacy in reducing cortisol levels in mental health have reported both pre- and post-intervention decreases (Field, Diego, Delgado, & Medina, 2012; Naveen et al., 2016; Thirthalli, Naveen et al., 2013). These studies also report reductions in stress. Other important biochemicals may also be influenced by yoga and underpin its beneficial effects in mental health. Yoga may potentially upregulate depressed levels of serotonin and dopamine; however, to date research regarding yoga's effects on these neurotransmitters is too sparse to draw clear conclusions (Kjaer et al., 2002; Lee, Moon, & Kim, 2014).

Brain-derived neurotrophic factor (BDNF) is a protein that promotes neuroplasticity. Depression of BNDF is present in many mental health conditions, which prevents the genesis of neurons and new neural pathways. Low BDNF is effectively a biological correlate of cognitive inflexibility. A handful of studies reveal that yoga practice increased BDNF in those suffering from depression and was associated with symptom reduction (Thirthalli et al., 2013; Naveen et al., 2016). The upregulation of BDNF may play a crucial role in the various mechanisms through which yoga exerts its neuroplastic effects.

Conclusions

Given that yoga developed as an all-inclusive methodology for mental refinement, it isn't surprising that both practitioners and professionals find the comprehensive practice of yoga and certain aspects of it to be attractive tools for managing mental health. Supporting this are research studies and academic literature that delineate clear physiological, psychological, and philosophical reasons for yoga's efficacy in promoting mental wellbeing. Concurrently, there are unique reasons and benefits associated with yoga practice germane to particular mental health disorders, and these are articulated in the following chapters of this book. We hope that as readers progress through the book a theme will emerge, that yoga may—and presumably should—have a significant role to play in mental healthcare in the future. As Doriswamy, professor of psychiatry at Duke University has said: "If the promise of yoga on mental health was found in a drug, it would be the best selling medication world-wide" (EurekAlert!, 2013). Finding parity with Doriswamy, we believe that there is a growing trend in which yoga will become an integral part of mental health treatment. This book is both a testament to this trend as well as a springboard to bolster greater interest and appreciation of the field. By detailing how and why yoga is being used in mental healthcare, along with best practice and precautions, this book aims to enhance awareness of yoga's inclusion in the

There are unique reasons and benefits associated with yoga practice germane to particular mental health disorders.

management of and the recovery from mental health conditions, and therefore to intelligently promote the growing field of yoga within mental healthcare.

References

Akers, B. D. (trans.) (2002). *The hatha yoga Pradipika, The Original Sanskrit: Svatmarama.* Woodstock, NY: Yoga Vidya.

Alter, J. S. (2004). *Yoga in Modern India: The Body between Science and Philosophy.* Princeton: Princeton University Press.

Arnfred, S., Raballo, A., Morup, M., & Parnas, J. (2015). Self-disorder and brain processing of proprioception in schizophrenia spectrum patients: A re-analysis. *Psychopathology, 48*(1), 60–64.

Arnsten, A. (2009). Stress signalling pathways that impair prefrontal cortex structure and function. *Nature Reviews Neuroscience, 10*(6), 410–422.

Balasubramaniam, M., Telles, S., & Doraiswamy, P. (2013). Yoga on our minds: A systematic review of yoga for neuropsychiatric disorders. *Frontiers in Psychiatry, 3.*

Barnes, P. M., Bloom, B., & Nahin, R. L. (2008). Complementary and alternative medicine use among adults and children: United States, 2007. *National Health Statistics Reports, 10*(12), 1–23.

Brown, R., & Gerbarg, P. (2005). Sudarshan kriya yogic breathing in the treatment of stress, anxiety, and depression: Part I—neurophysiologic model. *The Journal of Alternative and Complementary Medicine, 11*(1), 189–201.

Brown, R., & Gerbarg, P. (2012). *The Healing Power of the Breath. Simple Techniques to Reduce Stress and Anxiety, Enhance Concentration, and Balance Your Emotions.* Colorado: Shambhala.

Büssing, A., Michalsen, A., Khalsa, S., Telles, S., & Sherman, K. (2012). Effects of yoga on mental and physical health: A short summary of reviews. *Evidence-Based Complementary and Alternative Medicine.*

Chalmers, J., Quintana, D., Abbott, M., & Kemp, A. (2014). Anxiety disorders are associated with reduced heart rate variability: A meta-analysis. *Frontiers in Psychiatry, 5.*

Chand, D. (1982). *The Atharvaveda: Sanskrit text with English translation.* New Delhi: Munshiram Manoharlal.

Clarke, T. C., Black, L. I., Stussman, B. J., Barnes, P. M., & Nahin, R. L. (2015). Trends in the use of complementary health approaches among adults: United States, 2002–2012. *National Health Statistics Reports, 10*(79), 1–16.

Cohen, M., & Tyagi, A. (2016). Yoga and heart rate variability: A comprehensive review of the literature. *International Journal of Yoga, 9*(2), 97.

Cornwell, E., & Waite, L. (2009). Social disconnectedness, perceived isolation, and health among older adults. *Journal of Health and Social Behavior, 50*(1), 31–48.

Craig, A. D. (2009). How do you feel—now? The anterior insula and human awareness. *Nature Reviews Neuroscience, 10*(1), 59–70.

Cramer, H., Hall, H., Leach, M., Frawley, J., Zhang, Y., & Leung, B., Adams, J., & Lauche, R. (2016). Prevalence, patterns, and predictors of meditation use among US adults: A nationally representative survey. *Scientific Reports, 6.*

Decety, J., & Moriguchi, Y. (2007). The empathic brain and its dysfunction in psychiatric populations: Implications for intervention across different clinical conditions. *Biopsychosocial Medicine, 1*(1), 22.

Diamond, A. (2000). Close interrelation of motor development and cognitive development and of the cerebellum and prefrontal cortex. *Child Development, 71*(1), 44–56.

Downar, J., Blumberger, D., & Daskalakis, Z. (2016). The neural crossroads of psychiatric illness: An emerging target for brain stimulation. *Trends in Cognitive Sciences, 20*(2), 107–120.

Drevets, W., Price, J., & Furey, M. (2008). Brain structural and functional abnormalities in mood disorders: Implications for neurocircuitry models of depression. *Brain Structure and Function, 213*(1–2), 93–118.

Elwy, A. R., Groessl, E. J., Eisen, S. V., Riley, K., Maiya, M., Lee, J. P., & Park, C. L. (2014). A systematic scoping review of yoga intervention components and study quality. *American Journal of Preventive Medicine, 47*(2), 220–232.

Etkin, A., & Wager, T. (2007). Functional neuroimaging of anxiety: A meta-analysis of emotional processing in PTSD, social anxiety disorder, and specific phobia. *American Journal of Psychiatry, 164*(10), 1476–1488.

EurekAlert! (2013, January 25). *Frontiers publishes systematic review on the effects of yoga on major psychiatric disorders.* Retrieved from: https://www.eurekalert.org/pub_releases/2013-01/f-fps012213.php.

Farb, N., & Mehling, W. (2016). Editorial: Interoception, contemplative practice, and health. *Frontiers in Psychology, 7.*

Farb, N., Segal, Z., & Anderson, A. (2013). Mindfulness meditation training alters cortical representations of interoceptive attention. *Social Cognitive and Affective Neuroscience, 8*(1), 15–26.

Feuerstein, G. (trans.) (1989). *The Yoga-Sūtra of Patanjali: A New Translation and Commentary.* Vermont: inner traditions international.

Feuerstein, G. (trans.) (2011). *The Bhagavad Gita: A New Translation* (1st ed.). Boston and London: Shambala.

Field, T., Diego, M., Delgado, J., & Medina, L. (2012). Yoga and social support reduce prenatal depression, anxiety and cortisol. *Journal of Yoga & Physical Therapy, 2,* 124.

Gard, T., Noggle, J., Park, C., Vago, D., & Wilson, A. (2014). Potential self-regulatory mechanisms of yoga for psychological health. *Frontiers in Human Neuroscience, 8.*

Gard, T., Taquet, M., Dixit, R., Hölzel, B. K., Dickerson, B. C., & Lazar, S. W. (2015). Greater widespread functional connectivity of the caudate in older adults who practice kripalu yoga and vipassana meditation than in controls. *Frontiers in Human Neuroscience, 9*, 137.

Government of India (2015, June 19). *Yoga brings harmony in all walks of life and prevents disease & promotes health.* Retrieved from: http://www.pib.nic.in/newsite/mbErel.aspx?relid=122626.

Guendelman, S., Medeiros, S., & Rampes, H. (2017). Mindfulness and emotion regulation: Insights from neurobiological, psychological, and clinical studies. *Frontiers in Psychology, 8.*

Heinze, K., Lin, A., Reniers, R., & Wood, S. (2016). Longer-term increased cortisol levels in young people with mental health problems. *Psychiatry Research, 236*, 98–104.

Hendriks, T., de Jong, J., & Cramer, H. (2017). The effects of yoga on positive mental health among healthy adults: A systematic review and meta-analysis. *The Journal of Alternative and Complementary Medicine, 23*(7), 505–517.

Hölzel, B., Lazar, S., Gard, T., Schuman-Olivier, Z., Vago, D., & Ott, U. (2011). How does mindfulness meditation work? Proposing mechanisms of action from a conceptual and neural perspective. *Perspectives on Psychological Science, 6*(6), 537–559.

Inami, T., Shimizu, T., Baba, R., & Nakagaki, A. (2014). Acute changes in autonomic nerve activity during passive static stretching. *American Journal of Sports Science and Medicine, 2*(4), 166–170.

Izawa, J., Pekny, S., Marko, M., Haswell, C., Shadmehr, R., & Mostofsky, S. (2012). Motor learning relies on integrated sensory inputs in ADHD, but over-selectively on proprioception in autism spectrum conditions. *Autism Research, 5*(2), 124–136.

Jadhav, S., Rothschild, G., Roumis, D., & Frank, L. (2016). Coordinated excitation and inhibition of prefrontal ensembles during awake hippocampal sharp-wave ripple events. *Neuron, 90*(1), 113–127.

Janig, W. (2006). Functional anatomy of the peripheral sympathetic and parasympathetic system. In: *The Integrative Action of the Autonomic Nervous System: Neurobiology of Homeostasis* (pp. 13–34). Cambridge, UK: Cambridge University Press.

Jeter, P., Slutsky, J., Singh, N., & Khalsa, S. (2015). Yoga as a therapeutic intervention: A bibliometric analysis of published research studies from 1967 to 2013. *The Journal of Alternative and Complementary Medicine, 21*(10), 586–592.

Jung, C., & Shamdasani, S. (1999). *The psychology of Kundalini Yoga.* Notes on seminar given in 1932 by C. G. Jung, 2nd ed. Princeton: Bollingen [Imprint].

Kawachi, I. (2001). Social capital for health and human development. *Development, 44*(1), 31–35.

Kerr, C., Sacchet, M., Lazar, S., Moore, C., & Jones, S. (2013). Mindfulness starts with the body: Somatosensory attention and top-down modulation of cortical alpha rhythms in mindfulness meditation. *Frontiers in Human Neuroscience, 7.*

Khalsa, S. B. S. (2016, July 11). [Public Lecture] Biomedical scientific research on yoga: Revolutionizing wellness and healthcare.

Kinser, P., Bourguignon, C., Taylor, A., & Steeves, R. (2013). "A feeling of connectedness": Perspectives on a gentle yoga intervention for women with major depression. *Issues in Mental Health Nursing, 34*(6), 402–411.

Kjaer, T., Bertelsen, C., Piccini, P., Brooks, D., Alving, J., & Lou, H. (2002). Increased dopamine tone during meditation-induced change of consciousness. *Cognitive Brain Research, 13*(2), 255–259.

Lee, M., Moon, W., & Kim, J. (2014). Effect of yoga on pain, brain-derived neurotrophic factor, and serotonin in premenopausal women with chronic low back pain. *Evidence-Based Complementary and Alternative Medicine.*

Lehrer, P., & Gevirtz, R. (2014). Heart rate variability biofeedback: How and why does it work? *Frontiers in Psychology, 5.*

Lutz, J., Brühl, A., Scheerer, H., Jäncke, L., & Herwig, U. (2016). Neural correlates of mindful self-awareness in mindfulness meditators and meditation-naïve subjects revisited. *Biological Psychology, 119*, 21–30.

Machleidt, W., & Ziegenbein, M. (2008). An appreciation of yoga-therapy in the treatment of schizophrenia. *Acta Psychiatrica Scandinavica, 117*(5), 397–398.

Mallinson, J., & Singleton, M. (2017). *Roots of Yoga.* London, UK: Penguin.

Manoliu, A., Meng, C., Brandl, F., Doll, A., Tahmasian, M., & Scherr, M., Schwerthöffer, D., Zimmer, C., Förstl, H., Bäuml, J., Riedl, V., Wohlschläger, A. M., & Sorg, C. (2013). Insular dysfunction within the salience network is associated with severity of symptoms and aberrant inter-network connectivity in major depressive disorder. *Frontiers in Human Neuroscience, 7*, 930.

Mason, H., Vandoni, M., deBarbieri, G., Codrons, E., Ugargol, V., & Bernardi, L. (2013). Cardiovascular and respiratory effect of yogic slow breathing in the yoga beginner: What is the best approach? *Evidence-Based Complementary and Alternative Medicine.* Advance publication online.

Morris, M., Rao, U., & Garber, J. (2012). Cortisol responses to psychosocial stress predict depression trajectories: Social-evaluative threat and prior depressive episodes as moderators. *Journal of Affective Disorders, 143*(1–3), 223–230.

Nasrallah, H. A. (2012). Impaired mental proprioception in schizophrenia. *Current Psychiatry, 11*(8), 4–5.

Naveen, G., Varambally, S., Thirthalli, J., Rao, M., Christopher, R., & Gangadhar, B. (2016). Serum cortisol and BDNF in patients with major depression—effect of yoga. *International Review of Psychiatry, 28*(3), 273–278.

Nyer, M., Nauphal, M., Roberg, R., & Streeter, C. (2018). Applications of yoga in psychiatry: What we know. *FOCUS, 16*(1), 12–18.

Olivelle, P. (1996). *Upanisads: A New Translation.* Oxford: Oxford University Press.

Paulus, M., & Stein, M. (2010). Interoception in anxiety and depression. *Brain Structure and Function, 214*(5–6), 451–463.

Penman, S., Stevens, P., Cohen, M., & Jackson, S. (2012). Yoga in Australia: Results of a national survey. *International Journal of Yoga, 5*(2), 92.

Porges, S. (2009). The polyvagal theory: New insights into adaptive reactions of the autonomic nervous system. *Cleveland Clinic Journal of Medicine*, *76*(Suppl_2), S86–S90.

Porges, S. (2011). *The Polyvagal Theory*. New York: W.W. Norton.

Rao, N., Varambally, S., & Gangadhar, B. (2013). Yoga school of thought and psychiatry: Therapeutic potential. *Indian Journal of Psychiatry*, *55*(6), 145.

Reddy, M., & Vijay, S. (2016). Yoga in psychiatry: An examination of concept, efficacy, and safety. *Indian Journal of Psychological Medicine*, *38*(4), 275.

Ross, A., Bevans, M., Friedmann, E., Williams, L., & Thomas, S. (2013). "I am a nice person when i do yoga!!!" *Journal of Holistic Nursing*, *32*(2), 67–77.

Ross, A., Friedmann, E., Bevans, M., & Thomas, S. (2012). Frequency of yoga practice predicts health: Results of a national survey of yoga practitioners. *Evidence-Based Complementary and Alternative Medicine.*, Advance publication online.

Ross, A., Friedmann, E., Bevans, M., & Thomas, S. (2014). National survey of yoga practitioners: Mental and physical health benefits. *Complementary Therapies in Medicine*, *21*(4), 313–323.

Routledge, F., Campbell, T., McFetridge-Durdle, J., & Bacon, S. (2010). Improvements in heart rate variability with exercise therapy. *Canadian Journal of Cardiology*, *26*(6), 303–312.

Schmalzl, L., Powers, C., & Henje Blom, E. (2015). Neurophysiological and neurocognitive mechanisms underlying the effects of yoga-based practices: toward a comprehensive theoretical framework. *Frontiers in Human Neuroscience*, *9*, 235.

ScienceDirect (2018). *Muscle Spindle – an overview*. Retrieved from: https://www.sciencedirect.com/topics/neuroscience/muscle-spindle.

Shaffer, F., & Ginsberg, J. (2017). An overview of heart rate variability metrics and norms. *Frontiers in Public Health*, *5*, 28.

Singleton, M. (2010). *Yoga Body: The Origins of Modern Posture Practice*. Oxford: Oxford University Press.

Sirey, J. (2008). The impact of psychosocial factors on experience of illness and mental health service use. *The American Journal of Geriatric Psychiatry*, *16*(9), 703–705.

Steffen, P., Austin, T., DeBarros, A., & Brown, T. (2017). The impact of resonance frequency breathing on measures of heart rate variability, Blood Pressure, and Mood. *Frontiers in Public Health*, *5*, 222.

Streeter, C., Gerbarg, P., Saper, R., Ciraulo, D., & Brown, R. (2012). Effects of yoga on the autonomic nervous system, gamma-aminobutyric-acid, and allostasis in epilepsy, depression, and post-traumatic stress disorder. *Medical Hypotheses*, *78*(5), 571–579.

Streeter, C., Jensen, J., Perlmutter, R., Cabral, H., Tian, H., & Terhune, D., Ciraulo, D. A., & Renshaw, P. F. (2007). Yoga asana sessions increase brain GABA levels: A pilot study. *The Journal of Alternative and Complementary Medicine*, *13*(4), 419–426.

Streeter, C., Whitfield, T., Owen, L., Rein, T., Karri, S., Yakhkind, A., Perlmutter, R., Prescot, A., Renshaw, P. F., Ciraulo, D. A., & Jensen, J. E. (2010). Effects of yoga versus walking on mood, anxiety, and brain GABA

levels: A randomized controlled MRS study. *The Journal of Alternative and Complementary Medicine*, *16*(11), 1145–1152.

Teasdale, J., Segal, Z., Williams, J., Ridgeway, V., Soulsby, J., & Lau, M. (2000). Prevention of relapse/recurrence in major depression by mindfulness-based cognitive therapy. *Journal of Consulting and Clinical Psychology*, *68*(4), 615–623.

Thayer, J., Hansen, A., Saus-Rose, E., & Johnsen, B. (2009). Heart rate variability, prefrontal neural function, and cognitive performance: The neurovisceral integration perspective on self-regulation, adaptation, and health. *Annals of Behavioral Medicine*, *37*(2), 141–153.

The International Association of Yoga Therapists (2017). *Learn about IAYT*. Retrieved from http://www.iayt.org/?page=LearnAbout.

Thirthalli, J., Naveen, G., Rao, M., Varambally, S., Christopher, R., & Gangadhar, B. (2013). Cortisol and antidepressant effects of yoga. *Indian Journal of Psychiatry*, *55*(7), 405.

Thirthalli, J., Rao, M., Varambally, S., Christopher, R., Gangadhar, B., & Naveen, G. (2013). Positive therapeutic and neurotropic effects of yoga in depression: A comparative study. *Indian Journal of Psychiatry*, *55*(7), 400.

Uebelacker, L., & Broughton, M. (2018). Yoga for depression and anxiety: A review of published research and implications for healthcare providers. *FOCUS*, *16*(1), 95–97.

Uebelacker, L., Epstein-Lubow, G., Gaudiano, B., Tremont, G., Battle, C., & Miller, I. (2010). Hatha yoga for depression: Critical review of the evidence for efficacy, plausible mechanisms of action, and directions for future research. *Journal of Psychiatric Practice*, *16*(1), 22–33.

Umberson, D., & Karas Montez, J. (2010). Social relationships and health: A flashpoint for health policy. *Journal of Health and Social Behavior*, *51*(1_suppl), S54–S66.

Varambally, S., & Gangadhar, B. (2016). Current status of yoga in mental health services. *International Review of Psychiatry*, *28*(3), 233–235.

Villemure, C., Ceko, M., Cotton, V., & Bushnell, M. (2014). Insular cortex mediates increased pain tolerance in yoga practitioners. *Cerebral Cortex*, *24*(10), 2732–2740.

Vreeburg, S., Zitman, F., van Pelt, J., DeRijk, R., Verhagen, J., van Dyck, R., Hoogendijk, W. J., Smit, J. H., & Penninx, B. W. (2010). Salivary cortisol levels in persons with and without different anxiety disorders. *Psychosomatic Medicine*, *72*(4), 340–347.

Wooten, S., Signorile, J., Desai, S., Paine, A., & Mooney, K. (2018). Yoga meditation (YoMed) and its effect on proprioception and balance function in elders who have fallen: A randomized control study. *Complementary Therapies in Medicine*, *36*, 129–136.

Yoga Alliance. (2016, January 13). 2016 Yoga in America study conducted by *Yoga Journal* and Yoga Alliance reveals growth and benefits of the practice. [Press Release] Retrieved from https://www.yogaalliance.org/Contact_Us/Media_Inquiries/2016_Yoga_in_America_Study_Conducted_by_Yoga_Journal_and_Yoga_Alliance_Reveals_Growth_and_Benefits_of_the_Practice.

Zucker, N., Merwin, R., Bulik, C., Moskovich, A., Wildes, J., & Groh, J. (2013). Subjective experience of sensation in anorexia nervosa. *Behaviour Research and Therapy*, *51*(6), 256–265.

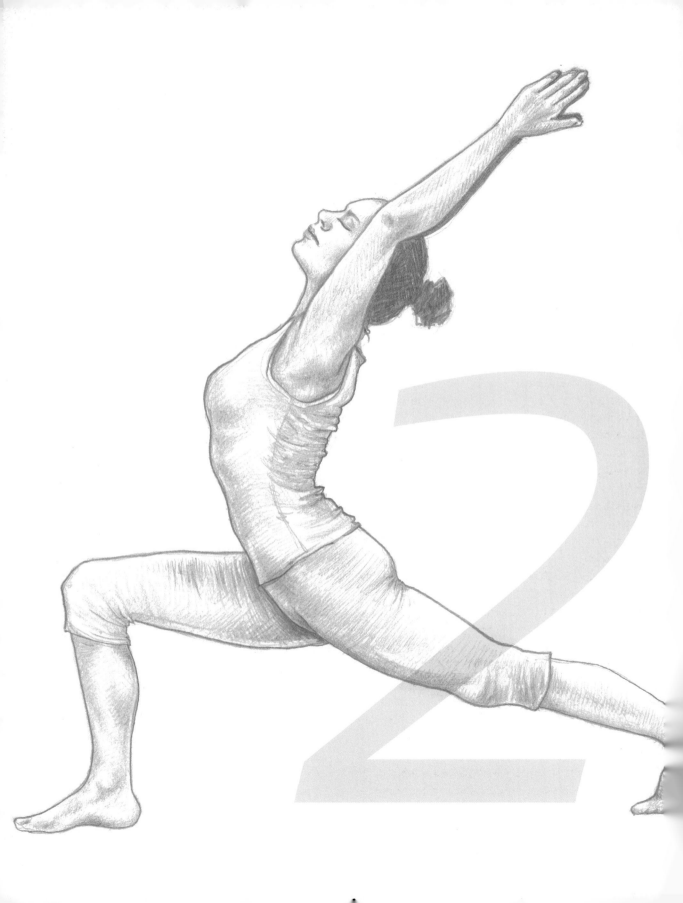

Anxiety

Heather Mason and Patricia Gerbarg

Overview

Anxiety is a mental and physical experience common to all human beings that initiates protective and defensive behavior. The anxiety response can be triggered acutely by external events (e.g., expected failure of an exam) or by internal events (e.g., thoughts, memories, beliefs, or sensations). On a spectrum of intensity, common symptoms include rapid heartbeat, trembling, shallow rapid breathing, a "knot" in the stomach, dread, repetitive negative anticipatory thoughts, heightened sensory awareness, and an urgent desire to escape. Anxiety can be distinguished from fear in that fear is expressed as a mobilizing response to an actual and imminent threat, whereas anxiety is defined as a reaction to a projected, but not necessarily actual, future threat (Fanselow & Lester, 1988; Quinn & Fanselow, 2006). Anxiety may have evolutionary survival value by helping us to notice and therefore avoid or escape potential dangers. In contrast, excessive anxiety can impair our ability to accurately evaluate a perceived threat or choose the best strategy for dealing with it (Nardi, Fontenelle, & Crippa, 2012). A distinction is made between *state anxiety*, anxiety that relates to a particular perceived threat and *trait anxiety*, which is associated with a generally anxious personality. Trait anxiety may trigger a chronic physiological cascade that over time has deleterious consequences for health. Longer and more frequently triggered anxiety responses can increase the intensity of the anxiety and the magnitude of the perceived threat. As anxiety becomes more maladaptive it may reach a level of clinical significance that meets the criteria for an anxiety disorder. The status of disorder is defined as "excessive and uncontrollable….and manifests with a wide range of physical and affective symptoms as well as changes in behaviour and cognition"; at this level it significantly impairs functioning at work or in school and/or in social relationships (Rowney, Hermida, & Malone, 2010).

> In 2007, the World Mental Health Survey Initiative reported that one in four individuals was likely to have (or previously have had) an anxiety disorder.

Although epidemiological studies report considerable variation in prevalence across different societies, anxiety disorders and depression are the prevailing global mental health problems with an estimated 10% of the world's population exhibiting a twelve-month prevalence of one or both (World Health Organization, 2016). In 2007, the World Mental Health Survey Initiative reported that one in four individuals was likely to have (or previously have had) an anxiety disorder (Kessler et al., 2007).

Diagnostics of anxiety spectrum disorders

According to the *Diagnostic and Statistical Manual of Mental Disorders* (DSM-5) (American Psychiatric Association, 2013), anxiety spectrum disorders share similar symptoms and traits such as distress, sleep disturbance, poor concentration, and compromised social and occupational functioning. The seven anxiety spectrum disorders are separation anxiety, selective mutism, specific phobia, social phobia, panic disorder (PD), agoraphobia, and generalized anxiety disorder (GAD). Previously, anxiety spectrum disorders included posttraumatic stress disorder (PTSD) and obsessive compulsive disorder (OCD), but these have been reclassified as belonging to other diagnostic categories, trauma and stress-related disorders and obsessive compulsive related disorders, respectively. Recent research shows that PTSD included an array of emotions (guilt, shame, and anger) that did not cor-relate with anxiety spectrum disorders (Pai, Suris, & North, 2017). However, many previously conducted anxiety disorder studies included PTSD and (to a lesser degree) OCD in their analyses; therefore data must be qualified with the proviso that it may not correspond to the current iteration of the diagnostic categories.

Social anxiety disorder (or social phobia) is one of the most intractable anxiety disorders, with a lifetime prevalence of 12% (National Institute for Health and Care Excellence, 2013). It is characterized by a persis-tent fear of social situations, in particular a dread of possible humiliation or embarrassment that is out of proportion to the actual threat posed. Selective mut-ism is a rare disorder usually witnessed in children and most often resolved in childhood; it is diagnosed when a person capable of speaking is consistently speechless for more than one month.

GAD is defined by excessive and persistent worry that is hard to control, causing significant distress or impairment. Data from the United States and Europe reveal a lifetime prevalence of between 4% and 5% with low levels of remission.

Agoraphobia, the fear of open public spaces and a percieved inability to escape from them, is a severe anxiety disorder that often renders a person house-bound and unable to work. Agoraphobia is often a response to the panic that emerges when an individual leaves home, explaining the high co-occurrence between agoraphobia and PD.

PD presents with persistent panic attacks and often a debilitating fear of future attacks. American and European data show a twelve-month prevalence of agoraphobia at 1% with 1.8% lifetime prevalence. For PD, there is a US lifetime prevalence of 4.7% with a twelve-month prevalence of just under 2%:

this suggests that people do remit from PD, but to a lesser extent from agoraphobia (Kessler et al., 2010; Goodwin, Faravelli, & Rosi, 2005).

A diagnosis of separation anxiety disorder is assigned to individuals who exhibit an inappropriate and excessive fear or anxiety concerning separation from those to whom they are attached. The diagnosis is applied when the distress is unusual for an individ-ual's developmental level or is prolonged and severe. For adults to receive this diagnosis, the anxiety must exceed a six-month period; for children the anxiety must exceed a four-month period. Lifetime prevalence estimates for children and adults are 4.1% and 6.6%, respectively, with a twelve-month prevalence of 1.9% (Shear, 2006).

Specific phobia is defined by a clinically significant fear of a particular object, animal, or situation that typically leads to avoidance behavior. Common pho-bias include fear of heights, snakes, and closed spaces. The prevalence within specific phobias is highly vari-able depending upon the etiology of the condition. United States statistics report specific phobia at 9.1%, with 12.2% for women and 5.8% for men (National Institute of Mental Health, 2017).

Neurophysiology and anxiety spectrum disorders

There is a high incidence of co-occurrence among anxiety spectrum disorders. For example, GAD, social phobia, and agoraphobia often present together (Bystritsky, Khalsa, Cameron, & Schiffman, 2013). One hypothesis based on this co-occurrence proposes that people with clinical levels of anxiety may share risk factors as well as an underlying propensity for an expansion of fear-based neural pathways, whereby an increasing array of stimuli is deemed as threatening (Hettema, Prescott, Myers, Neale, & Kendler, 2005). This theory of elaboration is consistent with the onset of most anxiety disorders in childhood or adolescence and with the increasing severity of symptoms over time, often reaching disorder status in early adulthood (Lijster et al., 2017). A host of interrelated factors such as genetic predisposition, early life adversity, and temperamental susceptibilities constitute vulnerabilities for the development of an anxiety disorder. Research has found that people whose parents had an anxiety or mood disorder are two to four times more likely to develop one themselves (Lieb, Isensee, Höfler, Pfister, & Wittchen, 2002). It is notable that some of these hereditary predispositions can be elicited or exacerbated by the environment provided by caregivers, including nutrition, neglect, abuse, low emotion regulation modeling, a proclivity to focus on negative ideation, cognitive framing of stressful events with excess attention to threat at the expense of other considerations, and low uncertainty tolerance. Childhood experiences associated with increased risk include an inconsistent attachment to a primary caregiver, parental divorce, financial strain, family illness, few peer relationships, and overly involved, critical parenting (Craske et al., 2017). Personality traits that may indicate predisposition to an anxiety disorder, particularly in the presence of the aforementioned risks, include low extroversion, neuroticism, and avoidance (Brandes & Bienvenu, 2006). Gender is also an influential factor in adulthood: women are one-and-a-half to two times more likely than men to present with an anxiety disorder, particularly GAD or PD (McLean et al., 2011).

> Research has found that people whose parents had an anxiety or mood disorder are two to four times more likely to develop one themselves.

As a complex mental and physical phenomenon, anxiety influences the cardiovascular, respiratory, gastrointestinal, immune, and endocrine systems, each of which is modulated by interactive feedback loops within the nervous and circulatory systems.

Although some studies report minor heterogeneity among anxiety disorders, their neural correlates show a high level of similarity (Martin, Ressler, Binder, & Nemeroff, 2009). Studies of anxiety disorders reveal dysfunctions in the central nervous system (CNS), autonomic nervous system (ANS), and hypothalamic-pituitary-adrenal (HPA) axis, a neuroendocrine component of the stress response. The two branches of the ANS, the PNS and the SNS, counterbalance each other.

The ANS and the HPA axis, the primary components of the stress response systems, can be triggered acutely in response to threat. Individuals with anxiety disorders are particularly vulnerable to overreactions to external and internal stressors and have greater difficulty calming down once they have been triggered. Such dysregulation is usually associated with reduced activity in the PNS and heightened activity of the SNS. This imbalance can lead to increased and chronic release of the excitatory neurotransmitters norepinephrine and epinephrine, with a consequent increase in arousal, alertness, vigilance, heart rate, respiratory rate, and other physiological functions (Thayer, Friedman, & Borkovec, 1996). Given the links between ANS dysfunction and stress-related medical conditions (e.g., cardiovascular disease, irritable bowel syndrome, and chronic skin conditions such as eczema and psoriasis), it is not surprising that individuals with anxiety disorders often present with these physical conditions (Azimi, Lerner, & Elmariah, 2015; Manabe, Tanaka, Hata, Kusunoki, & Haruma, 2009; Roy-Byrne et al., 2008).

Heightened activity of the HPA axis increases the release of cortisol, the most studied stress response hormone. Chronically elevated cortisol levels impede the production of immune cells and increase the risk of cardiovascular diseases, type 2 diabetes (Siddiqui, Madhu, Sharma, & Desai, 2015), cancer, cognitive impairment, and dementia. The sensitive neurons of the hippocampus, implicated in cognition, memory, and emotion regulation, are highly vulnerable to damage from excess cortisol. The association between hippocampal cell loss and conditions such as anxiety disorders and neurodegenerative disorders is an area of ongoing research (Lundberg, 2005).

Anxiety disorders are characterized by dysfunctions in emotion regulation circuits. The higher centers, such as the medial prefrontal cortex (mPFC), modulate activity in the lower subcortical centers, particularly the amygdala, via multiple pathways including the thalamus. The amygdala is the nexus of species-specific defensive reactions such as fear and anger, as well as their associated behaviors. In anxiety disorders, the amygdala, which generates the fear response, is typically overactive, while the mPFC, which inhibits this system, is underactive (Craske et al., 2017). The thalamus, a complex bilateral structure, projects to and communicates with the amygdala, mPFC, and vast areas of the cerebral cortex. When the thalamus provides input to the amygdala that it has previously encoded as threatening, the amygdala, in the absence of sufficient inhibition by the mPFC, triggers a fear response by recruiting various brain circuits, as well as activating the SNS and the HPA axis. Similarly, thoughts may activate the excitatory neurons in the PFC, which then projects to the amygdala, stimulating an integrated visceral response via the thalamus, resulting in physical symptoms of anxiety (Immordino-Yang, 2014, 2017). In anxiety disorders, these bottom-up and top-down pathways reciprocally and chronically activate each other augmenting the overall response (Bandelow et al., 2015; Porges, 2001, 2009; Venkatraman, Edlow, & Immordino-Yang, 2017).

The primary inhibitory neurotransmitter implicated in this pathology is GABA. Neurons in the PFC and other cortical structures as well as the thalamus release GABA, which inhibits overactivity in the amygdala. GABA attaches to receptor sites, for instance those in the central extended nucleus of the amygdala, thus inhibiting the overreactivity that generates anxiety reactions. Research reveals that individuals with anxiety disorders have lower levels of GABA, and that other biochemicals correlated with anxiety may block GABA receptor sites (Nuss, 2015). Numerous medications, for instance, benzodiazepines, gabapentin, and antidepressants, target the GABA system as a way of decreasing anxiety. Levels of serotonin are also attenuated in anxiety disorders, providing a rationale for the use of selective serotonin reuptake inhibitors (SSRIs) in treating anxiety disorders (Albert, Vahid-Ansari, & Luckhart, 2014).

Conventional treatment of anxiety spectrum disorders

Currently, treatment for anxiety spectrum disorders typically occurs first in primary care settings (Bystritsky et al., 2013) where individuals usually receive self-help strategies and medication or are referred for cognitive behavioral therapy (CBT). Pharmacological treatments include anxiolytics (benzodiazepines), antidepressants, beta-blockers (which block the action of epinephrine), and sometimes the anticonvulsant pregabalin.

Treatment varies depending on the type of anxiety disorder, but tends to follow a framework of psychotherapy and medication, or a combined approach that may include other techniques. The most commonly recommended form of psychotherapy, CBT for anxiety disorders, is multifaceted and involves cognitive restructuring; psychoeducation about anxiety; training in the awareness and regulation of cognitive, physiological, and behavioral cues; techniques to alter and replace unhelpful coping mechanisms; relaxation techniques; and more recently, mindfulness (Bystritsky et al., 2013; Crits-Christoph et al., 2011). Other treatments include group CBT, exposure therapy, psychodynamic psychotherapy, mindfulness-based psychotherapies, and exercise. A meta-analysis of interventions for anxiety found the greatest efficacy for medication, followed by mindfulness-based psychotherapies, CBT, relaxation techniques, and exercise (Bandelow et al., 2015). Other reviews comparing combinations of psychotherapy and medication to a mono-intervention yield inconsistent results, suggesting that responses may be individual and treatments should be tailored on a case-by-case basis (Bystritsky et al., 2013; Crits-Christoph et al., 2011).

This diversity in response may also be linked to the high co-occurrence between anxiety spectrum disorders and other mental health conditions. Specifically, anxiety disorders often present with major depressive disorder (MDD) due to underlying neurophysiological vulnerabilities as well as the disheartening impact of anxiety on an individual's personal and professional life. Additionally, addiction disorders often co-present with anxiety disorders. Childhood risk factors for addiction and anxiety disorders are analogous. Furthermore, those with chronic anxiety often self-medicate with addictive substances to dampen the crippling experience of the anxiety. Consequently, clinicians must take into account a constellation of symptoms that complicate the core anxiety diagnosis.

> Anxiety disorders often present with major depressive disorder (MDD) due to underlying neurophysiological vulnerabilities as well as the disheartening impact of anxiety on an individual's personal and professional life.

According to Baldwin and Polkinghorn (2005), 50% of those prescribed pharmacological interventions report symptom improvement. The popularity of CBT as a referral for treatment by primary care physicians may be due in part to clinical trials that claim a high degree of efficacy (Foa, Franklin, & Moser, 2002). There is controversy about the efficacy of CBT outside clinical trials. In their meta-analysis,

Stewart and Chambless (2009) found that the value of CBT in real life practice is slightly exaggerated, but still robust. However, a 2011 patient satisfaction survey of CBT treatment for anxiety disorders found that only 41.4% felt they had received adequate treatment (Baldwin & Polkinghorn, 2005; Stein et al., 2011; Stewart & Chambless, 2009). Dissatisfaction with treatment, concerns about side effects, and potential addiction to medication may explain why a high preponderance of those with anxiety disorders (56.7%) seek CAM (complementary and alternative medicine). Indeed, the diagnosis of an anxiety disorder is a predictor of CAM usage (Kessler et al., 2001; Nutt et al., 2007). Popular CAM treatments include herbs, nutrients, massage, acupuncture, homeopathy, and mind-body treatments such as mindfulness, yoga, qigong, and tai chi (Sarris et al., 2012).

Rationale for use of yoga for anxiety

The second line of Patanjali's Yoga Sutras (see Chapter 1, p. 5), "*Yoga citta vritti nirodhah*," is often translated as "Yoga leads to the cessation of the fluctuations (*vritti*) of the mind." A modern understanding is that the practice of yoga helps to ease the agitated parts of the mind. Clearly such calming effects can be beneficial in the management of anxiety. Remarkably, Patanjali's eightfold system of yoga contains many elements used in modern treatments for anxiety: cognitive reframing, behavioral recommendations, relaxation techniques focused on breath regulation, mindfulness of sensory input, as well as methods for greater cognitive flexibility, concentration, and downregulation of distress.

Nadis

Yoga also describes an energy system in which we may find congruence with our current understanding of the ANS. According to yogic philosophy, energy tracks, called *nadis*, course through the body carrying the lifeforce (*prana*). Free flow in all *nadis* is vital for health. However, three main *nadis* exert the most influence on wellbeing. Along the left side of the spinal cord up through the left nostril is the *ida*, the *nadi* associated with calming energy, which may be analogous to the PNS. On the right side of the spinal cord up through the right nostril runs the *pingala*, the active aspect, which could correspond to the SNS. In the center, running up the spinal cord, is the *sushumna nadi*. Specific yoga practices are intended to balance the forces of *ida* and *pingala*, causing *prana* to rise through the *sushumna*, leading to a positive shift in mental and physical experience giving rise to peace and clarity. Much of yoga is focused on balancing *ida* and *pingala*. Indeed, the term *hatha* is sometimes translated as "sun-moon": *pingala* refers to the sun and the moon corresponds to *ida*. Based on this transliteration of ancient ideas into modern scientific ones, yoga can be considered a practice that balances the ANS and is therefore uniquely suited to the treatment of anxiety and anxiety spectrum disorders.

Autonomic nervous system and heart rate variability

Numerous studies support a role for yoga in balancing the ANS. Researchers often measure autonomic balance using heart rate variability (HRV), derived from the rate of change in the number of heartbeats per minute occurring between inhaling and exhaling. Normally, whenever we inhale the heart rate slightly speeds up then slows down during exhalation; this is called normal sinus arrhythmia (RSA). It occurs because breathing in stimulates the sympathetic nerves, which release noradrenaline, increasing the rate of action potentials generated in the sinoatrial node (the heart's pacemaker). Conversely, breathing out stimulates the parasympathetic nerves, which release acetylcholine, decreasing the rate of sinoatrial node action potentials. HRV is a composite of the effects of breathing (and other factors) on vagal parasympathetic activity (slowing the heart) and sympathetic activity (speeding up the heart). In anxiety

disorders, the overactivity of the SNS and underactivity of the PNS lead to a reduction in HRV, which reflects a loss of flexibility and adaptability of the cardio-respiratory system. Even more crucial for anxiety disorders, low HRV indicates that the PNS, necessary for feeling safe and calm, is underactive, while the SNS is free to induce anxiety in all of its manifestations. The fact that respiratory rate is a major factor in determining SNS, PNS, and HRV gives us a powerful key to emotion regulation. Respiration is the only autonomic function that can be controlled voluntarily. Therefore, voluntarily regulated breathing practices (VRBPs) provide a portal of entry to the ANS, achieved by sending messages from the respiratory system to the brain, which influences emotional states (Brown & Gerbarg, 2017; Brown, Gerbarg, & Muench, 2013; Gerbarg & Brown, 2016). Research shows increases in HRV associated with integrated yoga programs and discrete yoga practices (Tyagi & Cohen, 2016); and studies also indicate that slow controlled breathing, a cornerstone of many styles of yoga, can significantly increase HRV (Brown et al., 2013; Brown & Gerbarg, 2012; Peng et al., 1999).

Notably, the vagally mediated parasympathetic branch of the ANS exerts a greater influence on HRV than the sympathetic branch (Beech et al., 2018). Based on his groundbreaking neuroanatomic studies, Stephen Porges developed the polyvagal theory, which proposes that the vagus nerves contain pathways from different levels of evolution. He noted that the majority of vagal fibers are unmyelinated (lacking the myelin sheaths found in later stages of evolution). Myelin forms a sheath that surrounds and insulates the nerve, enabling faster transmission of nerve impulses. Myelinated fibers comprise only 3% of vagal pathways, are found only in mammals, and are most developed in primates. Porges explains that the myelinated nerves within the vagus significantly influence prosocial behavior because they articulate to and permit greater control of those areas of the body that support social engagement. These include the larynx for voice control, facial muscles for emotion expression, neck muscles for turning toward another person, and the muscles controlling attunement of the ears to human voices. Furthermore, when vagal tone is higher, defensive reactivity is reduced, which allows positive social interactions to occur more easily (Porges, 2011). The effects may be further enhanced in a yoga group practice environment, which for the most part doesn't require conversation or eye contact. Practicing in this way while experiencing physiological shifts that support social engagement could potentially reduce anxiety and social anxiety in particular. Increased vagal tone is also linked to a decrease in symptoms of disorders in which autonomic dysfunction is implicated, such as anxiety spectrum disorders.

According to polyvagal theory (Porges, 2009):

- a physiological state characterized by increased vagal influence on HRV supports social engagement and bonding;

- any stimuli that result in a feeling of safety can recruit neural circuits which support the social engagement system and inhibit defensive limbic structures; and

- interoception (the perception of sensations arising from inside the body) enables social behavior by distinguishing between safe and dangerous situations.

Physical yoga practices provide abundant opportunities to stimulate interoceptive experiences through movement and breathing. Interoception is generally defined as the perception of sensations arising from inside the body, including the internal sensations associated with breathing. Every movement and every breath activate millions of internal receptors that transmit messages through neural pathways (afferents) to the brain (Figure 2.1). This bottom-up transmission from the body to the brain has been called "interoceptive messaging" by Gerbarg and Brown. Voluntarily regulated breathing practices (VRBPs) enable us to send bottom-up messages from the respiratory system to the brain, messages that can help us to regulate our emotions (Brown & Gerbarg, 2017). By studying changes in anxiety symptoms and biological markers (e.g., HRV, cortisol, inflammatory markers) and through brain imaging, it may be possible in the future to correlate yoga techniques with the effective treatment of anxiety spectrum disorders.

Changes in biochemicals implicated in anxiety have also been reported with yoga practice. For example, several studies found statistically significant reductions in cortisol pre- and post-yoga intervention (Field, Diego, Delgado, & Medina, 2013; Naveen et al., 2016; Riley & Park, 2015). Intriguingly, a 2014 randomized controlled trial (RCT) found statistically significant improvements in perceived stress and cortisol levels for a stretching yoga intervention, but not for a restorative yoga intervention (Corey et al., 2014). This preliminary finding indicates that for an anxious population, more stretching and movement may be preferable to long periods of stillness and silence, wherein anxious ruminations can emerge. Movement may engage the mind and activate bottom-up calming parasympathetic pathways, positively influencing the internal biochemical environment.

> Movement may engage the mind and activate bottom-up calming parasympathetic pathways, positively influencing the internal biochemical environment.

In a pilot study, Streeter et al. (2007) found that yoga increased GABA levels in the thalamus. A subsequent RCT by the same group demonstrated that yoga significantly increased GABA more than in a metabolically matched exercise intervention (Streeter et al., 2010). Drawing on these findings and on polyvagal theory, Streeter and colleagues proposed the

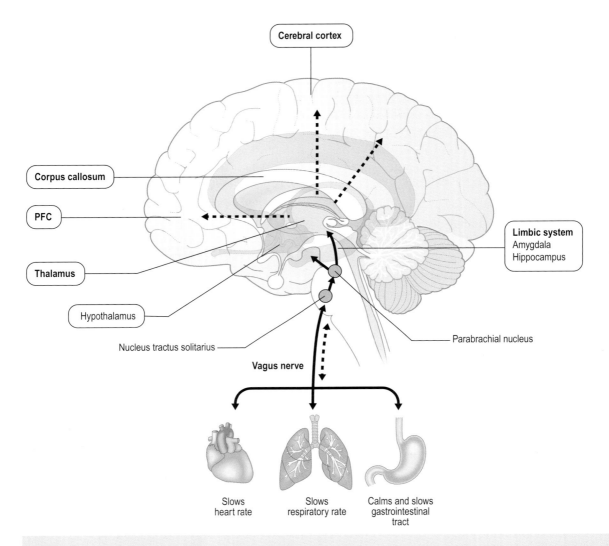

Figure 2.1

Afferent branches of the vagus nerve. Representation of vagal output to the brain. Redrawn with permission from Brown RP, Gerbarg PL, Muskin PR. *How to Use Herbs, Nutrients, and Yoga in Mental Health Care.* W.W. Norton. 2012

vagal-gaba theory, extending Porges's work to the potential effects of increased PNS activity on brain GABA (Streeter, Gerbarg, Saper, Ciraulo, & Brown, 2012). This offers an additional mechanism whereby certain movements and breathing practices could improve emotion regulation. Preliminary evidence suggests that during gentle slow breathing and yogic postures, increased vagal activity may upregulate GABAergic transmission along inhibitory pathways from the PFC and insular cortex to the amygdala

(Streeter et al., 2012). This in turn may reduce the overactivity of the amygdala occurring during anxiety. This theory is being evaluated via clinical investigation into the effects of yoga and coherent breathing (gentle breathing, inhaling for six seconds and exhaling for six seconds) in patients with depression, but it has yet to be tested with anxiety disorders (Nyer 2018; Streeter et al. 2017).

Downregulating amygdala activity

Other research has been conducted to examine different mechanisms that point to yoga's role in downregulating amygdala activity. One study comparing the chanting of the yoga mantra, OM, to making the sound "sssssssssssssssss" found greater deactivation of the amygdala during OM practice, signifying that OM chanting may help curb anxiety: researchers attributed this change to vibrational stimulation of the vagus (Kalyani et al., 2011).

Afonso (2017) found that long-term yoga practitioners had larger PFCs than age-matched controls. Given that reduced PFC activity and volume, as well as increased amygdala activity, have been found in anxiety disorders, this evidence correlating yoga with greater PFC volume is encouraging.

Research on yoga for anxiety

There is a growing corpus of research on yoga for anxiety in which anxiety may be the main complaint or be present in relationship to another disorder but does not meet criteria for an anxiety spectrum disorder. However, there is a paucity of research on yoga for individuals who do meet diagnostic criteria for anxiety spectrum disorders. Pilkington et al. (2016) reviewed research into yoga for anxiety consisting of three studies of yoga for GAD, one of yoga plus CBT, one of yoga and CBT for panic disorder, and two of yoga for anxiety neurosis (an earlier diagnosis that has been replaced by GAD and PD). Two open studies

investigated the effect on GAD of Sudarshan Kriya yoga (SKY), a breath-based yoga intervention that combines gentle calming breathing techniques with highly activating cyclical breathing. In the first trial, patients with severe treatment-resistant GAD with co-occurrences were taught SKY for five days, were asked to practice the technique each day for 20 minutes, and were given six weekly follow-up sessions: among the 31 individuals who completed the trial there was a 73% response rate and a 41% remission rate. In the second trial, 69 patients with GAD practiced SKY for six months: significant reductions in anxiety were measured by the Hamilton Anxiety Scale (Doria, de Vuono, Sanlorenzo, Irtelli, & Mencacci, 2015; Katzman et al., 2012). A small nonrandomized pilot study compared yoga with naturopathy in twelve patients with GAD (Gupta & Mamidi, 2013). Following three weeks of treatment, both groups had improved levels of anxiety. However, results from such a small study are preliminary at best (Gupta & Mamidi, 2013; Pilkington et al, 2016).

There is also interest in investigating yoga combined with CBT. A 2014 open study augmented CBT with Kundalini yoga for patients with GAD, during which the participants met for six 90-minute weekly sessions of a yoga-based CBT (Y-CBT) program. Statistically significant changes were reported for trait anxiety and also on the Treatment Outcome Package (TOP) scale measuring depression, panic, sleep, and quality of life. Although researchers suggested that Y-CBT might have added value over CBT, these preliminary findings need to be confirmed by a randomized controlled study (Khalsa, Greiner-Ferris, Hofmann, & Khalsa, 2015).

One study in PD compared yoga to yoga combined with group CBT. The interventions lasted for ten months and were administered at weekly 100-minute sessions. Both types of intervention significantly reduced anxiety, panic beliefs, and panic regarding bodily sensations. The yoga enriched with CBT showed additional reductions for all of these symptoms (Vorkapic & Rangé, 2014). Further investigation into the value of comparing yoga with CBT and other therapies for enhanced outcomes is warranted. This could also support the role of top-down mechanisms present in yoga in combination with its bottom-up effects.

Two studies on yoga for anxiety neurosis were conducted in Indian hospitals. One found that yoga breath practices improved anxiety more than a placebo control. It was also reported that a comprehensive yoga intervention led to greater improvement in anxiety in comparison to diazepam (Sahasi, Mohan, & Kacker, 1989; Sharma, Azmi, & Settiwar, 1991). However, when reviewing these trials, Kirkwood et al. (2005) observed poor methodology and follow-up work for both.

Since 2005, several reviews have evaluated the effects of yoga on anxiety in individuals who were not diagnosed with anxiety spectrum disorders. One briefly reviewed research evidence and offered a rationale for using yoga to promote self-efficacy and comprehensive transformation (Joshi & Desousa, 2012). A review of 35 trials found that 25 of them showed significant improvements in stress and/or anxiety. Although this evidence was promising, it was marred by inconsistencies: interventions varied widely and the methodologies were not rigorous (Li & Goldsmith, 2012). A review of 25 studies, including sixteen RCTs and seven prospective, controlled, non-randomized studies, reported yoga's role in reducing state anxiety in certain situations (Chugh-Gupta, Baldassarre, & Vrkljan, 2013). Two reviews of yoga efficacy in depression and anxiety found superior evidence for depression, with promising albeit inconsistent results for anxiety (Duan-Porter et al., 2016; Uebelacker & Broughton, 2013). A review of 32 articles on yoga efficacy for anxiety in children and

adolescents found that yoga reduced anxiety in every study, but unfortunately poor methodology and high heterogeneity among the interventions precluded clear conclusions (Weaver & Darragh, 2015). There is general agreement that yoga has value for the treatment of anxiety, but that better study design and clarity regarding the efficacy of different interventions are necessary to understand which practices should be employed, and whether yoga should be used as a monotherapy or as part of a multimodal protocol.

Exploring appropriate dosage and best practices for anxiety, de Manincor and colleagues surveyed 24 yoga teachers with expertise in applying yoga to mental health conditions (de Manincor, Bensoussan, Smith, Fahey, & Bourchier, 2015). The consensus indicated that practice should be conducted over five 30–40 minute sessions per week for at least six weeks. Breath-regulation techniques, relaxing postures, relaxation techniques, and meditation were identified as best practices for improving anxiety. Teachers also suggested avoiding stimulating practices such as rapid breathing or breath holding, or practices involving complicated instructions or a heated environment (de Manincor et al., 2015). Some of the recommendations conflicted with protocols in other studies. Certain interventions focus on practices that may stimulate and then calm the nervous system, theoretically promoting physiological flexibility. In contrast, other studies focus on the vital role of calming practices without stimulating techniques.

Recommendations for practice

Yoga teachers/therapists offer yoga for anxiety classes to individuals with self-reported anxiety as well as to those with diagnosed anxiety spectrum disorders. Such classes can offer techniques described below) that are useful for anxiety in general. Alternatively, classes for anxiety spectrum disorders are most appropriately taught by a yoga therapist, who should have a higher level of training to develop cumulative skills from one week to the next. Based on the survey by de Manincor et al. (2015), as well as on the experience gained by this author (Heather Mason) from delivering yoga courses for people with anxiety spectrum disorders, we recommend that courses be six to eight weeks long, that sessions occur at least biweekly, and that each session lasts for 90 minutes.

Developing safety

Coming to a yoga class to confront feelings of mental discomfort takes great courage, and it is very affirming for students with anxiety to be congratulated for taking an active role in improving their wellbeing.

When offering anxiety-focused classes, cultivating an environment of safety is paramount. There are basic safety tenets common to any yoga class for anxiety. For example, the space should be quiet with very limited interference. Individuals with anxiety tend to be on high alert, such that unexpected sounds or events can be jarring; and due to ANS dysfunction, a person with chronic anxiety will often have more difficulty calming down once they become agitated.

> When offering anxiety-focused classes, cultivating an environment of safety is paramount.

Ample space between the mats is important. When people are chronically anxious the mind feels full, and there is often a correlated feeling of limited physical space, creating a greater need for such space. Specifically, the gaps between mats should be wide enough to prevent anyone from accidentally touching another participant, for example, when lying on the mat with arms spread out to the sides or with arms reaching overhead.

Because heat in the body often accompanies the stress response, a hot room may trigger anxiety. However, the room should not be too cold. People with anxiety tend to have cold hands and feet, because when the sympathetic drive is increased small blood vessels in the hands, feet, and gut constrict. Simultaneously, the body redirects blood and oxygen to large muscles and the brain. Finding a temperature that keeps most of the group comfortable is important. For temperature variations, providing blankets and allowing those with cold feet to keep their socks on is comforting. If the yoga class has mats with good traction, students should not be asked to remove socks. However, physical safety overrides the importance of warm feet, so if slipping is a risk, socks cannot stay on.

Because the vagally mediated social engagement network is underactive when anxiety is present, eye contact can be uncomfortable for people with anxiety, especially for those with social phobia. The mats should be set up in rows rather than a semicircle so that students are not facing one other. Teachers should be be mindful about their eye contact with students. Providing options for a downward gaze in poses during which the teacher will be facing students, or attending to a *dristi* (a specific point of focus for the eyes) as is done in classical yoga, provides a structured focal point that helps to diminish uneasiness. Note this does not mean that the teacher must avoid a student's gaze, rather just to be aware of individual reactions to eye contact.

Specific safety needs can best be gauged in yoga therapy classes, when a therapist has obtained background information from each student. For a drop-in anxiety-focused class, intake forms are important, and they are essential when running a program for anxiety or anxiety spectrum disorders (see example intake form in Appendix). As students provide information about what may distress them in a class environment, they may lower their guard a little, knowing that the teacher/therapist will be more aware of their sensitivities. Most importantly, intake forms allow the teacher to effectively tailor the class to accommodate individual needs and concerns.

Uncertainty tolerance tends to be very low for people with anxiety. Explaining what you are going to do before you do it helps reduce anxiety. This applies to a brief overview at the start of class as well as teaching movements. For example, informing a student that you are going to adjust their arm position before you do so may avoid causing an excess startle or fear reaction. Providing information about the flow of the class, about how long a pose is going to be held, and what is expected fosters certainty and allows students to relax. Teachers must be consistent and stick to what they say. This means keeping minor promises such as class time boundaries, length of time in poses, and what will be offered in class. If students sign up for an extended course, teachers can gradually provide less information, gently guiding students to tolerate some uncertainty, a helpful skill for them to take into daily life.

Class sequencing

Although inducing relaxation for someone with anxiety is of primary importance, there is often a misunderstanding of what this entails. People with high anxiety are not usually able to begin class with what are traditionally deemed relaxation practices. When there is high sympathetic drive and the mind is racing, sitting silently in gentle, restorative poses may kindle rumination and distress.

> People with high anxiety are not usually able to begin class with what are traditionally deemed relaxation practices.

Starting class with dynamic movement and short holds (45–60 seconds) in challenging poses, especially standing postures, help keeps the mind in the present. As needs may vary, students should be cued to go at their own pace, and honor what they feel they need. Knowing that a yoga teacher/therapist is providing the opportunity to tend to their own comfort, rather than expecting them to conform to expectations, often helps to reduce anxiety.

Dynamic movement could include inhaling while raising hands overhead and exhaling while bringing the arms down, shoulder rolls, cats and cows, and joint rotations; or if the group is physically strong, it might involve sun salutations and *vinyasa* flow. Make sure not to include breath holding, because breathlessness is a common feature of heightened anxiety and therefore holding the breath may increase anxiety. Likewise, the level of challenge for poses depends on the physical capacity of the class. For one group this might mean a very gentle lunge or a chair-assisted standing posture; for another group it might be a sequence of warrior postures. As neck and shoulder tension commonly occur with anxiety, be sure to teach postures that help release these areas. These should be practiced with a pranayama to relax and balance the ANS (see later for focal points of practice).

After about 30–40 minutes of melding dynamic moving and standing poses with pranayama, the body is usually tired, some of the nervous energy has been expended, and the nervous system is generally calmer. This is the perfect time to bring students down to the mat for longer holds in gentle and relaxing poses. Forward bends that stretch the hamstrings are particularly useful, because stretching large muscle groups can be quite relaxing and can release physical tension.

Savasana (a supine resting pose) should be taught with care when students are exhibiting symptoms of anxiety. Although the intent of *savasana* is generally understood as time for relaxation, for those with anxiety disorders, *savasana* provides the greatest space for rumination. Therefore, long *savasanas* are not advisable. To avoid this problem, *savasana* should either be kept short (five to seven minutes), or it should be replaced by a guided relaxation practice, for example, yoga nidra.

Focal points of practice

There are three main focal points to help reduce anxiety during yoga:

1. The development of self-regulation through relaxation-based practices.

2. The cultivation of resiliency.

3. The development of mindfulness in conjunction with 1 and 2.

Self-regulation and relaxation

Self-regulation includes the ability to modulate anxious responses by actively working to induce parasympathetic drive and by cognitive reappraisal. Yoga for anxiety programs should devote the first few sessions to teaching students to notice signals of sympathetic activity and how to reduce them. Many methods can be added for class relaxation such as stretching poses, OM chanting, and the basic class sequencing discussed earlier. However, the influence of breath on the ANS is profound and immediate, and hence pranayama practices that increase parasympathetic activity are a core and primary focus. Two of the most effective techniques are elongated exhalation and conscious slow, gentle abdominal breathing. As mentioned in the rationale section, during exhalation there is increased vagal transmission to the heart, reducing the heart rate. Students with anxiety spectrum disorders can find relief when they learn how to slow their breath and slow their pounding heart. The parasympathetic, calming effects can be further enhanced with *ujjayi* (a form of breathing that involves gentle contraction of throat muscles and leads to an ocean-like sound) during exhalation. It is preferable to teach anxious students ujjayi on the exhalation rather than on the inhalation because they will tend to *pull in* the inhalation, which may increase sympathetic drive—possibly even triggering the stress response—thus undoing the calming effects associated with the breath. Therefore, the technique should be performed softly with a barely audible sound and without any strain or forcefulness in moving the air in or out. After the student has mastered ujjayi on the exhalation, they can try it as they inhale as well. To really benefit from this practice, and for it to become embodied learning for off-the-mat emotion regulation, students should be taught to elongate the exhale in every posture until *savasana*. In more challenging poses, the teacher can prompt students to see how elongating exhalation helps them stay present in the posture. Learning how to stay present during uncomfortable feelings and situations is excellent preparation for dealing with fear and stress in daily life.

> Individuals with anxiety tend to breathe primarily into the chest and at a faster rate than other people.

Abdominal breathing is equally important as learning to elongate the exhalation. Individuals with anxiety tend to breathe primarily into the chest and at a faster rate than other people. Rapid chest breathing (known clinically as accessory breathing because it relies on the effort of a group of muscles in the upper chest and neck collectively known as accessory muscles) activates the sympathetic response. Reciprocally, sympathetic activity promotes rapid accessory breathing. Those with chronic anxiety and anxiety spectrum disorders are prone to breathing this way, which maintains a bidirectional feedback loop of mounting threat. Teaching students slow breathing and relaxing abdominal muscles to allow freer movement of the breath curbs this habit through respiratory signals that activate vagal parasympathetic pathways, calming the body and mind, reducing defensiveness, and supporting social engagement.

Additional benefits of *ujjayi*

Ujjayi may enhance the calming effect of slow breathing and prolonged exhalation by adding vibrational components to the vagal stimulation (Brown & Gerbarg, 2005, 2012; Gerbarg & Brown 2015). The vagus nerve enervates the respiratory tract from the lungs up through the larynx and pharynx. Breathing against the resistance created by vocal cord contraction increases stimulation of the vagus (Brown & Gerbarg, 2005).

Cultivating resiliency

Resiliency refers to the capacity to respond to stressors adaptively, that is, the ability to bounce back, recover, and function well following an adverse event. The practice of relaxation and regulation techniques helps develop resiliency by increasing the range and flexibility of the stress response systems. Resiliency fosters the ability to appropriately respond to the challenges of life; mobilizing for action when necessary and seamlessly returning to a state of peace and ease when action is no longer needed. It is a comprehensive capacity that includes cognitive, neurological, emotional, and physiological flexibility, all of which are influenced by the ANS and reflected in HRV (Thayer, 2000). Flexibility in the ANS includes the ability to downregulate quickly when sympathetic activity isn't necessary, and to move from a relaxed state to a more energetic one if a situation calls for it. Relaxation-based practices theoretically tone the vagus and enhance HRV and resiliency. Furthermore, specific techniques that tone both the sympathetic and parasympathetic branches of the ANS also cultivate resiliency. For example, alternating between a calming and an activating pranayama, which could be a brief rapid breath (*bhastrika* or *kapalabhati*) followed by a slow *ujjayi* breath. Another example is the cyclical breathing (no pause between inhalation and exhalation) at varying rates, slow, medium, fast, and slow again, as is practiced in Sudarshan Kriya yoga (discussed in the section covering research on yoga for anxiety). The basis of resiliency is the capacity to shift, adapt, and balance activity of the SNS and the PNS in response to changing demands and challenges, which

can be trained through these techniques. Because introducing a breath that increases sympathetic drive can induce anxiety, it needs to be done with caution; please refer to the Additional Precautions section for specific guidance.

Research on the respiratory system aligns with the yogic idea of balancing the *ida* and *pingala nadis*, namely that right nostril breathing is associated with sympathetic drive, while left nostril breathing promotes greater parasympathetic activity (Pal, Agarwal, Karthik, Pal, & Nanda, 2014). Teaching alternate-nostril breathing (ANB) may therefore balance these systems (Lee & Ghiya, 2012). Because airflow is reduced during this practice, it is best to build up to it gradually, reducing the risk of causing panic. People with PD may associate the slight breathlessness that usually occurs in the learning stages with symptoms of a panic attack. Therefore, yoga teachers should tread lightly and use careful discernment regarding when and how to introduce alternate-nostril breathing.

Teaching coherent breathing, which involves gently inhaling for six seconds and gently exhaling for six seconds, is one of the most effective ways to enhance HRV. For most adults, excluding significant respiratory or other medical conditions, optimal HRV occurs when the individual does coherent breathing at 4.5–6 breaths per minute (bpm). Adults who are more than six feet tall reach optimal HRV between 3–4.5 bpm. The influence of breathing on HRV is most amplified at this rate (Brown & Gerbarg, 2012). Students can practice coherent breathing as a stand-alone technique during class, or can be guided to keep this breathing rhythm throughout the entire posture practice. Pacing the breath with a soundtrack of a chime once every six seconds to cue inhalation and exhalation assures the ideal breath rate and eliminates the sympathetically activating effect of mental counting. Students can download a breath-pacing chime track (or other appealing tones) to use during home practice, during the day when they feel stressed or anxious, and at night to quell the worried ruminations that often prevent sleep (Brown & Gerberg, 2012).

Threading mindfulness through the practice

A state of mindfulness may naturally arise as postures direct students' attention to sensations in the body; this will engage cortical structures without effort. Specific mindfulness teaching can enrich this practice, further recruiting top-down processes through explicit attention to body sensations and cognitive reframing.

Mindfulness techniques can be integrated into self-regulating practices. For example, the yoga teacher/therapist can ask students to notice where the breath is felt in the body, to notice the specific sensation of breathing into this area, and then to consciously bring the breath into the abdomen. Offering very basic psychoeducation regarding how chest (accessory) breathing increases sympathetic response while belly (diaphragmatic) breathing invokes parasympathetic activation, followed by a recommendation to notice how mood and thoughts elicit respiratory changes (throughout the practice), can help students to observe this process in daily life. In fact, students may learn to prevent a mounting sympathetic response by developing awareness of the location of the breath; if they notice they are chest breathing they can immediately engage in abdominal breathing, thus curbing anxiety. Similarly, teaching students to notice the length of breath, sense if anxiety is present, and then elongate the exhalation, is another way to bring mindfulness and regulation together.

Building tolerance

Yoga teachers/therapists can use challenging poses as a form of mindful exposure therapy. For example, students can be asked to maintain an intense position such as *utkatasana* (chair, or powerful, pose) while noticing their mental reactions. Classic reactions include a desire to escape, self-judgment, and fear, especially concerning how long the experience will last. The teacher/therapist can explicitly name such responses to help students notice them.

> Reminding students that the class is a safe space to explore thoughts and reactions may strengthen their resolve to try.

Another way to build tolerance and also self-awareness is to take a student into a challenging pose and ask them to notice exactly which sensations are arising and driving their desire to escape the pose, and also what thoughts and beliefs arise in connection with these sensations. Through careful use of humor, the teacher can mention common mental and physical experiences to normalize them (assuring students that their experiences may be different and unique). Reminding students that the class is a safe space to explore thoughts and reactions may strengthen their resolve to try. Mentioning that any physical distress can be easily alleviated by simply exiting the posture—as opposed to in daily life, where distress is not so easily relieved—inspires a greater willingness to explore. By remaining present with the experience, students can build greater tolerance and a different relationship to uncomfortable feelings. This enhanced awareness can be transposed onto uncomfortable experiences and responses as they occur outside the yoga class.

Managing emotionally challenging experiences in yoga classes

It is not uncommon for people with high anxiety to have anxiety responses triggered in class or individual yoga therapy sessions. The experience of doing something new, coupled with a host of sensations that arise through poses and the tendency to easily panic, may elevate levels of anxiety, even in classes that are tailored to reduce anxiety. This is not something for the yoga teacher/therapist to worry about. Such reactions provide opportunities for students to learn how to manage their anxiety reactions in a safe and accepting environment. The following considerations are helpful in calming down a student and recontexualizing the experience: normalizing the experience for the student can reduce embarrassment and fear, and explaining how this reaction in a yoga class provides an opportunity to alter responses can reframe the experience as useful in managing anxiety. This can be done in a group setting as well as in individual yoga therapy sessions (albeit it with only a brief explanation as other students may need attention). The student can then be asked if there is a pose they would prefer. To further downregulate anxiety, the yoga teacher/therapist might stand or kneel by the student and breathe with them at a slow controlled rate to help the student slow down their breathing. This may be enhanced by suggesting the student looks at the teacher, potentially engaging the mirror neuron system to help guide the way to a slower respiratory rate. Another method is to hold a challenging or empowering pose that redirects attention (unless this was the cause of distress) and mitigates feelings of helplessness or vulnerability.

Scope of practice for yoga therapists

Given the higher level of distress for individuals with anxiety disorders compared to those with trait anxiety, we recommend that classes targeting anxiety spectrum disorders be taught by yoga therapists. Techniques to manage emotionally overwhelming reactions require greater knowledge and understanding of general anxiety and anxiety spectrum disorders, the therapeutic relationship, and the potentially harmful adverse reactions in clients. These are beyond the scope of practice of most yoga teachers.

Yoga therapists are also best prepared to offer individual sessions for people with anxiety disorders because their training specifically covers the use of yoga in anxiety management. Through a thorough clinical intake, yoga therapists can understand factors contributing to anxiety and design a therapeutic plan that uniquely suits the student, as the following case report illustrates.

CASE REPORT

Dan suffered from PD (panic disorder). Participating in a yoga class for anxiety management reduced his anxiety overall, but panic attacks continued to plague him. Dan was nervous about his performance at work and would often have panic attacks on the way to the office. In the initial session with the yoga therapist he explained that his experience of panic included a rapid change in breathing and limpness in his legs that would render him unable to walk or even stand. Incapacitated by this experience, Dan was despondent and self-loathing and often did not make it to work, which only worsened the problem. Through mindful inquiry during yoga therapy, Dan was able to identify the cascade of thoughts that would precede a full-blown panic attack. As Dan only lived two miles from work, the yoga therapist suggested that he walk rather than take public transport. The intention was that the act of walking would prevent Dan's legs from going limp. Therefore, Dan was instructed that whenever he felt nervous during his walk, he should speed up to prevent his legs from buckling and simultaneously elongate his *ujjayi* exhale (Dan already knew *ujjayi* breathing from his yoga class). Whenever the thought cascade began, even before his anxiety arose, Dan was to speed up and elongate his exhalation.

In later sessions, Dan identified aspects of his life in which he felt inadequate. He learned to overcome feelings of inadequacy by the same techniques: elongated *ujjayi* exhalation and fast walking. An assessment of Dan's movement and strength revealed weakness in his shoulders and lack of tone in his leg muscles. A yoga therapy sequence was designed to strengthen Dan's legs and shoulder muscles, as well as to open his chest to give him a sense of confidence. Over the course of four months Dan's body began to change, his panic attacks subsided, and he started to feel competent at work, which in turn enhanced other aspects of his life.

Yoga in clinical practice

Integrating yoga practices with psychotherapy and other forms of mental health treatment can significantly support therapeutic progress. With specific training, clinicians can learn how to integrate breath practices, basic movements, and yogic relaxation techniques into a wide array of treatments.

Breathing techniques that cultivate self-regulation and promote resiliency, which supports client self-efficacy, can be integrated into both therapy sessions and home practices. Many psychology students are already taught breath-regulation techniques to help clients manage distress. Through yoga training, clinicians can refine these skills. Similarly, psychiatric nurses, psychiatrists, general practitioners, dentists, social workers, counselors, and other therapists can be trained to teach breathing techniques to anxious patients. Anxiety often arises during therapy sessions as the client tries to talk about painful, frightening experiences. The fear of this anxiety can inhibit the client from thinking or talking about such issues. Anxiety-disordered patients frequently rely on avoidance, including avoidance of their own memories and thoughts, to prevent the discomfort of overwhelming emotions.

Teaching patients to do calming practices during therapy sessions as needed provides a way for them to work on anxiety-related issues and to make progress. Knowing that they can control anxiety emboldens patients to tackle issues they would otherwise avoid.

> Anxiety-disordered patients frequently rely on avoidance, including avoidance of their own memories and thoughts, to prevent the discomfort of overwhelming emotions.

Sometimes during a session, after exploring difficult issues, a patient may feel upset. Encouraging the patient to do three to five minutes of calming breath practices at the end of the session reduces distress and facilitates transition out into the world.

Mental health professionals can also learn to teach techniques like yoga nidra to help clients to deeply relax and better understand the roots of their anxiety. Traditionally, yoga nidra was used to induce a deep relaxation to uncover and transform unconscious tendencies. Its careful use in therapeutic work can be highly valuable in helping clients to accept and integrate previously intolerable feelings and emotions. Teaching yoga nidra does require specific training, because it differs from the techniques generally used by mental health providers. Many guided yoga nidra downloads are available, but students with acute anxiety disorders should be referred to teachers with expertise in applying yoga nidra to this population, rather than directed to use recordings without therapeutic supervision.

The worldview offered by yoga may also support therapeutic work. Rather than focusing on pathology, yoga sees the person as a dynamic interplay of arising tendencies, some of which have been cultivated and others that have been ignored, and most of which derive from forces outside the client's realm of responsibility. Through self-development, calm and ease can emerge while fear and worry can move into the background. People need not suppress aspects of themselves, but rather notice the spectrum of experiences, aspects of the self, wherein constant change is the norm. This broader view can help patients re-envision themselves on a trajectory of possibility rather than to identify solely with a diagnosis. Clients who are interested in yoga philosophy may also benefit from the comprehensive view of reality expressed in yoga where daily concerns can be held by the background container of the cosmos. Many people with anxiety disorders feel isolated and disconnected. The experience of meaningful connection to oneself and to others, which sometimes occurs during yoga practice, can mitigate isolation and greatly enhance the quality of life.

Additional precautions

People with anxiety spectrum disorders can be exquisitely sensitive to physical sensations, social interactions, perceived criticisms, tones of voice, or other stimuli that they may perceive or misperceive as unsafe. Although it is impossible to eliminate all potential anxiety triggers, being mindful of the client's vulnerabilities enables the teacher/therapist to minimize adverse reactions (see the section covering developing safety in yoga in clinical practice).

The most specific precautions exist around teaching any kind of rapid breathing. In a one-on-one session, the client should be asked about the nature of their anxiety, including the duration and intensity of anxiety, and the presence of symptoms such as panic, phobias, and specific triggers. The yoga teacher/therapist should also find out what (if any) methods have helped the client control their anxiety in the past, so that the client's strengths and skills can be integrated into their treatment plan.

> The most specific precautions exist around teaching any kind of rapid breathing.

In an anxiety-focused yoga class, it is important to avoid bringing attention or exposure to individual students by making general suggestions to the whole class, for instance, "As we do more rapid breathing, if you begin to feel anxious, just slow your breathing and breathe gently until it subsides." Given that people with anxiety may struggle to calm down from excess sympathetic drive, teaching a calming pranayama, such as gentle *ujjayi*, followed by an activating one, such as a very brief *kapalabhati*, and then returning to *ujjayi*, is safer than teaching only rapid or forceful breathing, particularly at the beginning.

Future directions

Research on yoga for anxiety, studies exploring discrete mechanisms, and an increasing trend toward using yoga in anxiety management, collectively indicate that the inclusion of yoga in the treatment of anxiety disorders is on the rise. Although yoga is widely used for everyday anxiety, a gap exists in knowledge about the efficacy of yoga programs for anxiety spectrum disorders. Better studies are needed to bridge this gap, particularly to develop evidence-based guidelines for integrating yoga into clinical mental health practice. Such guidelines would include information about the expected benefits as well as the potential risks inherent in each practice. Mental healthcare professionals and facilities need to match treatments with specific diagnoses. Yoga programs will need to adapt to the constraints (e.g., treatment time, staff time, and facilities) of clinics, hospitals, and other institutions. Requiring adherence to complex, time-consuming regimens will make integrative treatment more difficult. Yoga teachers and researchers will do well to listen and take into account the needs and limitations of mental healthcare providers. By the same token, mental healthcare professionals will need time to learn about the many possibilities for enhancing patient outcomes by integrating yoga into their treatment regimens or by referring to yoga therapists who are qualified to work with severely anxious patients.

The emergence of research on integrating yoga with treatments such as CBT and other psychotherapies opens a new domain for helping a significant proportion of patients who do not respond adequately to conventional intellect-based approaches. Once the evidence is sufficiently robust to establish significant anxiolytic effects with yoga, consumers, mental healthcare professionals, and mental health policy leaders should welcome the arrival of new approaches that are less expensive and free of the side effects and possible addictions associated with pharmaceuticals.

In summary, anxiety spectrum disorders can provide a point of entry for yoga into mental healthcare. The popularity of classes and training in yoga for anxiety indicates that this aspect of treatment could lay the groundwork for how yoga will be adapted for other mental health conditions. With such growth, there will ideally be increased knowledge sharing and availability of resources for research, resulting in the development of best practices based on clinical experience and solid research. Practice guidelines could include a menu of yoga options or combinations of practices best suited for specific anxiety symptoms and specific anxiety spectrum disorders, how to safely tailor practices for different levels of symptom severity, how to modify practices in the presence of comorbidities, and how best to integrate yoga with other psychological interventions for the benefit of the patient.

References

Afonso, R.F., Balardin, J.B., Lazar, S., Sato, J.R., Igarashi, N., Danilo F. Santaella, D.N., Lacerda, S.S., Amaro Jr., E., & Kozasa, E.H. (2017). Greater cortical thickness in elderly female yoga practitioners: A cross-sectional study. *Frontiers in Aging Neuroscience*, 9, 201.

Albert, P. R., Vahid-Ansari, F., & Luckhart, C. (2014). Serotonin-prefrontal cortical circuitry in anxiety and depression phenotypes: Pivotal role of pre- and post-synaptic 5-HT1A receptor expression. *Frontiers in Behavioral Neuroscience*, 8, 199.

American Psychiatric Association (2013). *Diagnostic and Statistical Manual of Mental Disorders* (5th edn). Arlington, VA: American Psychiatric Publishing.

Azimi, E., Lerner, E. A., & Elmariah, S. B. (2015). Altered manifestations of skin disease at sites affected by neurological deficit. *British Journal of Dermatology, 172*(4), 988–993.

Baldwin, D. S., & Polkinghorn, C. (2005). Evidence-based pharmacotherapy of generalized anxiety disorder. *International Journal of Neuropsychopharmacology, 8*(2), 293–302.

Bandelow, B., Reitt, M., Röver, C., Michaelis, S., Görlich, Y., & Wedekind, D. (2015). Efficacy of treatments for anxiety disorders: A meta-analysis. *International Clinical Psychopharmacology, 30*(4), 183–92.

Beech, A.R., Carter, A.J., Mann, R.E., Rotshtein, P. (Eds.) (2018). *The Wiley Blackwell Handbook of Forensic Neuroscience.* New Jersey: Wiley-Blackwell.

Brandes, M., & Bienvenu, O. J. (2006). Personality and anxiety disorders. *Current Psychiatry Reports, 8*(4), 263–269.

Brown, R. P., & Gerbarg, P.L. (2005). Sudarshan Kriya yogic breathing in the treatment of stress, anxiety, and depression: Part I-neurophysiologic model. *Journal of Alternative and Complementary Medicine, 11*(1), 189–201.

Brown, R. P., & Gerbarg, P.L. (2012). *The Healing Power of Breath.* New York: Shambhala Press.

Brown, R. P., Gerbarg, P. L., & Muench, F. (2013). Breathing practices for treatment of psychiatric and stress-related medical conditions. *Psychiatric Clinics of North America, 36,* 121–140.

Brown, R. P., & Gerbarg, P. L. (2017). Breathing techniques in psychiatric treatment. In P.L. Gerbarg, R.P. Brown & P.R. Muskin (Eds.), *Complementary and Integrative Treatments in Psychiatric Practice* (pp. 241–250). Washington D.C.: American Psychiatric Association Publishing.

Bystritsky, A., Khalsa, S. S., Cameron, M. E., & Schiffman, J. (2013). Current diagnosis and treatment of anxiety disorders. *Pharmacy and Therapeutics, 38*(1), 30–57.

Chugh-Gupta, N., Baldassarre, F. G., & Vrkljan, B. H. (2013). A systematic review of yoga for state anxiety: Considerations for occupational therapy. *Canadian Journal of Occupational Therapy, 80*(3), 150–170.

Corey, S. M., Epel, E., Schembri, M., Pawlowsky, S. B., Cole, R. J., Araneta, M. R. G., Barrett-Connor, E., & Kanaya, A. M. (2014). Effect of restorative yoga vs. stretching on diurnal cortisol dynamics and psychosocial outcomes in individuals with the metabolic syndrome: The PRYSMS randomized controlled trial. *Psychoneuroendocrinology, 49,* 261–270.

Craske, M. G., Stein, M. B., Eley, T. C., Milad, M. R., Holmes, A., Rapee, R. M., & Wittchen H. U. (2017). Anxiety disorders. *Nature Reviews Disease Primers, 4,* 3.

Crits-Christoph, P., Newman M. G., Rickels, K., Gallop, R., Gibbons M. B. C., Hamilton, J. L., Ring-Kurtz, S., & Pastva, A. M. (2011). Combined medication and cognitive therapy for generalized anxiety disorder. *Journal of Anxiety Disorders, 25*(8), 1087–1094.

De Manincor, M., Bensoussan, A., Smith, C., Fahey, P., & Bourchier, S. (2015). Establishing key components of yoga interventions for reducing depression and anxiety, and improving well-being: A Delphi method study. *BMC Complementary and Alternative Medicine, 15,* 85.

Doria, S., de Vuono, A., Sanlorenzo, R., Irtelli, F., & Mencacci, C. (2015). Anti-anxiety efficacy of Sudarshan Kriya Yoga in general anxiety disorder: A multicomponent, yoga based, breath intervention program for patients suffering from generalized anxiety disorder with or without comorbidities. *Journal of Affective Disorders, 184,* 310–317.

Duan-Porter, W., Coeytaux, R. R., McDuffie, J. R., Goode, A. P., Sharma, P., Mennella, H., Nagi, A., & Williams J. W. Jr. (2016). Evidence map of yoga for depression, anxiety, and posttraumatic stress disorder. *Journal of Physical Activity and Health, 13*(3), 281–288.

Fanselow, M. S., & Lester, L. S. (1988). A functional behavioristic approach to aversively motivated behavior: predatory imminence as a determinant of the topography of defensive behavior. In R. C. Bolles (Ed.), *Evolution and Learning* (pp. 185–212). Hillsdale, New Jersey: Lawrence Erlbaum Associates.

Field, T., Diego, M., Delgado, J, & Medina, L. (2013). Yoga and social support reduce prenatal depression, anxiety and cortisol. *Journal of Bodywork and Movement Therapies, 17*(4), 397–403.

Foa, E. B., Franklin, M. E., & Moser, J. (2002). Context in the clinic: How well do cognitive-behavioral therapies and medications work in combination? *Biological Psychiatry, 52*(10), 987–997.

Gerbarg, P.., Jacob, V. E., Stevens, L., Bosworth, B. P., Chabouni, F., DeFilippis, E. M., Warren, R., Trivellas, M., Patel, P. V., Webb, C. D., Harbus, M. D., Christos, P. J., Brown, R. P., & Scherl, E. J. (2015). The effect of breathing, movement, and meditation on psychological and physical symptoms and inflammatory biomarkers in inflammatory bowel disease: A randomized controlled trial. *Inflammatory Bowel Diseases*, 21(12), 2886–2896,

Gerbarg, P. L., & Brown, R. P. (2016). Neurobiology and neurophysiology of breath practices in psychiatric care. *Psychiatric Times*, 33(11), 22–25.

Goodwin, R. D., Faravelli, C., Rosi, S., Cosci, F., Truglia, E., de Graaf, R., Wittchen, H.U. (2005). The epidemiology of panic disorder and agoraphobia in Europe. *European Neuropsychopharmacology, 15*(4), 435–443.

Gupta, K., & Mamidi, P. (2013). A pilot study on certain yogic and naturopathic procedures in generalized anxiety disorder. *International Journal of Research in Ayurveda and Pharmacy, 4,* 858–861.

Hettema, J. M., Prescott, C. A., Myers, J. M., Neale, M. C., & Kendler, K. S. (2005). The structure of genetic and environmental risk factors for anxiety disorders in men and women. *Archives of General Psychiatry, 62*(2), 182–189.

Immordino-Yang, M.H., & Yang, X.F., & Damasio, H. (2014). Correlations between social-emotional feelings and anterior insula activity are independent from visceral states but influenced by culture. *Frontiers in Human Neuroscience, 168,* 728.

Immordino-Yang, M.H., & Yang, X.F. (2017). Cultural differences in the neural correlates of social-emotional feelings: an interdisciplinary, developmental perspective. *Current Opinion in Psychology, 17,* 34–40.

Joshi, A., & Desousa, A. (2012). Yoga in the management of anxiety disorders. *Sri Lanka Journal of Psychiatry, 3*(1), 3–9.

Kalyani, B. G., Venkatasubramanian, G., Arasappa, R., Rao, N. P., Kalmady, S. V., Behere, R. V., Rao, H., Vasudev, M. K., & Gangadhar, B. N. (2011). Neurohemodynamic correlates of 'OM' chanting: A pilot functional magnetic resonance imaging study. *International Journal of Yoga, 4*(1), 3–6.

Katzman, M. A., Vermani, M., Gerbarg, P. L., Brown, R. P., Iorio, C., Davis, M., Cameron, C., & Tsirgielis, D. (2012). A multicomponent yoga-based, breath intervention program as an adjunctive treatment in patients suffering from generalized anxiety disorder with or without comorbidities. *International Journal of Yoga, 5*(1), 57–65.

Kessler, R.C., Berglund, P., Demler, O., Jin, R., Merikangas, K.R., Walters, E.E. (2005). Lifetime prevalence and age-of-onset distributions of DSM-IV disorders in the National Comorbidity Survey Replication. *Archives of General Psychiatry, 62,* 593–602.

Kessler, R. C., Angermeyer, M., Anthony, J. C., de Graaf, R., Demyttenaere, K., Gasquet, I., de Girolamo, G., Gluzman, S., Gureje, O., Haro, J. M., Kawakami, N., Karam, A., Levinson, D., Mora, M. E. M.,

Browne, M. A. O., Posada-Villa, J., Stein, D. J., Tsang, C. H. A., Aguilar-Gaxiola, S., Alonso, J., Lee, S., Heeringa, S., Pennell, B.-E., Berglund, P., Gruber, M. J., Petukhova, M., Chatterji, S., & Üstün, T. B. (2007). Lifetime prevalence and age-of-onset distributions of mental disorders in the World Health Organization's World Mental Health Survey Initiative. *World Psychiatry, 6,* 168–176.

Kessler, R. C., Soukup, J., Davis, R. B., Foster, D. F., Wilkey, S. A., van Rompay, M. I., & Eisenberg, D. M. (2001). The use of complementary and alternative therapies to treat anxiety and depression in the United States. *American Journal of Psychiatry, 158,* 289–294.

Khalsa, M. K., Greiner-Ferris, J. M., Hofmann, S. G., & Khalsa, S. B. (2015). Yoga-enhanced cognitive behavioural therapy (y-cbt) for anxiety management: A pilot study. *Clinical Psychology & Psychotherapy, 22*(4), 364–371.

Kirkwood, G., Rampes, H., Tuffrey, V., Richardson, J., Pilkington, K., & Ramaratnam, S. (2005). Yoga for anxiety: A systematic review of the research evidence. *British Journal of Sports Medicine, 39*(12), 884–891.

Lee, C., & Ghiya, S. (2012). Influence of alternate nostril breathing on heart rate variability in non-practitioners of yogic breathing. *International Journal of Yoga, 5*(1), 66.

Li, A. W., & Goldsmith, C. A. (2012). The effects of yoga on anxiety and stress. *Scientific Review of Alternative Medicine, 17*(1), 21–35.

Lieb, R., Isensee, B., Höfler, M., Pfister, H., & Wittchen, H.-U. (2002). Parental major depression and the risk of depression and other mental disorders in offspring: A prospective-longitudinal community study. *Archives of General Psychiatry, 59,* 365–374.

Lijster, J. M., Dierckx, B., Utens, E. M., Verhulst, F. C., Zieldorff, C., Dieleman, G. C., & Legerstee, J. S. (2017). The age of onset of anxiety disorders. *The Canadian Journal of Psychiatry, 62*(4), 237–246.

Lundberg, U. (2005). Stress hormones in health and illness: The roles of work and gender. *Psychoneuroendocrinology, 30,* 1017–1021.

Manabe, N., Tanaka, T., Hata, J., Kusunoki, H., & Haruma, K. (2009). Pathophysiology underlying irritable bowel syndrome--from the viewpoint of dysfunction of autonomic nervous system activity. *Journal of Smooth Muscle Research, 45*(1), 15–23.

Martin, E. I., Ressler, K. J., Binder, E., & Nemeroff, C. B. (2009). The Neurobiology of Anxiety Disorders: Brain Imaging, Genetics, and Psychoneuroendocrinology. *The Psychiatric Clinics of North America, 32*(3), 549–575.

McLean, C.P., Asnaani, A., Litz, B.T., & Hofmann, S.G. (2011). Gender differences in anxiety disorders: Prevalence, course of illness, comorbidity and burden of illness. *Journal of Psychiatric Research, 45*(8), 1027–1035.

Nardi, A. E., Fontenelle, L. F., & Crippa, J. A. S. (2012). New trends in anxiety disorders. *Revista Brasileira de Psiquiatria, 34(Suppl. 1),* 5–6.

National Institute for Health and Care Excellence (2013, May). *Social anxiety disorder: recognition, assessment and treatment* (NICE Clinical Guidelines No. 159). Retrieved from https://www.nice.org.uk/guidance/cg159.

National Institute of Mental Health (2017, November). *Specific Phobia*. Retrieved from: https://www.nimh.nih.gov/health/statistics/specific-phobia.shtml.

Naveen, G. H., Varambally, S., Thirthalli, J., Rao, M., Christopher, R., & Gangadhar, B. N. (2016). Serum cortisol and BDNF in patients with major depression-effect of yoga. *International Review of Psychiatry, 28*(3), 273–278.

Nuss, P. (2015). Anxiety disorders and GABA neurotransmission: A disturbance of modulation. *Neuropsychiatric Disease and Treatment, 11,* 165–175.

Nutt, D. J., Kessler, R. C., Alonso, J., Benbow, A., Lecrubier, Y., Lépine, J. P., Mechanic, D., & Tylee, A., (2007). Consensus statement on the benefit to the community of ESEMeD (European Study of the Epidemiology of Mental Disorders) survey data on depression and anxiety. *Journal of Clinical Psychiatry, 68*(2), 42–48.

Nyer, M., Gerbarg, P. L., Silveri, M. M., Johnston, J., Scott, T.M., Nauphal, M., Owen, L., Nielsen, G.H., Mischoulon, D., Brown, R. P., Fava, M., & Streeter, C.C. (2018). A randomized controlled dosing study of Iyengar yoga and coherent breathing for the treatment of major depressive disorder: Impact on suicidal ideation and safety findings. *Complementary Therapies in Medicine*, 37, 136–142.

Pai, A., Suris, A. M., & North, C. S. (2017). Posttraumatic stress disorder in the DSM-5: Controversy, change, and conceptual considerations. *Behavioral Sciences, 7*(1).

Pal, G., Agarwal, A., Karthik, S., Pal, P., & Nanda, N. (2014). Slow yogic breathing through right and left nostril influences sympathovagal balance, heart rate variability, and cardiovascular risks in young adults. *North American Journal of Medical Sciences, 6*(3), 145.

Peng, C. K., Mietus, J. E., Liu, Y., Khalsa, G., Douglas, P. S., Benson, H., & Goldberger, A. L. (1999). Exaggerated heart rate oscillations during two meditation techniques. *International Journal of Cardiology, 70*(2), 101–107.

Pilkington, K., Gerbarg, P. L., & Brown, R.P. (2016). Yoga therapy for anxiety. In S. B. S. Khalsa, L. Cohen, T. McCall, S. Telles (Eds.), *The Principles and Practice of Yoga in Health Care* (pp. 95–115). East Lothian, UK: Handspring Publishing.

Porges, S. W. (2009). The polyvagal theory: New insights into adaptive reactions of the autonomic nervous system. *Cleveland Clinic Journal of Medicine, 76(Suppl 2),* S86–S90.

Porges, S. W. (2001). The polyvagal theory: Phylogenetic substrates of a social nervous system. *International Journal of Psychophysiology, 42*(2), 123–146.

Porges, S. W., & Furman, S. A. (2011). The early development of the autonomic nervous system provides a neural platform for social behavior: A polyvagal perspective. *Infant and Child Development*, 20(1), 106–118.

Porges, S. W., Carter, C.S. (2017). Polyvagal Theory and the social engagement system. In P.L. Gerbarg, R.P. Brown & P.R. Muskin (Eds.), *Complementary and Integrative Treatments in Psychiatric Practice* (pp. 221–240). Washington D.C.: American Psychiatric Association Publishing.

Quinn, J. J., & Fanselow, M. S. (2006). Defenses and memories: Functional neural circuitry of fear and conditional responding. In M.G. Craske, D. Hermans, & D. Vansteenwegen (Eds.), *Fear and Learning: from basic processes to clinical implications* (pp. 55–74). Washington, DC: American Psychological Association.

Riley, K. E., & Park, C. L. (2015). How does yoga reduce stress? A systematic review of mechanisms of change and guide to future inquiry. *Health Psychology Review, 9*(3), 379–396.

Rowney, J., Hermida, T., & Malone, D. (2010, August). *Anxiety Disorders*. Retrieved from: http://www.clevelandclinicmeded.com/medicalpubs/diseasemanagement/psychiatry-psychology/anxiety-disorder/.

Roy-Byrne, P. P., Davidson, K. W., Kessler, R. C., Asmundson, G. J., Goodwin, R. D., Kubzansky, L., Lydiard, R. B., Massie, M. J., Katon, W., Laden, S. K., & Stein, M. B. (2008). Anxiety disorders and comorbid medical illness. *General Hospital Psychiatry, 30*(3), 208–225.

Sahasi, G., Mohan, D., & Kacker, C. (1989). Effectiveness of yogic techniques in the management of anxiety. *Journal of Personality Clinical Studies, 5,* 51–55.

Sarris, J., Moylan, S., Camfield, D. A., Pase, M. P., Mischoulon, D., Berk, M., Jacka, F. N., & Schweitzer, I. (2012). Complementary medicine, exercise, meditation, diet, and lifestyle modification for anxiety disorders: A review of current evidence. *Evidence-Based Complementary and Alternative Medicine, 420,* 809653.

Sharma, I., Azmi, S. A., & Settiwar, R. M. (1991). Evaluation of the effect of pranayama in anxiety state. *Alternative Medicine, 3,* 227–235.

Shear, K. (2006). Prevalence and correlates of estimated DSM-IV Child and Adult Separation Anxiety Disorder in the National Comorbidity Survey Replication. *American Journal of Psychiatry, 163*(6), 1074–1083.

Siddiqui, A., Madhu, S. V., Sharma, S. B., & Desai, N. G. (2015). Endocrine stress responses and risk of type 2 diabetes mellitus. *Stress, 18*(5), 498–506.

Stein, M. B., Roy-Byrne, P. P., Craske, M. G., Campbell-Sills, L., Lang, A. J., Golinelli, D., Rose, R. D., Bystritsky, A., Sullivan, G., & Sherbourne, C. D. (2011). Quality of and patient satisfaction with primary health care for anxiety disorders. *Journal of Clinical Psychiatry, 72*(7), 970–976.

Stewart, R. E., & Chambless, D.L. (2009). Cognitive-behavioral therapy for adult anxiety disorders in clinical practice: A meta-analysis of effectiveness studies. *Journal of Consulting and Clinical Psychology, 77*(4), 595–606.

Streeter, C. C., Gerbarg, P. L., Saper, R. B., Ciraulo, D. A., & Brown, R. P. (2012). Effects of yoga on the autonomic nervous system, gamma-aminobutyric-acid, and allostasis in epilepsy, depression, and post-traumatic stress disorder. *Medical Hypotheses, 78*(5), 571–579.

Streeter, C. C., Gerbarg, P. L., Whitfield, T. H., Owen, L., Johnston, J., Silveri, M. M., Gensler, M., Faulkner, C. L., Mann, C., Wixted, M., Hernon, A. M., Nyer, M. B., Brown, E. R., & Jensen, J. E. (2017). Treatment of major depressive disorder with Iyengar yoga and coherent breathing: A randomized controlled dosing study. *Journal of Alternative and Complementary Medicine, 23*(3), 201–207.

Streeter, C., Jensen, J., Perlmutter, R., Cabral, H., Tian, H., Terhune, D., Ciraulo, D. A, & Renshaw, P. F. (2007). Yoga asana sessions increase brain GABA levels: A pilot study. *The Journal of Alternative And Complementary Medicine, 13*(4), 419–426.

Streeter, C., Whitfield, T., Owen, L., Rein, T., Karri, S., Yakhkind, A., Perlmutter, R., Prescot, A., Renshaw, P. F., Ciraulo, D. A., & Jensen, J. E. (2010). Effects of yoga versus walking on mood, anxiety, and brain GABA levels: A randomized controlled MRS study. *The Journal of Alternative and Complementary Medicine, 16*(11), 1145–1152.

Thayer, J. F., Friedman, B. H., & Borkovec, T. D. (1996). Autonomic characteristics of generalized anxiety disorder and worry. *Biological Psychiatry, 39*(4), 255–266.

Thayer, J. (2000). A model of neurovisceral integration in emotion regulation and dysregulation. *Journal of Affective Disorders, 61*(3), 201–216.

Tyagi, A., & Cohen, M. (2016). Yoga and heart rate variability: A comprehensive review of the literature. *International Journal of Yoga, 9*(2), 97–113.

Uebelacker, L. A., & Broughton, M. K. (2013). Yoga for depression and anxiety: A review of published research and implications for healthcare providers. *Rhode Island Medical Journal, 99*(3), 20–22.

Venkatraman, A., Edlow, B. L., & Immordino-Yang, M. H. (2017). The brainstem in emotion: A review. *Frontiers in Neuroanatomy, 11*, 15.

Vorkapic, C. F., & Rangé, B. (2014). Reducing the symptomatology of panic disorder: The effects of a yoga program alone and in combination with cognitive-behavioral therapy. *Frontiers in Psychiatry, 5*, 177.

Weaver, L. L., & Darragh, A. R. (2015). Systematic review of yoga interventions for anxiety reduction among children and adolescents. *The American Journal of Occupational Therapy, 69*(6).

World Health Organization (2016). Investing in treatment for depression and anxiety leads to fourfold return [News Release]. Retrieved from http://www.who.int/en/news-room/detail/13-04-2016-investing-in-treatment-for-depression-and-anxiety-leads-to-fourfold-return

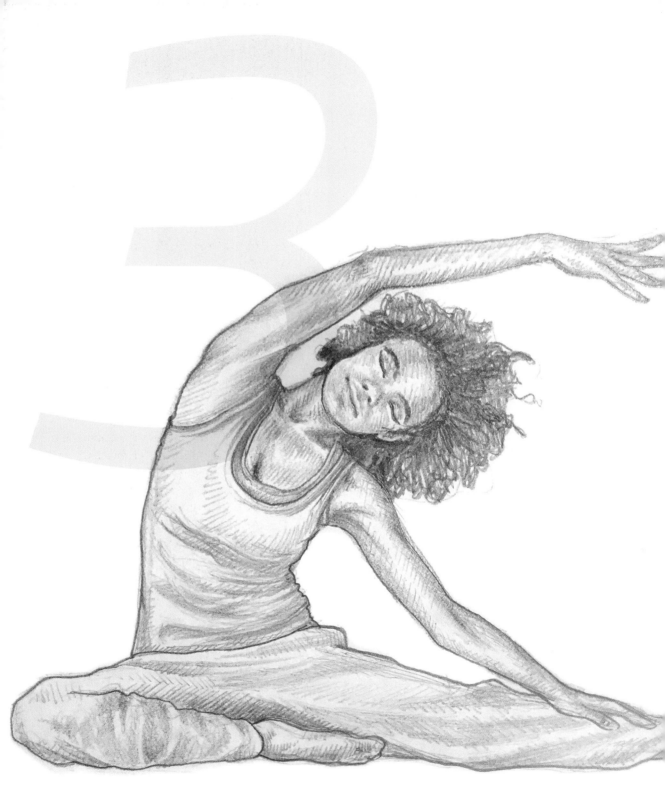

Depression

Holger Cramer and Amy Weintraub

(with contributions from Heather Mason)

Overview

In contrast to common mood fluctuations, depression is a serious health condition. According to the World Health Organization (WHO), more than 300 million individuals are affected worldwide. The WHO cites suicide from depression as occurring throughout the lifespan and as the second leading cause of death among 15- to 29-year-olds (World Health Organization, 2017). The WHO predicts that depression will be the leading cause of disease globally by 2030. The reasons for this prevalence are manifold, and cross-cultural studies suggest that modernization may be a driving force (Hidaka, 2012). Increases in social inequality and loneliness are implicated, but it is also argued that malnutrition, sedentary lifestyles, and sunlight-deficiency increase prevalence rates.

> WHO predicts that depression will be the leading cause of disease globally by 2030.

Depressive disorders as defined by the *Diagnostic and Statistical Manual of Mental Disorder* (DSM-5) include a number of conditions, including major depressive disorder (MDD), dysthymia, premenstrual dysphoric disorder, substance/medication-induced depressive disorder, depressive disorder due to another medical condition, and disruptive mood dysregulation disorder. Those disorders have been grouped together because they are characterized by the presence of sad, empty, or irritable mood, which is accompanied by somatic and cognitive changes (American Psychiatric Association, 2013).

The classic depressive disorder is MDD, a condition that is characterized by at least one (but often far more) depressive episode(s) lasting for at least two weeks (but often far longer). During these episodes individuals are almost continually depressed; interest and pleasure are strongly reduced. The mood is often described as sad and hopeless, but individuals sometimes report themselves as not feeling anything (emotional numbness). In almost all cases this is accompanied by a loss of interest, enjoyment, and desire (anhedonia). People can be fatigued, feel worthless or guilty, and experience rumination and recurrent thoughts of death. The latter can range from passive wishes to die to suicide ideation—concrete thoughts of suicide that may also include a plan for implementing an attempt—and suicide attempts. Sleep behavior changes with either insomnia or hypersomnia; psychomotor agitation or retardation are common. An important diagnostic criterion is that the condition is causing distress and/or marked impairments of quality of life. A minority of people experience only a single episode in their lifetime while a majority experience several episodes that are separated by phases of remission (American Psychiatric Association, 2013). The lifetime prevalence of major depression has been estimated to vary widely across countries, ranging from 1.5% in Taiwan to 19% in Beirut (Weissman et al., 1996).

Another widespread depressive disorder is dysthymia: a persistently depressed mood lasting for at least two years, but composed of a lower intensity than MDD. Major depressive episodes often precede or interrupt dysthymia, and dysthymia is a major risk factor for subsequent MDD. Chronic major depression—symptoms of a major depressive episode that persist for two years or more— results in a diagnosis of both major depression and dysthymia, and is three times more common than dysthymia on its own (American Psychiatric Association, 2013). The other

Chapter 3

depressive disorders named by the DSM-5 are mainly characterized by their specific causes: premenstrual dysphoric disorder is characterized by the presence of depressed, irritable, and/or anxious mood in women that begins following ovulation and remits with the onset of the menses. Diagnoses of substance/medication-induced depressive disorders as well as of depressive disorders due to other medical conditions reflect the presence of depressed mood and other symptoms of depressive disorders due to substance abuse, as side effects of pharmacotherapy or as a co-occurrence of other somatic or mental health conditions. All of these are common causes of depressive symptoms. Disruptive mood disorder is quite different to the other depressive disorders since it is only diagnosed in children and is characterized by chronic severe irritability, that is, frequent temper outbursts that alternate with chronic, persistent irritable or angry mood.

Depression is thought to be caused by a combination of different neurophysiological and neuropsychological factors (American Psychiatric Association, 2013). Depression has been described as reflecting a primary disorder of biochemical and neurophysiological functions, and there is evidence that alterations in the metabolism of monoamine neurotransmitters (primarily noradrenaline, serotonin, and dopamine), specifically an insufficiency in monoamine concentrations, play a major role in the pathophysiology of depression (Syvälahti, 1994). Based on those proposed pathomechanisms, as well as on scientific evidence of effectiveness and on clinical experience, pharmacotherapy—consisting mainly of SSRIs, serotonin-norepinephrine reuptake inhibitors (SNRIs), or (in treatment-resistant cases) nonselective monoamine oxidase inhibitors—is recommended for those patients in the acute phases of depressive disorders (Gelenberg et al., 2010). SSRIs and SNRIs are thought to inhibit the uptake of serotonin or norepinephrine in the synapse, increasing the availability of the respective neurotransmitter. There are also medications like

bupropion, which have been characterized as a norepinephrine-dopamine reuptake inhibitor. However, bupropion has been shown to occupy only a few dopamine transporter sites during in vivo studies (Meyer et al., 2002), indicating there are other mechanisms at play. However, monoamine oxidase inhibitors block the activity of the enzyme monoamine oxidase, which catalyzes the oxidation of monoamines: therefore, levels of monoamines are nonselectively increased.

Low levels of other central neurotransmitters such as GABA are associated with depression.

Low levels of other central neurotransmitters such as GABA are associated with depression (Kalueff & Nutt, 2007; Streeter, Gerbarg, Saper, Ciraulo, & Brown, 2012). Another important factor is BDNF (brain-derived neurotrophic factor), which is associated with the protection of existing, and the growth and differentiation of new neurons and synapses in the CNS: it is often referred to as "fertilizer for neuroplasticity." BDNF levels are low in people with major depression, which may explain problems they tend to have with cognitive shifting, if neurological change is inhibited. BDNF is increased by a number of antidepressant drugs, potentially associated with plastic changes in the CNS (Lee & Kim, 2010). Another functional change associated with depression is dysregulation in the HPA axis, known as the stress response (Carroll et al., 2012; Streeter et al., 2012). Many patients with depression present with increased levels of plasma cortisol that decrease to normal levels after effective treatment (Thase, Jindal, & Howland, 2002). Findings on salivary cortisol levels in patients with depression are inconsistent, with some studies finding a higher cortisol awakening response (Vreeburg et al., 2009), while others show flatter diurnal cortisol slopes (Gartside, Leitch, McQuade, & Swarbrick, 2003; Jarcho, Slavich, Tylova-Stein, Wolkowitz, & Burke, 2013). This indicates that there is a general dysregulation of the HPA axis in patients with depression, which can present in a variety of ways. In a healthy person, cortisol is highest in the morning, but within a normative range, and in the evening it will decrease as melatonin increases.

From a cognitive psychology viewpoint, depression is associated with biased information processing, mainly attentional bias and memory, rumination, and dysfunctional thoughts and schemas (Beck, 2008; Disner, Beevers, Haigh, & Beck, 2011). These psychological mechanisms appear to be associated with specific neurophysiological changes: an overactive influence of subcortical emotional systems that includes the amygdala, and a reduced top-down control of those subcortical influences, mainly characterized by a hypoactive PFC (Beck, 2008; Disner et al., 2011). Psychotherapy, mainly cognitive-behavioral, interpersonal, or psychodynamic therapy, is therefore recommended in combination with pharmacotherapy (or instead of it), because it may help to increase activity of the frontal lobe structures implicated in the downgrading of subcortical regions associated with fear and negative thinking. Both treatment strategies are typically adequate for maintenance during remission phases (Gelenberg et al., 2010). Specifically during remission, meditation-based psychotherapy such as Mindfulness-based Cognitive Therapy (MBCT) can be a useful alternative to other, more traditional, forms of cognitive therapy approaches (MacKenzie & Kocovski, 2016); and regular exercise is also generally recommended due to its at least moderate antidepressant effects.

Review of the research on yoga for depression

Research has shown that adults with depression are much less physically active than non-depressed adults (Hallgren et al., 2016), and that precipitating depressed individuals into action is an effective way to counteract their depressed mood. Recommending that depressed individuals exercise regularly can be at least as effective as prescribing antidepressant medica-

tion (Schuch et al., 2016). A meta-analysis showed that drug–placebo differences in antidepressant efficacy increase as a function of baseline depression severity. For patients with only moderate depression, the analysis found virtually no difference in efficacy between antidepressant drugs and placebo. Only in cases of very severe depression were there small differences between drugs and placebo that could be considered clinically relevant (Kirsch et al., 2008). This might be interpreted to mean that antidepressant drugs are mainly effective for patients with really severe depression. On the other hand, exercise can also be effective for mild-to-moderately depressed mood (Schuch et al., 2016). Beyond exercise, other types of physical activity, such as work-related or leisure-time physical activities are considered even more important, mainly because they are done more frequently and contribute strongly to overall daily levels of activity (Hallgren et al., 2016). Yoga is believed by many to be a form of exercise or physical activity, and it may be considered a more accessible first step for clients suffering from depression rather than a workout at a gym. Individuals with depression may lack the motivation to commit to a prescribed exercise program, and the high co-occurring of depression with chronic pain might further reduce their ability to exercise. Given that yoga offers a wide range of practices that differ in their intensity of physical activity, yoga might be a useful alternative for patients who are not adherent to other forms of exercise. If patients are not motivated to perform more vigorous forms of physical activity, then gentle forms of yoga (if shown to be effective) could be considered a viable alternative.

> Yoga is believed by many to be a form of exercise or physical activity, and it may be considered a more accessible first step for clients suffering from depression rather than a workout at a gym.

Improving symptoms of depression has always been one of the main aims of clinical yoga research.

However, many trials include depression as a secondary target when studying the effects of yoga on physical or other mental health conditions. Yoga has been shown to improve depressive symptoms in patients with cancer (Cramer, Lange, Klose, Paul, & Dobos, 2012), chronic pain (Büssing, Ostermann, Ludtke, & Michalsen, 2012), multiple sclerosis (Cramer, Lauche, Azizi, Dobos, & Langhorst, 2014), and heart disease (Cramer, Lauche, Haller, Dobos, & Michalsen, 2015). While depression often presents as co-occurring with physical diseases, to the best of our knowledge, none of those yoga trials assessed patients with a formal diagnosis of "depressive disorder due to another medical condition" as previously defined, but simply measured whether yoga was effective on potential depressive symptoms that could be present in some patients but absent in others. Consequently, those trials can inform treatment decisions concerning mild depressive symptoms in physically ill individuals. However, the treatment of depressive disorders requires a very different approach, and must take into account the neurophysiological mechanisms, as well as the mental and social consequences of the disease.

Although research trials assessing the effects of yoga in patients with depressive disorders are relatively sparse, there is more evidence in this domain than for most other yoga research. Seven RCTs have investigated the effects of yoga on DSM-diagnosed depressive disorders (Butler et al., 2008; Janakiramaiah et al., 1998; Kinser, Bourguignon, Whaley, Hauenstein, & Taylor, 2013; Rohini, Pandey, Janakiramaiah, Gangadhar, & Vedamurthachar, 2000; Sarubin et al., 2014; Schuver & Lewis, 2016; Sharma, Das, Mondal, Goswampi, & Gandhi, 2005); each of these used DSM-IV diagnostic criteria, which are very similar to DSM-5 criteria. For example, in a sample of 45 individuals with a long-term diagnosis of dysthymia and/or major depression, 77% of patients participating in a ten-week meditation and yoga plus psychoeducation program experienced a remission

(that is, they fell below the cut-off for clinically relevant symptoms) at the nine-month follow-up, compared to only 36% of patients who only received psychoeducation. The effects of yoga were comparable to those of a group psychotherapy with hypnosis plus psychoeducation program (Butler et al., 2008). Likewise, other trials demonstrated that yoga is equally effective in reducing depressive symptoms or in increasing remission rates in patients with major depression as health education (Kinser et al., 2013), exercise (Schuver & Lewis, 2016), relaxation (Rohini et al., 2000), electroconvulsive therapy, or tricyclic antidepressants (Janakiramaiah et al., 1998). Specifically, rumination was strongly reduced by yoga interventions, suggesting a potential psychological mechanism of the intervention (Kinser et al., 2013; Schuver & Lewis, 2016). However, while most of the aforementioned RCTs allowed the use of antidepressant medication, a recent RCT did not find any additional effects of combining atypical antipsychotic drugs with antidepressant properties and SSRIs with an additional five-week yoga program (Sarubin et al., 2014). This is in contrast to another RCT of 25 patients with major depression, which found that adding Sudarshan Kriya yoga (a yoga style focused on breathing and meditation) to antidepressant medication was more effective in decreasing the severity of depression than medication on its own. The number of patients who reached remission were more than three times as high in the yoga group compared to the medication only group (Sharma, Barrett, Cucchiara, Gooneratne, & Thase, 2017).

Another focus of research in recent years, driven mainly by Dr. Tiffany Field's research group at the Fielding Graduate University in Florida, is the effectiveness of yoga for prenatal depression. In a series of RCTs, Field and her team demonstrated that yoga effectively reduced depression and co-occurring anxiety in DSM-IV-diagnosed pregnant women (Field, Diego, Delgado, & Medina, 2013a, 2013b; Field et al., 2012; Mitchell et al., 2012). Through further research by this group and other groups, yoga was shown to be equally effective in this patient population as social support, massage (Field et al., 2013b; Field et al., 2012), or health education (Uebelacker, Battle, Sutton, Magee, & Miller, 2016). Comparable effects were found in a trial on postpartum women with depressive symptoms (but without a formal diagnosis of a depressive disorder), where yoga was more effective than usual care in improving depressive and anxiety symptoms (Buttner, Brock, O'Hara, & Stuart, 2015).

As previously discussed, slow breathing techniques are considered to be a vital part of yoga practice for alleviating depression. Yogic breathing and meditation have been shown to increase PNS activity (Markil, Whitehurst, Jacobs, & Zoeller, 2012; Mourya, Mahajan, Singh, & Jain, 2009; Telles et al., 2013), which is helpful in depression even if the person is feeling lethargic. People who are depressed may feel tired but not rested. Increased parasympathetic response activates the body's natural healing reserves and consequently supports an increase in energy. Aligned with this greater parasympathetic activity is an increase in GABA levels (Streeter, 2012), which may be mediated by an increase in certain kinds of stimulation of the vagus nerve that occur through slow breathing (Kinser, 2012; Streeter et al., 2012) and, over time, increased HRV (Patil, 2013; Tyagi, 2016). HRV indicates a flexibility to move between the PNS and the SNS, thereby supporting psychological resiliency.

> Increased parasympathetic response activates the body's natural healing reserves and consequently supports an increase in energy.

Finally, a number of trials have investigated the effects of yoga on otherwise healthy individuals with depressive mood as measured by depression questionnaires, but without a formal diagnosis of a depressive disorder. These studies generally found that yoga was more effective than no treatment or unspecific relaxation in decreasing depressive symptoms (Khumar, Kaur, & Kaur, 1993; Lavretsky et al., 2013; Shahidi et al., 2011; Woolery, Myers, Sternlieb, & Zeltzer, 2004); and that yoga was equally effective as aerobic exercise (Shahidi et al., 2011; Veale et al., 1992).

Based on the available RCTs, meta-analyses pooling the statistical data on this specific topic concluded that yoga effectively improved depression in a variety of populations including healthy individuals with depressed mood, patients with a diagnosis of a depressive disorder, and pregnant women with prenatal depression (Cramer, Lauche, Langhorst, & Dobos, 2013; Gong, Ni, Shen, Wu, & Jiang, 2015).

The exact mechanisms of the action of yoga in treating depression remain under debate; however, there are indications of specific physiological effects that relate to depression. For example, preliminary evidence from imaging studies shows that yoga practice can increase endogenous dopamine release in the ventral striatum (Kjaer et al., 2002) and thalamic GABA levels (Streeter et al., 2007, 2010). Furthermore, yoga practice was associated with increased plasma serotonin in patients with depression (Devi, Chansauria, & Udupa, 1986). In addition, yoga can raise BDNF levels as much as antidepressant drugs, and increases in BDNF after yoga practice correlate with decreases in depression severity (Naveen et al., 2013). Further studies suggest that yoga can decrease depression-associated dysregulation in the HPA axis: yoga can reduce subjective stress in healthy adults as well as levels of plasma cortisol in individuals with depression (Devi et al., 1986) or alcohol abuse (Vedamurthachar et al., 2006). In cancer patients, reduced morning salivary cortisol levels have been found after a yoga intervention (Vadiraja et al., 2009) together with a steeper diurnal salivary cortisol slope (Banasik, Williams, Haberman, Blank, & Bendel, 2011), meaning less stress in the morning and an easier time accessing sleep in the evening, something many cancer patients struggle with. However, a recent RCT in patients with major depression found no additional effects of yoga on HPA function when it was combined with strong antidepressant medication (Sarubin et al., 2014). In accordance with its nonsignificant effects on depression, this trial and others (described earlier) indicate that yoga might have its strongest neuromodulating and antidepressant effects when no or only low-level antidepressant agents are additionally used.

Although yoga is often regarded as an alternative form of exercise, it is more than that. Indeed, RCTs have shown that while yoga is effective in reducing depression and increasing remission rates in both mild and more severe depression, asana-based yoga interventions that included no or only very few breathing or meditation components showed little evidence for effectiveness. In contrast, interventions that used breathing and/or meditation as the primary focus of their yoga program showed strong positive effects: in the two trials adding yoga to antidepressant medication, only the one using a breathing/meditation-based yoga form was effective; the more asana-based yoga form in the other trial was not (Sarubin et al., 2014; Sharma et al., 2017). This finding was confirmed in a meta-analysis of twelve RCTs with a total of more than 600 depressed individuals, which demonstrated significant antidepressant effects for breathing/meditation-based yoga interventions, but not for more asana-based forms of yoga (Cramer, Lauche, Langhorst, & Dobos, 2013). Therefore, limiting yoga to an alternative form of exercise cannot be regarded as evidence-based, while using a more holistic approach incorporating large components of breathing and meditation can.

Yoga philosophy and depression

No matter what yoga lineage or school, there is a shared philosophical foundation that supports optimal mental health and mitigates the sense of isolation that is common in depression: that we as human beings are interconnected. In fact, yoga teaches that suffering is based on the false perception of separateness. The practices of yoga remove the constrictions, physically and emotionally, so that we are able to feel that connection, even if momentarily, to a sense of a whole and undamaged self, to each other, and to something larger than who we are as individuals (Weintraub, 2004). Although the field of yoga therapy and schools offering training specific to mental health concerns may be varied in terms of the philosophies underlying their approaches to depression, all of the philosophical models address and foster this sense of interconnectedness. Likewise, yoga teaches that because we are multilayered beings, the experience of depression is not an identity—it is not "who we are"—but is simply an arising experience that can be changed through various practices that cultivate other ways of perceiving and allowing energy to flow. Additionally, many schools adhere to the *kosha* model, first introduced in the *Taittiriya Upanishad* more than 3000 years ago. This doctrine is the foundation for the understanding that we are composed of many elements: body, mind, breath, and consciousness. It allows for a multidimensional way of understanding how depression influences all parts of the person, and how working with depression can work on any of these parts.

> Yoga teaches that suffering is based on the false perception of separateness.

To better understand the *kosha* model, imagine a set of Russian nesting dolls. Within this metaphor you can treat any one of the dolls, and all the dolls will reap the benefit because they are interdependent. The outermost sheath, the densest doll, is the *annamaya kosha*, or food sheath, which refers to the physical body. Depression is experienced in this sheath as physical block and constrictions, which may show up as lethargy or soreness in muscles or joints. Working with physical postures and movement may help to alleviate some of these constrictions. The next sheath is the *pran-amaya kosha*, often defined as the lifeforce, energy, or breath body. Depression is experienced in this sheath as shallow breathing that does not fully engage the diaphragm and as a corresponding lack of vitality; therefore, facilitating deeper breathing may allow for an experience of ease to emerge. The next sheath surrounding the first two is the *manomaya kosha*, which is the *kosha* of mind. Depression may be experienced in this sheath as rumination and negative self-talk, and techniques to redirect attention and bring the mind into the body may be helpful. The fourth sheath surrounding the first three is the *vijnana-maya kosha*, often defined as awareness, containing our core beliefs (true or not) about ourselves and the world. Depression at this level may be experienced as a self-limiting belief system, and we can use yoga philosophy to support a wider vista of self-perception. The fifth and final sheath is the *anandamaya kosha*, known as the bliss body. From the yogic perspective, the bliss body is always available to us. It is transcendent reality, or pure awareness. But when depression constricts any one of the other four *kosha*, access to wellbeing (joy, bliss, connectedness, our own true nature) is correspondingly limited. The goal of yoga therapy and practice in all traditions is to offer clients practices that, when tailored for them, remove depression in all the *koshas*, so that they return to a state of wellbeing, balanced mood, and their own sense of wholeness.

Rationale for yoga in treating depression

Whether a yoga teacher/therapist or mental health professional, there are techniques appropriate for each setting that can be used to help alleviate depression. Practices to manage mood include simple breathing practices, secular mantra tones, asana, hand gestures, and yoga meditations that anchor the ruminative mind in the present moment. These practices can individually, or collaboratively with a teacher/therapist, open a window out of the depressed mood, even if only momentarily (Weintraub, 2012).

Furthermore, by learning these tools and practicing them at home, the client/student becomes able to cultivate present-moment awareness themselves, which can increase feelings of self-efficacy, an important factor in the recovery from depression. What yoga does, more than many medical-based models of treatment, is to give people the tools for managing their depressive symptoms, thus encouraging what psychology calls an "internal locus of control" or "self-efficacy," and which we may commonly think of as empowerment (Lauche, Langhorst, Paul, Dobos, & Cramer, 2014). Studies show that the more we can elevate a client's sense of self-control, the more we see a drop in depressive symptoms (Astin, Shapiro, Lee, & Shapiro, 1999; Bandura, 1994).

Domains of consideration for working with people with depression

The key to working with mood disorders is to follow a three-step process: (1) assess the client's current state, (2) offer appropriate practices, and (3) consider how these practices can best be offered. From a yoga perspective, this necessitates a variety of considerations; for instance, is the client *rajasic* (overstimulated, as, for example, in an anxiety-based depression) or *tamasic* (depressed, lethargic)? Although ultimately the key to working with depression is balancing a person's mood, in the beginning it is vital that the presenting anxiety or lethargy is attended to. For those who are anxiously depressed, therapeutic yoga often begins with practices that might otherwise be used in the management of anxiety alone. This could mean starting a session with some fast movements that dispel anxious energy then moving to some long holds in relaxing poses. Working with anxious energy might also require slow controlled breathing that accompanies asana—not everyone is the same, and the key is to find something that helps a person relax. For a more *tamasic*/lethargic person who is lacking in energy, it may be useful to include a standing practice that incorporates several stronger standing poses, and some uplifting practices such as breath of joy and more stimulating breath like *kapalabhati*. However, first of all it is important to address the mood of the client; it is possible that beginning with breath of joy or fast-paced *kapalabhati* breathing might not be acceptable to them. A good way to assess the client's willingness to do a practice and to support their sense of self-efficacy is to (whenever possible) encourage the client to set the pace, building their ability to deepen the breath. Similarly, *kapalabhati* would likely be the second practice, after meeting the slower breath and more lethargic state. It might then be practiced slowly, allowing the client to lead an increase in speed, as tolerated.

Whether primarily characterized by anxiety or lethargy, depression leaves a person depleted, so ending with relaxation that might include yoga nidra, or any other guided form of relaxation in a reclining, resting position, can be useful. Given that the mind tends to be attached to negative thinking during depressive episodes, long periods of silent *savasana* should be substituted with guided relaxation techniques where the person can be anchored through the yoga teacher/therapist's voice.

In addition to viewing and managing depression from the perspective of anxious versus lethargic, the *kosha* model is a useful way to consider individual needs that can be addressed through yogic lifestyle. Typically, the individualized, in-depth approach described here will be performed by a yoga therapist. Through a detailed case history, the yoga therapist can assess the different *koshas* and consider ways to bring more energy and balance to each one. For example, to address imbalance in the *annamaya kosha* (the physical body), a yoga therapist would explore what the client eats, how they sleep, the way the client holds

their body, any present aches and pains and areas of stiffness, and then suggest practices that can address issues in each of these domains. Likewise, the yoga therapist might consider what the client already does, if anything, to support the physical body, then help further cultivate this skill. The same approach can be used with the other four *kosha*, allowing the yoga therapist to consider how the client breathes, what the nature of the client's thoughts are, how the client connects to their surroundings, and the client's social support systems. Finally, when examining the *anandamaya kosha*, it can be singularly helpful to discover what brings the client joy as an antidote to depressive mood, and to determine whether the client practices this regularly, and if not, how to motivate the client to do so.

In addition to the overall approach in using yoga to support the management of depression, there are other important overall considerations that support safety and wellbeing and allow the person to benefit from the practice, such as the use of language, the therapeutic environment, and the qualities of attentive listening and positive regard the yoga teacher/therapist brings to the client.

Language

There are general considerations with language that are very important, as well as those that are more specific to the individual. In a general yoga class it is common that a teacher/therapist will suggest that students might have a specific experience related to yoga practices, often with the assumption that the experience is a positive one, such as the "ahhh" feeling of letting go. However, for an individual managing depression, such a response may be rare or absent. It is therefore preferable to suggest that students explore with interest what is actually occurring for them, rather than adding a value to feeling. This fosters an attitude of curiosity, which can be a balm for the self-judgment often present in depression. This in turn promotes the ability to accept and welcome all internal states, whether they are pleasant or unpleasant.

Another consideration is when working with a *sankalpa* (aspiration); for example, "I am joyful" or "may I be at peace," which helps some clients to release negative thinking. However, for others it may feel like a suppression of real feelings and a forced attempt to pretend one feels OK. Furthermore, people with acute depression may not be able to imagine something positive, safe, or nurturing in developing a *sankalpa*. Therefore, when working with people experiencing depression, it's important to consider that mindful attention to what is present may be more helpful than imagining life in a different way. Rather than risking a client feeling alienated by trying to engage in aspirational thinking, present-moment attention can facilitate a cognitive shift regarding how they approach the nature of their actual experience.

The yoga teacher/therapist should be aware that an individual in a depressed mood may perceive even neutral language as a personal attack or an indication of inadequacy. Spending time encouraging acceptance of all feelings and emotions, as well as minimizing attention to exacting detail in postures, is therefore important. This approach can help to avoid activating the student/client's inner critic, which can hijack the ability to just be with the body and breath as they are—an important reprieve from negative thinking that yoga can offer.

> The yoga teacher/therapist should be aware that an individual in a depressed mood may perceive even neutral language as a personal attack or an indication of inadequacy.

Finally, it is not advisable to regularly refer to the experience of depression with clients. This can feed the client's sense of identification with depression and reify the client's concept that "I am a depressed person." Instead, it is helpful to talk about working with emotional wellbeing and to recognize that sadness is part of life, while appreciating that it can be overwhelming. Likewise, being playful with language and keeping the mood light can be restorative for depressed mood, perhaps introducing joy to people who may usually find it inaccessible.

Environment

Whether working with groups or individuals, the space should be neutral and quiet. Quiet is especially important because people with depression often have low serotonin levels, which can cause them to be more sensitive to sound. Wherever possible, the space should be spacious and bright, as light can help to lift mood.

Specific practices

Given that several trials with varying yogic protocols show encouraging results, it is likely that yoga in general may be useful. Furthermore, a yoga professional would usually want to design a class that includes all movements, including forward, back, side to side, and twisting.

Nonetheless, there are specific practices that are likely to be helpful and others that would not be ideal for most people with depression. Often these practices seem to be most effective in combination, but first of all we will look at the individual categories of practice, beginning with asana.

A research trial found that backbends elevated mood more than other postures (Shapiro & Cline, 2004), which aligns with traditional understanding in yoga teaching that many backbends are stimulating. Research has not yet identified the precise mechanisms of action, but there are several possible explanations for their role in alleviating depression.

Physiologically, there may be some correlates. For example, the thoracic part of the spine is replete with sympathetic nerve fibers. By arching the spine, these nerves are stimulated, which may help to lift a person out of lethargy. If the depression is anxiety-based, then the application of the backbend would include a longer hold, perhaps in a supported posture using props, and with encouragement of yogic three-part breath (*dirga pranayama*). In this way the lift that might occur is less likely to provoke anxiety. As mentioned earlier there should be other postures that would precede a hold in a backbend. It is important to initially meet the agitated state with a slightly more dynamic practice, such as a sun salutation or other warm-ups for the spine, before slowing down for the longer holding of a backbend.

If anxiety is not co-occurring with depression, then the backbend could be performed dynamically, moving in and out of a *bhujangasana* (cobra) or a more challenging pose like *urdva danurasana* (upward-facing bow/wheel), if the person has this capacity.

Poses like *viparita karani* (legs up the wall) are excellent poses for an anxiety-based depression. It tends to be very relaxing, and by promoting lymphatic flow it is healthy for the body and may improve its functioning, leading to a sense of greater wellbeing. It is important, though, to be cautious with long holds in gentle poses. In the absence of intensity in poses, the individual is left to try and relax, and a depressed mind may return to its personal tirade of negative thinking. This is one reason that although restorative yoga poses can be very useful in helping a person to relax and offer respite from negative mood, they also have the potential to feed it. The use of these poses should be decided on an individual basis within the context of the group.

Dynamic mantras such as *"di ri ha"* can help to release emotions. When said vigorously, this mantra evokes a mild pumping action at the solar plexus, which, like *kapalabhati* and other vigorous *kriya* breathing practices, is excellent for self-empowerment

and for releasing anger. Because depression is sometimes the result of anger turned toward self, this can be an important way to transform that experience.

Another consideration in *tamasic*, or lethargic, depression is the breath of joy. Usually done standing, this traditionally involves three strong inhalations with arms lifting forward, to the side and then up in front on each inhale, followed by a strong releasing exhale as the person bends forward in an almost falling action (see Figures 3.1 to 3.4). For safety, it is suggested that for practitioners who are older or who suffer back discomfort, *utkatasana* (chair, or powerful, pose) with arms back should be substituted for the forward-falling action on the exhale. For more vulnerable individuals a modified version is useful, during which individuals engage in the same practice, but in a chair.

As inhalation is uplifting, this kind of breathing with movement helps to enliven someone feeling sluggish. The root chakra mantra, *"lum,"* may be added to the exhale to increase vitality and grounding. Breath practices like *kapalabhati* and *bhastrika* are also uplifting and can be useful for someone feeling sluggish. However, if a person's depression is co-occurring with anxiety, then care must be taken when introducing such practices since they could increase nervousness. Instead, paying attention to slow controlled breathing practices, and practices with elongated exhalation can help to curb nervous feelings.

For people whose breathing is shallow, three-part inhalation quickly expands the lungs in all directions, and supports fuller breathing.

Regardless of the type of depression, most people with depression will likely benefit from *dirga* breath and alternate-nostril breathing. The three-part inhalation is not stressful for the lungs but requires them to work, thereby increasing wakefulness and lifting energy. For people whose breathing is shallow,

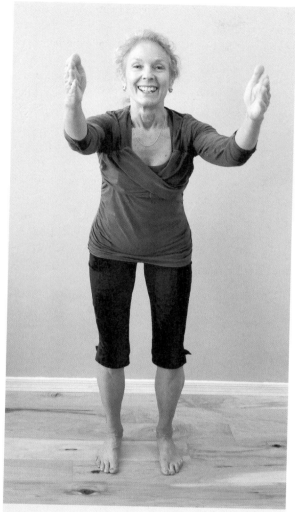

Figure 3.1

Inhale one-third and swing arms forward and upward in front of the body

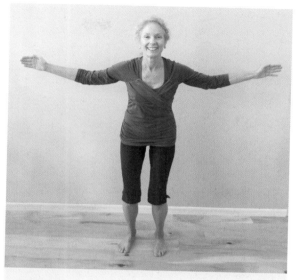

Figure 3.2

Inhale another third and swing arms out to the side

can cause agitation and emotional upheaval. It may also trigger a sense of inadequacy and feelings of "not good enough" in those unable to accomplish it. In this case, a focus on gentle *ujjayi* breathing along with suggestions such as "welcoming the breath wherever it's landing" is recommended (Weintraub, 2012).

Once students are comfortable with some of the breathing and postures already suggested then mantras, mudras, and meditations can be included. Likewise, students can be taught to choose poses based on their particular need on a given day. For example, a yoga teacher/therapist might say, "If you are feeling revved up, try, on a 4–6 count breath, slowing down your exhalation to reduce any anxiety or agitation. If you're feeling sluggish, try a 4–4 count breath as you move, as this will help to balance your nervous system." Or they might propose, "If you're feeling lethargic, you may wish to come in and out of cobra or sphinx, using your breath. If you're feeling agitated, hold sphinx for several 4–6 count breaths, and then

three-part inhalation quickly expands the lungs in all directions, and supports fuller breathing. The long exhalation that follows can be deeply relaxing. For those who struggle with breathing or who are chest breathers, it is important that the breath is guided gently and that inhalation is not forced, otherwise this

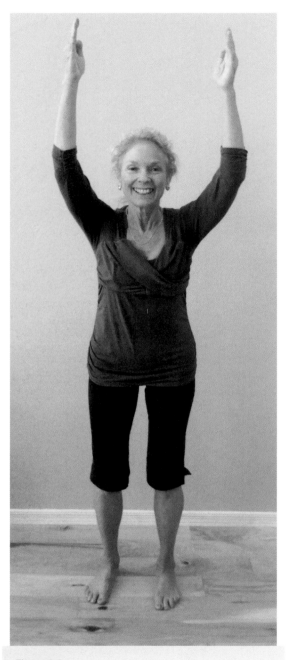

Figure 3.3
Inhale the final third and swing arms forward and upward and in front of the body once again

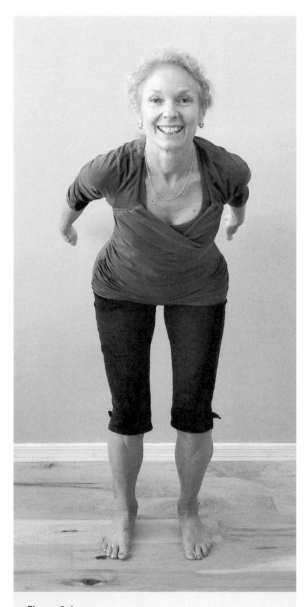

Figure 3.4
Exhale with the mantra *lum* into chair pose, with the arms swung back
Photographer: Liz Payne Merideth

come back to child pose, using the *mmm* sound, as you roll across your brow point. We'll all meet in child pose." The aim is to empower the client or group to understand their needs and to respond to them accordingly.

In addition to asana and pranayama, chanting is usually well received by people who are depressed. It tends to lift mood, and when done collectively, creates a feeling of joyful connection. Depending upon your unique style as a yoga teacher/therapist, you may choose to chant OM, use a mantra that is meant to invoke particular effects that are meaningful to the person or group, or even rely on the chakra model of healing and chant the sounds of each of these. From a yogic perspective, people with depression might have blocks in any or all of the chakras, for example, in the *muladhara* (at the root) there may be a feeling of a lack of groundedness or of basic needs not being met; in the *manipura* (at the solar plexus), where a person's sense of power might be weakened; in the *anahata*, where the heart feels wounded and closed; in the *anjana* chakra, where too much mental energy may be sabotaging the ability to feel the body. Chanting tones associated with each chakra in succession can feel empowering and may open up areas of blockage. Likewise, the sound of chanting may support a person's feeling of self-expression and expansiveness. Once a person learns the relationship between the sounds, the chakras, and their meaning, then they can be invited to chant the sound of the chakra that they feel needs attention at different times during the practice.

Integrating yoga practices into mental healthcare settings

Breathing practices

There are many non–mat-based practices that can easily be integrated into mental healthcare settings. It is suggested that clinicians find practices that work for a client and begin each session this way. This kind of ritual may support a conditioned response of safe-

ty, positive experience, and relaxation, each of which provides a supportive container for therapeutic work.

> The aim is to empower the client or group to understand their needs and to respond to them accordingly.

For example, beginning a session with a simple breathing practice, a secular tone, a cue to an image for peace or calm, and/or a calming hand gesture, can facilitate the nonverbal work of therapy.

Simple yogic breathing practices that can be easily integrated into therapeutic work include slow breathing with an even inhale and exhale. A rate of 5–6 bpm has been shown to be an ideal rate for increasing HRV in research trials (Lehrer, Vaschillo, & Vaschillo, 2000). As previously mentioned, an elongated exhalation can be remarkably helpful, especially when anxiety is present. This might include breathing in for 4 and out for 6, or for greater effect, in a 1:2 ratio. Both of these practices can be taught with or without *ujjayi* breathing.

Another common yogic breath that works well in clinical practice is yogic three-part breath (*dirga*), which is sometimes taught with victory ocean-sounding breath (*ujjayi*). The typical breathing pattern of a person suffering from depression may be shallow, and *dirga* expands the lungs and deepens the breath, thus encouraging an increase in oxygen consumption and a release of carbon dioxide (Telles & Desiraju, 1991; Telles, Nagarathna, & Nagendra, 1996). Therefore, practices such as *dirga* that promote deep breathing may induce short-term feelings of activation and vitality. However, a deep breath to the bottom of the lungs is not always accessible to someone suffering from depression. In such a case, the teacher/therapist should start with other breathing methods that meet the chest breathing first, such as a staged inhalation like stair-step breath (*analoma krama*), accompanied by a smooth exhalation.

There are two reasons why a yoga teacher/therapist should take a gradual approach to *dirga pranayama*. First, many people with depression are upper-chest breathers who may not yet be able to breathe deeply and fully, so beginning with an expectation to breathe to the bottom of the lungs (as in *dirga*) may be setting the student up to fail in the very first session. An alternative for someone unable to breathe deeply is to practice slow breathing with the arms hugged around the chest: this will naturally encourage belly breathing (since it contracts the muscles necessary for chest breathing by effortlessly moving the breath downward) and so can help the client to later access this breath with ease. Second, some upper-chest breathers are tamping down a lot of negative emotions—for example, anger, shame, and grief—for a very good reason: they may not yet have the resources to deal with the repressed material. When someone who, for self-protection, has been a shallow breather starts to breathe deeply, there can be an eruption of emotion as the walls of defense tumble down. Catharsis may feel good when there is an established therapeutic relationship and the client has the resources to deal with the emotion that arises. But if emotional flooding occurs too early in the work together, the client may feel frightened or ashamed. They may not return or could develop an antipathy toward yoga (Weintraub, 2012).

Other practices

In addition to breathing, there are various other techniques that can be incorporated into a therapy session. For instance, if the client appreciates the role of affirmations, a short guided yoga nidra practice with a *sankalpa* can be taught to strengthen client resolve.

Affirmations can also be used without yoga nidra in conjunction with additional yogic practices, which may amplify the effects. One could add a mudra, a mantra, a pranayama, or possibly a visual image of empowerment. For example: "See an image for courage, maybe from nature, or a time when you've felt strong and clear—inhale the arms out in front of the heart, see that image or the word *courage*. Draw the hands into the heart with the mantra, 'soham' (I am that)."

Yoga in a mental health setting

Many psychotherapists and other health professionals are beginning to integrate yoga into clinical work to help their clients relax, focus, and self-regulate. All of these aspects cultivate a sense of safety in the client and may promote a better therapeutic bond, setting the stage for deeper therapeutic work while also promoting self-efficacy and self-reliance in the client, core features of wellbeing. Additionally, yoga practices, even those that do not involve asana, can develop greater interoceptive awareness. This can help a client to better understand what they are experiencing in the context of their cognitive narrative, which is a first step to reframing unhelpful thoughts and beliefs.

Giving clients cues to notice sensations, for example, in their faces or hands after guiding a practice, enables them to safely begin to feel grounded in somatic sensation, and in some cases, reoccupy a body that has been disavowed. Client-created affirmations that arise from a brief meditation may also foster the goals of therapy.

Future directions

While psychopharmacology remains the cornerstone of the treatment of depressive disorders, its relatively weak effects with patients who are mildly to moderately depressed suggest a need for additional avenues of exploration. Given that yoga offers a variety of tools to work with the mind and support the body toward better mental health, it may well represent one such avenue. We take heart from the growing body of scientific evidence examining yoga's efficacy, which suggests that although more rigorous research is required, yoga could play an important role in the treatment of depression. In some cases, this may include yoga as a preventive measure for a patient with dysthymia who would like to seek alternative methods such as yoga as primary intervention, before MDD presents. In other cases yoga might serve as an adjunct intervention to support greater self-reliance and overall health.

According to the WHO, depression is the fourth-largest contributor to the global burden of disease. As beautifully stated by Doriswamy, "The search for improved treatments, including non-drug based, to meet the holistic needs of patients is of paramount importance and we call for more research into yoga as a global priority—if the promise of yoga on mental health was found in a drug, it would be the best selling medication world-wide" (Balasubramaniam, Telles, & Doraiswamy, 2013).

It should be noted that as levels of depression are expected to rise, yoga may play an important part in its management. Yoga is multidimensional and can manage a host of depressive symptoms ranging from psychological, to physiological, to behavioral. Yoga gives back power to people who feel hopeless, offers community through sangha to those who feel isolated, and provides a value system that provides meaning and purpose to those in despair.

References

American Psychiatric Association (2013). *Diagnostic and Statistical Manual of Mental Disorder* (5th edn*)*. Arlington, VA: American Psychiatric Association.

Astin, J. A., Shapiro, S. L., Lee, R. A., & Shapiro, D. H., Jr. (1999). The construct of control in mind-body medicine: Implications for healthcare. *Alternative Therapies in Health and Medicine, 5*(2), 42–47.

Balasubramaniam, M., Telles, S., & Doraiswamy, P. M. (2013). Yoga on our minds: A systematic review of yoga for neuropsychiatric disorders. *Frontiers in Psychiatry*. Article publication online.

Banasik, J., Williams, H., Haberman, M., Blank, S. E., & Bendel, R. (2011). Effect of Iyengar yoga practice on fatigue and diurnal salivary cortisol concentration in breast cancer survivors. *Journal of the American Academy of Nurse Practitioners, 23*(3), 135–142.

Bandura, A. (1994). Self-efficacy. In V. S. Ramachaudran (Ed.), *Encyclopedia of human behavior* (vol. 4). New York: Academic Press.

Beck, A. T. (2008). The evolution of the cognitive model of depression and its neurobiological correlates. *American Journal of Psychiatry, 165*(8), 969–977.

Büssing, A., Ostermann, T., Ludtke, R., & Michalsen, A. (2012). Effects of yoga interventions on pain and pain-associated disability: A meta-analysis. *The Journal of Pain, 13*(1), 1–9.

Butler, L. D., Waelde, L. C., Hastings, T. A., Chen, X. H., Symons, B., Marshall, J., Kaufman, A., Nagy, T. F., Blasey, C. M., Seibert, E. O., & Spiegel, D. (2008). Meditation with yoga, group therapy with hypnosis, and psychoeducation for long-term depressed mood: A randomized pilot trial. *Journal of Clinical Psychology, 64*(7), 806–820.

Buttner, M. M., Brock, R. L., O'Hara, M. W., & Stuart, S. (2015). Efficacy of yoga for depressed postpartum women: A randomized controlled trial. *Complementary Therapies in Clinical Practice, 21*(2), 94–100.

Carroll, B. J., Iranmanesh, A., Keenan, D. M., Cassidy, F., Wilson, W. H., & Veldhuis, J. D. (2012). Pathophysiology of hypercortisolism in depression: Pituitary and adrenal responses to low glucocorticoid feedback. *Acta Psychiatrica Scandinavica, 125*(6), 478–491.

Cramer, H., Krucoff, C., & Dobos, G. (2013). Adverse events associated with yoga: A systematic review of published case reports and case series. *PLoS One, 8*(10), e75515.

Cramer, H., Lange, S., Klose, P., Paul, A., & Dobos, G. (2012). Yoga for breast cancer patients and survivors: A systematic review and meta-analysis. *BMC Cancer, 12*, 412.

Cramer, H., Lauche, R., Azizi, H., Dobos, G., & Langhorst, J. (2014). Yoga for multiple sclerosis: A systematic review and meta-analysis. *PLoS One, 9*(11), e112414.

Cramer, H., Lauche, R., Haller, H., Dobos, G., & Michalsen, A. (2015). A systematic review of yoga for heart disease. *European Journal of Preventive Cardiology, 22*(3), 284–295.

Cramer, H., Lauche, R., Langhorst, J., & Dobos, G. (2013). Yoga for depression: A systematic review and meta-analysis. *Depression and Anxiety, 30*(11), 1068–1083.

Cramer, H., Ward, L., Saper, R., Fishbein, D., Dobos, G., & Lauche, R. (2015). The safety of yoga: A systematic review and meta-analysis of randomized controlled trials. *Am J Epidemiol, 182*(4), 281–293.

Devi, S. K., Chansauria, J. P., & Udupa, K. N. (1986). Mental depression and kundalini yoga. *Ancient Science of Life, 6*(2), 112–118.

Disner, S. G., Beevers, C. G., Haigh, E. A., & Beck, A. T. (2011). Neural mechanisms of the cognitive model of depression. *Nature Reviews Neuroscience, 12*(8), 467–477.

Field, T., Diego, M., Delgado, J., & Medina, L. (2013a). Tai chi/yoga reduces prenatal depression, anxiety and sleep disturbances. *Complementary Therapies in Clinical Practice, 19*(1), 6–10.

Field, T., Diego, M., Delgado, J., & Medina, L. (2013b). Yoga and social support reduce prenatal depression, anxiety and cortisol. *Journal of bodywork and movement therapies, 17*(4), 397–403.

Field, T., Diego, M., Hernandez-Reif, M., Medina, L., Delgado, J., & Hernandez, A. (2012). Yoga and massage therapy reduce prenatal depression and prematurity. *Journal of bodywork and movement therapies, 16*(2), 204–209.

Gartside, S. E., Leitch, M. M., McQuade, R., & Swarbrick, D. J. (2003). Flattening the glucocorticoid rhythm causes changes in hippocampal expression of messenger RNAs coding structural and functional proteins: Implications for aging and depression. *Neuropsychopharmacology, 28*(5), 821–829.

Gelenberg, A. J., Freeman, M. P., Markowitz, J. C., Rosenbaum, J. F., Thase, M. E., Trivedi, M. H., & van Rhoads, R. S. (2010). Practice guideline for the treatment of patients with major depressive disorder. *American Journal of Psychiatry, 167*(10), 1–3,9–11,13–118.

Gong, H., Ni, C., Shen, X., Wu, T., & Jiang, C. (2015). Yoga for prenatal depression: A systematic review and meta-analysis. *BMC Psychiatry, 15*, 14.

Hallgren, M., Herring, M. P., Owen, N., Dunstan, D., Ekblom, O., Helgadottir, B., Nakitanda, O. A., & Forsell, Y. (2016). Exercise, physical activity, and sedentary behavior in the treatment of depression: Broadening the scientific perspectives and clinical opportunities. *Frontiers in Psychiatry, 7*, 36.

Hidaka, B. H. (2012). Depression as a disease of modernity: Explanations for increasing prevalence. *Journal of Affective Disorders, 140*(3), 205–214.

Janakiramaiah, N., Gangadhar, B., Murthy, P. J. N. V., Harish, M. G., Shetty, K. T., Subbakrishna, D. K., Meti, B. L., Raju, T., & Vedamurthachar, A. (1998). Therapeutic efficacy of Sudarshan Kriya Yoga (SKY) in dysthymic disorder. *NIMHANS J, 17*, 21–28.

Jarcho, M. R., Slavich, G. M., Tylova-Stein, H., Wolkowitz, O. M., & Burke, H. M. (2013). Dysregulated diurnal cortisol pattern is associated with glucocorticoid resistance in women with major depressive disorder. *Biological Psychology, 93*(1), 150–158.

Kalueff, A. V., & Nutt, D. J. (2007). Role of GABA in anxiety and depression. *Depression and Anxiety, 24*(7), 495–517.

Khumar, S. S., Kaur, P., & Kaur, S. (1993). Effectiveness of Shavasana on depression among university students. *Indian Journal of Clinical Psychology, 20*, 82–87.

Kinser, P. A., Goehler, L. E., Taylor, A. G. (2012). How might yoga help depression? A neurobiological perspective. *Explore (NY), 8*(2), 118–126.

Kinser, P. A., Bourguignon, C., Whaley, D., Hauenstein, E., & Taylor, A. G. (2013). Feasibility, acceptability, and effects of gentle hatha yoga for women with major depression: Findings from a randomized controlled mixed-methods study. *Archives of Psychiatric Nursing, 27*(3), 137–147.

Kirsch, I., Deacon, B. J., Huedo-Medina, T. B., Scoboria, A., Moore, T. J., & Johnson, B. T. (2008). Initial severity and antidepressant benefits: A meta-analysis of data submitted to the Food and Drug Administration. *PLoS Med, 5*(2), e45.

Kjaer, T. W., Bertelsen, C., Piccini, P., Brooks, D., Alving, J., & Lou, H. C. (2002). Increased dopamine tone during meditation-induced change of consciousness. *Brain research. Cognitive brain research, 13*(2), 255–259.

Lauche, R., Langhorst, J., Paul, A., Dobos, G., & Cramer, H. (2014). Self-reported health and satisfaction of patients with chronic diseases who meditate: A case-control study. *Quality of Life Research, 23*(9), 2639–2644.

Lavretsky, H., Epel, E. S., Siddarth, P., Nazarian, N., Cyr, N. S., Khalsa, D. S., Lin, J., Blackburn, E., & Irwin, M. R. (2013). A pilot study of yogic meditation for family dementia caregivers with depressive symptoms: Effects on mental health, cognition, and telomerase activity. *International Journal of Geriatric Psychiatry, 28*(1), 57–65.

Lee, B. H., & Kim, Y. K. (2010). The roles of BDNF in the pathophysiology of major depression and in antidepressant treatment. *Psychiatry Investigation, 7*(4), 231–235.

Lehrer, P. M., Vaschillo, E., & Vaschillo, B. (2000). Resonant frequency biofeedback training to increase cardiac variability: Rationale and manual for training. *Applied Psychophysiology and Biofeedback, 25*(3), 177–191.

MacKenzie, M. B., & Kocovski, N. L. (2016). Mindfulness-based cognitive therapy for depression: Trends and developments. *Psychology Research and Behavior Management, 9*, 125–132.

Markil, N., Whitehurst, M., Jacobs, P. L., & Zoeller, R. F. (2012). Yoga Nidra relaxation increases heart rate variability and is unaffected by a prior bout of hatha yoga. *Journal of Alternative and Complementary Medicine, 18*(10), 953–958.

Meyer, J. H., Goulding, V. S., Wilson, A. A., Hussey, D., Christensen, B. K., & Houle, S. (2002). Bupropion occupancy of the dopamine transporter is low during clinical treatment. *Psychopharmacology (Berl), 163*(1), 102–105.

Mitchell, J., Field, T., Diego, M., Bendell, D., Newton, R., & Pelaez, M. (2012). Yoga reduces prenatal depression symptoms. *Psychology, 3*(9A), 782–786.

Mourya, M., Mahajan, A. S., Singh, N. P., & Jain, A. K. (2009). Effect of slow- and fast-breathing exercises on autonomic functions in patients with essential hypertension. *Journal of Alternative and Complementary Medicine, 15*(7), 711–717.

Naveen, G. H., Thirthalli, J., Rao, M. G., Varambally, S., Christopher, R., & Gangadhar, B. N. (2013). Positive therapeutic and neurotropic effects of yoga in depression: A comparative study. *Indian Journal of Psychiatry, 55*(Suppl 3), S400–404.

Patil, S. G., Mullur, L. M., Khodnapur, J. P., Dhanakshirur, G. B., & Aithala, M. R. (2013) Effect of yoga on short-term heart rate variability measure as a stress index in subjunior cyclists: A pilot study. *Indian Journal of Physiological Pharmacology, 57*(2), 153–158

Rohini, V., Pandey, R. S., Janakiramaiah, N., Gangadhar, B. N., & Vedamurthachar, A. (2000). A comparative study of full and partial SudarshanKriya Yoga (SKY) in major depressive disorder. *NIMHANS J, 18*, 53–57.

Sarubin, N., Nothdurfter, C., Schule, C., Lieb, M., Uhr, M., Born, C., Zimmermannc, R., Bühner, M., Konopka, K., Rupprecht, R., & Baghai, T. C. (2014). The influence of hatha yoga as an add-on treatment in major depression on hypothalamic-pituitary-adrenal-axis activity: A randomized trial. *Journal of Psychiatric Research, 53*, 76–83.

Schuch, F. B., Vancampfort, D., Richards, J., Rosenbaum, S., Ward, P. B., & Stubbs, B. (2016). Exercise as a treatment for depression: A meta-analysis adjusting for publication bias. *Journal of Psychiatric Research, 77*, 42–51.

Schuver, K. J., & Lewis, B. A. (2016). Mindfulness-based yoga intervention for women with depression. *Complementary Therapies in Medicine, 26*, 85–91.

Shahidi, M., Mojtahed, A., Modabbernia, A., Mojtahed, M., Shafiabady, A., Delavar, A., & Honari, H. (2011). Laughter yoga versus group exercise program in elderly depressed women: A randomized controlled trial. *International Journal of Geriatric Psychiatry, 26*(3), 322–327.

Shapiro, D., & Cline, K. (2004). Mood changes associated with Iyengar yoga practices: A pilot study. *International Journal of Yoga Therapy, 14*(1), 35–44.

Sharma, A., Barrett, M. S., Cucchiara, A. J., Gooneratne, N. S., & Thase, M. E. (2017). A breathing-based meditation intervention for patients with major depressive disorder following inadequate response to antidepressants: A randomized pilot study. *Journal of Clinical Psychiatry, 78*(1), e59–e63.

Sharma, V. K., Das, S., Mondal, S., Goswampi, U., & Gandhi, A. (2005). Effect of Sahaj yoga on depressive disorders. *Indian Journal of Physiology and Pharmacology, 49*(4), 462–468.

Streeter, C. C., Jensen, J. E., Perlmutter, R. M., Cabral, H. J., Tian, H., Terhune, D. B., Ciraulo, D. A., & Renshaw, P. F. (2007). Yoga asana sessions increase brain GABA levels: A pilot study. *Journal of Alternative & Complementary Medicine, 13*(4), 419–426.

Streeter, C. C., Whitfield, T. H., Owen, L., Rein, T., Karri, S. K., Yakhkind, A., Perlmutter, R., Prescot, A., Renshaw, P. F., Ciraulo, D. A., & Jensen, J. E. (2010). Effects of yoga versus walking on mood, anxiety, and brain GABA levels: A randomized controlled MRS study. *Journal of Alternative & Complementary Medicine, 16*(11), 1145–1152.

Streeter, C. C., Gerbarg, P. L., Saper, R. B., Ciraulo, D. A., & Brown, R. P. (2012). Effects of yoga on the autonomic nervous system, gamma-aminobutyric-acid, and allostasis in epilepsy, depression, and post-traumatic stress disorder. *Medical Hypotheses, 78*(5), 571–579.

Syvälahti, E. K. (1994). Biological aspects of depression. *Acta Psychiatrica Scandinavica Supplement, 377*, 11–15.

Telles, S., & Desiraju, T. (1991). Oxygen consumption during pranayamic type of very slow-rate breathing. *The Indian Journal of Medical Research, 94*, 357–363.

Telles, S., Nagarathna, R., & Nagendra, H. R. (1996). Physiological measures of right nostril breathing. *Journal of Alternative and Complementary Medicine, 2*(4), 479–484.

Telles, S., Raghavendra, B. R., Naveen, K. V., Manjunath, N. K., Kumar, S., & Subramanya, P. (2013). Changes in autonomic variables following two meditative states described in yoga texts. *Journal of Alternative and Complementary Medicine, 19*(1), 35–42.

Thase, M. E., Jindal, R., & Howland, R. H. (2002). Biological aspects of depression. In I. H. Gotlib & C. Hammen (Eds.), *Handbook of Depression* (pp. 192–218). New York, NY: Guilford Press.

Tyagi, A., Cohen, M., Reece, J., Telles, S., & Jones, L. (2016). Heart rate variability, flow, mood and mental stress during yoga practices in yoga practitioners, non-yoga practitioners and people with metabolic syndrome. *Applied Psychophysiology and Biofeedback, 41*(4), 381–393.

Uebelacker, L. A., Battle, C. L., Sutton, K. A., Magee, S. R., & Miller, I. W. (2016). A pilot randomized controlled trial comparing prenatal yoga to perinatal health education for antenatal depression. *Archives of Women's Mental Health, 19*(3), 543–547.

Vadiraja, H. S., Raghavendra, R. M., Nagarathna, R., Nagendra, H. R., Rekha, M., Vanitha, N., Gopinath, K. S., Srinath, B. S., Vishweshwara, M. S., Madhavi, Y. S., Ajaikumar, B. S., Ramesh, B. S., Nalini, R., & Kumar, V. (2009). Effects of a yoga program on cortisol rhythm and mood states in early breast cancer patients undergoing adjuvant radiotherapy: A randomized controlled trial. *Integrative Cancer Therapies, 8*(1), 37–46.

Veale, D., Le Fevre, K., Pantelis, C., de Souza, V., Mann, A., & Sargeant, A. (1992). Aerobic exercise in the adjunctive treatment of depression: A randomized controlled trial. *Journal of the Royal Society of Medicine, 85*(9), 541–544.

Vedamurthachar, A., Janakiramaiah, N., Hegde, J. M., Shetty, T. K., Subbakrishna, D. K., Sureshbabu, S. V., & Gangadhar, B. N. (2006). Antidepressant efficacy and hormonal effects of Sudarshana Kriya Yoga (SKY) in alcohol dependent individuals. *Journal of Affective Disorders, 94*(1–3), 249–253.

Vreeburg, S. A., Hoogendijk, W. J., van Pelt, J., Derijk, R. H., Verhagen, J. C., van Dyck, R., Smit, J. H., Zitman, F. G., & Penninx, B. W. (2009). Major depressive disorder and hypothalamic-pituitary-adrenal axis activity: Results from a large cohort study. *Archives of General Psychiatry, 66*(6), 617–626.

Weintraub, A. (2012). *Yoga Skills for Therapists: Effective Practices for Mood Management*. W. W. Norton.

Weintraub, A. (2004). *Yoga for Depression: A Compassionate Guide to Relieve Suffering through Yoga*. Broadway Books

Weintraub, A. (2012). *Yoga Skills for Therapists: Effective Practices for Mood Management*. W. W. Norton.

Weintraub, A. (2016). *LifeForce Yoga Practitioner Manual*, 43–44.

Weissman, M. M., Bland, R. C., Canino, G. J., Faravelli, C., Greenwald, S., Hwu, H. G., Joyce, P. R., Karam, E. G., Lee, C. K., Lellouch, J., Lépine, J. P., Newman, S. C., Rubio-Stipec, M., Wells, J. E., Wickramaratne, P. J., Wittchen, H., & Yeh, E. K. (1996). Cross-national epidemiology of major depression and bipolar disorder. *JAMA, 276*(4), 293–299.

Woolery, A., Myers, H., Sternlieb, B., & Zeltzer, L. (2004). A yoga intervention for young adults with elevated symptoms of depression. *Alternative therapies in health and medicine, 10*(2), 60–63.

World Health Organization (2017, March). *Depression* (fact sheet). Retrieved from: http://www.who.int/mediacentre/factsheets/fs369/en/.

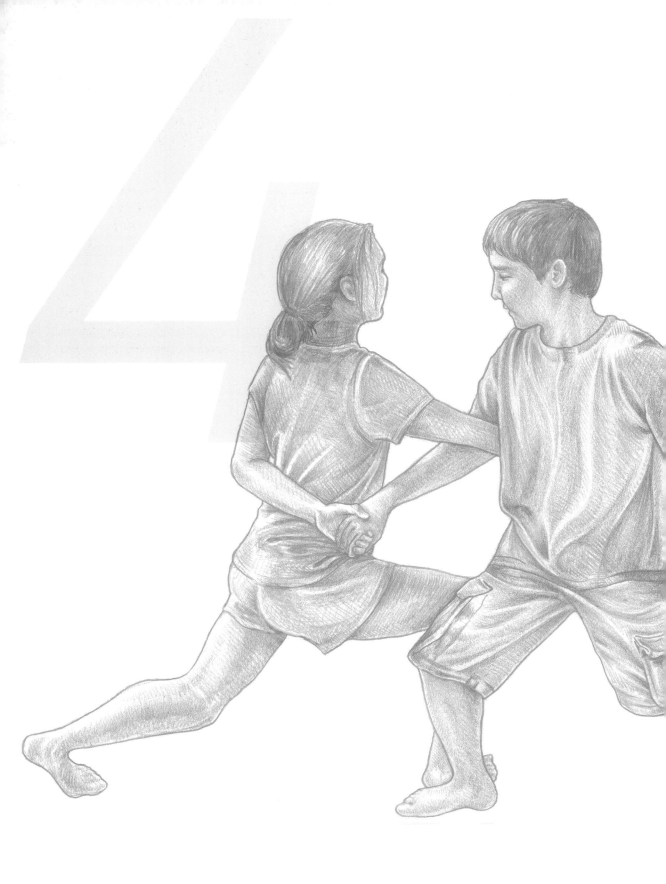

Attention-Deficit Hyperactivity Disorder

Lana Jackson and Lucy Arnsby-Wilson

4

Overview

Attention-deficit hyperactivity disorder (ADHD) is classified as a neurodevelopmental disorder in the *Diagnostic and Statistical Manual of Mental Disorders* (DSM-5) (American Psychiatric Association, 2013) and is characterized by persistent overactivity, impulsivity, and difficulties with sustaining attention. It is one of the most commonly diagnosed childhood conditions, although possibly still one of the most controversial. Many adults with ADHD were diagnosed during their childhood or adolescent years, and it is suggested that up to 60% of children with ADHD retain their symptoms into adulthood (Sibley et al., 2017). The estimated worldwide prevalence of ADHD varies across studies, reported as 5.29–7.1% in children and adolescents (American Psychiatric Association, 2013; Polanczyk et al., 2007; Thomas et al., 2015; Willcutt, 2012) and at 3.4% (1.2–7.3%) in adults (Centers for Disease Control and Prevention, 2010; Fayyad et al., 2007). These differences may be due to a number of factors including cultural, social, and environmental differences, as well as variations in both definitions and diagnoses across countries and studies (Faraone, Sergeant, Gillberg & Biederman, 2003).

> The key issues seen in ADHD are inattention, hyperactivity, and impulsivity.

In order to receive a diagnosis of ADHD, children or adults must have displayed the difficulties listed in the DSM-5 for at least six months (American Psychiatric Association, 2013). The key issues seen in ADHD are inattention, hyperactivity, and impulsivity. The symptoms of inattention include difficulties listening and following instructions, making careless mistakes, being easily distracted, appearing forgetful, and

having difficulties with organization and time management; children and adults report "busy minds" and "mental disorganization." In terms of hyperactivity and impulsivity, the symptoms include constant fidgeting and tapping of hands and feet, talking excessively, being constantly "on the go" or acting as if "driven by a motor," frequently interrupting others playing games or conversing, and experiencing difficulties waiting their turn. Many individuals describe feelings of inner restlessness and an inability to relax.

Such behaviors are at times found in most children and adults, but those diagnosed with ADHD will display them more frequently and severely. In order to receive a diagnosis, the symptoms must be present in more than one setting (home, school, or workplace) and must interfere with everyday functioning. Because ADHD is considered a childhood neurodevelopmental issue, for older adolescents or adults to be diagnosed, the symptoms must have been present before the age of 12 and should not be explainable by any other condition, such as psychosis or substance misuse.

Based on the criteria above, three presentations of ADHD are identified in the DSM-5: (1) ADHD Combined Presentation, when children and adults display both the inattentiveness and hyperactive-impulsive behaviors described earlier; (2) ADHD Predominantly Inattentive Presentation, where only the criteria for inattention difficulties are met (a worldwide meta-analysis of 86 studies showed that this was the most common presentation of ADHD across school-age children and adults (Willcutt, 2012)); and (3) ADHD Predominantly Hyperactive-Impulsive Presentation, where only the hyperactive-impulsive criteria are met. These outward behaviors are often more noticeable to parents and carers, and preschool children are more likely to be diagnosed with this presentation (Willcutt, 2012).

There can be many secondary issues for children living with ADHD, which may be observed within education, the home, and the community. Difficulties with sustaining attention, managing emotions, and regulating emotions and behavior can lead to poor attainment in school and problems with peer relationships (Hoza, 2007; Voigt et al., 2017). Some adolescents and young adults with poor impulse control are more likely to engage in risk-taking behaviors with associated complications such as substance misuse and involvement in the criminal justice system (Huntley & Young, 2012). Adults with ADHD have similar challenges, which can result in disproportionately high levels of unemployment (Barkley, Murphy, & Fischer, 2007; Shifrin, Proctor, & Prevatt, 2010).

Around 30% of children and 60%–80% of adults with ADHD report symptoms of sleep problems such as difficulties getting to sleep, insomnia, night-time waking, restless legs syndrome, sleep-disordered breathing, and excessive daytime sleepiness.

As well as the challenges described earlier, it is common for children and adults with ADHD to suffer from other mental and emotional health issues such as low self-esteem, anxiety, and low mood (Jensen, Shervette, Xenakis, & Richters, 1993). Children with ADHD are more likely to have associated learning difficulties, communication issues, and sleep problems (Curatolo, D'Agati, & Moavero, 2010; Hvolby, 2015). Around 30% of children and 60%–80% of adults with ADHD report symptoms of sleep problems such as difficulties getting to sleep, insomnia, night-time waking, restless legs syndrome, sleep-disordered breathing, and excessive daytime sleepiness (Yoon, Jain, & Shapiro, 2012). It has been estimated that approximately 50% of individuals with ADHD have poor motor skills, including sensorimotor coordination problems,

difficulties with balance, clumsiness, and poor handwriting (Goulardins, Marques, & De Oliveira, 2017; Piek, Pitcher, & Hay, 1999; Shum & Pang, 2009). For adults, common co-occurring conditions include bipolar disorder, generalized anxiety disorder, obsessive-compulsive disorder, major depressive disorder, and substance misuse (Kessler et al., 2006). ADHD has also been associated with other social and psychological factors such as attachment difficulties and childhood trauma and abuse, including physical and sexual abuse (Rucklidge, Brown, Crawford, & Kaplan, 2006). It has been argued that other conditions such as PTSD might be misdiagnosed as ADHD due to the overlap in symptoms, including problems with attentiveness and concentration at school or work, hyperactivity, restlessness, and difficulties sleeping (Siegfried & Blackshear, 2016; Weinstein, Staffelbach, & Biaggio, 2000).

There is much controversy around the diagnosis of ADHD. There are no physical tests for ADHD and the process of assessment and diagnosis is complex and subjective, relying on standardized self-report measures and clinical judgment. Some authors suggest that children are overdiagnosed and overmedicated for what could be seen as normal traits and behaviors in increasingly restrictive environments (Baughman, 2006). It has been argued that from an evolutionary viewpoint these traits might even be seen as beneficial within a different cultural context; for example, in a hunter-gatherer community an ability to scan the environment quickly, to be able to hyperfocus on something of interest (e.g., prey), to have the confidence to take risks, and to sustain physical energy levels would all benefit a hunter. For some this makes the validity of ADHD as a discrete disorder questionable (Hartmann, 2003). In contrast, others argue that ADHD is a neurobiological disorder residing in structural and functional brain changes and that this is evidenced by research showing differences in the brains of children and adults with ADHD compared to controls (Castellanos & Proal, 2012; Ellison-Wright, Ellison-Wright & Bullmore, 2008).

Studies have found that the overall brain size of children with ADHD is around 5% smaller than in healthy controls (Castellanos & Proal, 2012). Some research suggests that children with ADHD have delayed cortical development and reductions in both gray and white matter (Ellison-Wright et al., 2008). Several brain regions have been found to be of reduced volume in children and adults with ADHD. These include the prefrontal cortex (PFC), associated with executive functioning, directing attention, developing and pursuing goals, and inhibiting behavior, thoughts and actions; the striatum and basal ganglia, involved in movement, motor planning, reward, and motivation; the dorsal anterior cingulate cortex (ACC), involved in reward-based decision making and learning; the corpus callosum, which facilitates communication between the two hemispheres of the brain; and the cerebellum, associated with movement and motor coordination (Curatolo et al., 2010; Emond, Joyal, & Poissant, 2009).

White matter changes, shown by functional magnetic resonance imaging (fMRI), also suggest that neural connectivity in the brain is affected in those with ADHD. It is now postulated that ADHD is likely due to disruptions in neural networks in the brain, rather than solely abnormalities in isolated brain regions (Castellanos & Proal, 2012). In addition, fMRI studies have linked ADHD to underactivity in the frontal striatal circuitry, neural pathways that connect frontal lobe regions with the basal ganglia and striatum (Emond et al., 2009). This network is thought to be responsible for "cool" executive functions such as inhibiting responses, resisting interference from irrelevant stimuli, and working memory tasks (Vaidya & Stollstorff, 2008). The mesolimbic circuitry is also thought to be affected (Emond et al., 2009; Vaidya & Stollstorff, 2008). This circuit, also known as the reward circuit, links the ventromedial prefrontal regions of the brain with medial–temporal limbic regions of the amygdala and hippocampus. This circuit is involved in "hot" executive functions, such as decisions and reactions linked to emotional responses involved in pleasure and reward. Compared to controls, individuals with ADHD have been found to have hypoactivation of brain systems involved in executive functioning (frontal parietal control network) and attention (ventral attentional network) and hyperactivation of the default mode network (DMN), ventral attentional network, somatomotor network, and visual networks (Castellanos & Proal, 2012; Cortese & Castellanos, 2012). Dysfunctional modulation of the DMN is correlated with several psychiatric conditions including ADHD (Metin et al., 2015). The DMN is normally active when the mind is in a passive resting state and is associated with daydreaming, mind-wandering, mental unrest, and ruminative activity. ADHD is linked to an inability to suppress the DMN and focus the mind on a specific task.

As well as these structural and functional brain changes, ADHD has been associated with differences in the activity of neurotransmitters in the CNS. The two main neurotransmitters currently implicated are dopamine and norepinephrine (Pliszka, 2005; Volkow et al., 2009, 2011). Norepinephrine is an excitatory neurotransmitter that increases arousal and alertness and helps to focus attention; low levels may therefore contribute to the attentional difficulties seen in ADHD. Dopamine, which activates many brain structures, plays a role in attention, cognition, reward, desire, and motivation, as well as in movement and cognition. Dopamine helps to regulate and inhibit emotional and behavioral reactions. Reduced levels of dopamine in the PFC, a structure associated with inhibition control, may underscore the hyperactive and impulsive behaviors seen in ADHD, such as blurting out an answer in class. Some people with ADHD describe being able to hyperfocus (concentrate intensely) on information or tasks that interest them, but have great difficulty being able to concentrate on tasks they find uninteresting or mundane. Levels of dopamine naturally increase in the brain when we anticipate that an activity or object will be rewarding or salient. Dopamine acts to motivate us to take action to move toward that object or task. This may be why some people with ADHD gravitate toward highly stimulating and/or rewarding activities and high-risk situations, in an attempt to elevate levels of dopamine and norepinephrine and achieve a better level of cognitive control and focus (Volkow et al., 2011).

Whether these neurological differences are the cause or the consequence of ADHD is debatable, and the precise causes of ADHD are still unknown. Curatolo et al. (2010) suggest that ADHD is a result of a complex combination of prenatal and postnatal factors that interact in early development to cause a person to be more susceptible to developing a neurobiological vulnerability to ADHD.

> Although some researchers have disregarded the connection between nutrition and ADHD, there have been some studies suggesting links between additives and preservatives in food and hyperactivity.

Environmental factors may play a role, such as exposure to certain toxins (including nicotine, lead, alcohol and drug use, and maternal stress) during the prenatal and postnatal period (Linnet et al., 2003; Mick et al., 2002), being born prematurely (before the 37th week), oxygen deprivation in utero, a low birthweight, and early brain injury (Botting, Powls, Cooke & Marlow, 1997; Getahun et al., 2012). Although some researchers have disregarded the connection between nutrition and ADHD, there have been some studies suggesting links between additives and preservatives in food and hyperactivity (McCann et al. 2007). There is also some supportive evidence for the use of dietary supplements for ADHD, in particular omega 3 fatty acids (Millichap & Yee, 2012). Social factors, such as low economic status, low maternal education, and exposure to family discord might also contribute to the onset of ADHD (Biederman et al., 1995; Hjern, Weitoft, & Lindblad, 2010).

Data from the United States suggest that the rate of ADHD is increasing in the general population (Centers for Disease Control and Prevention, 2010). It has been proposed that this could be due to an increase in potential risk factors, such as toxins in the environment. Others have suggested that it is attributable to modern western lifestyles, including a decrease in outdoor activities and exercise, a lack of connection with nature, an increase in the consumption of processed food, and a rise in the time spent engaging with television and mobile devices (Kuo & Faber Taylor, 2004; Swing, Gentile, Anderson, & Walsh, 2010). Another factor may be an increase in public and professional awareness of ADHD, with the consequence that these difficulties are more easily recognized and diagnosed today (National Institute of Health and Clinical Excellence, 2018).

Current treatments

The most commonly recommended treatment for ADHD is a combination of parental support and behavior management (for children), psychological therapy (mainly CBT) and medication (American Academy of Pediatrics, 2011; National Institute of Health and Clinical Excellence, 2018; World Health Organization, 2012). Medication tends to be offered as the first line of treatment to adults and children over 6 years of age who are severely challenged by their ADHD symptoms. Drug treatments are not recommended for preschoolers (American Academy of Pediatrics, 2011; National Institute of Health and Clinical Excellence, 2018). The Food and Drug Administration (FDA) has approved two types of medication for ADHD: (1) stimulants such as methylphenidate, which are thought to affect dopamine levels; and (2) nonstimulants such as serotonin-norepinephrine reuptake inhibitors (SNRIs) (for instance, atomoxetine), which affect serotonin and norepinephrine levels (Bymaster et al., 2002; Easton, Steward, Marshall, Fone, & Marsden, 2007). As previously mentioned, dopamine and norepinephrine are believed to play important roles in regulating attention and impulsivity and have been found to be underactive in people with ADHD. These medications can help young people and adults to control their symptoms of ADHD and can improve attention, behavior, family functioning, and self-esteem (Remschmidt, 2005). However, it should be noted that not all individuals respond positively to drug treatment and its effects, therefore, they need to be monitored carefully. There are potentially harmful side effects, including loss of appetite, sleep difficulties, weight loss, abdominal pain, and heart problems; and in some instances liver damage, suicidal thinking, and self-harming behavior have been reported in connection with medication diagnosed for ADHD (National Institute of Health and Clinical Excellence, 2018; World Health Organization, 2012).

Many children with ADHD benefit from clear and consistent boundary setting and positive reinforcement for the things they have done well.

Many parents and caregivers are offered psychoeducation and group-based parent training (American Academy of Pediatrics, 2011; Centers for Disease Control and Prevention, 2010; National Institute of Health and Clinical Excellence, 2018). These interventions aim to support parents and caregivers in understanding and supporting their child with ADHD symptoms. Many children with ADHD benefit from clear and consistent boundary setting and positive reinforcement for the things they have done well. Group CBT and social skills training may also be offered to adolescents and adults with ADHD (Centers for

Disease Control and Prevention, 2010; National Institute of Health and Clinical Excellence, 2018). These approaches support a person to understand their thoughts, feelings, and behaviors; to discern more clearly any unhelpful patterns; and to learn strategies to help them manage their difficulties more effectively.

Research

Research on yoga as an intervention for ADHD

Although some research does exist on yoga as an intervention for ADHD, it is fairly sparse; there are currently only three controlled studies looking specifically at the effectiveness of yoga on the symptoms of ADHD with children and young people (Chou & Huang, 2017; Haffner, Roos, Goldstein, Parzer, & Resch, 2006; Jenson & Kenny, 2004). No studies have been conducted with adults.

The most recently published study was carried out in Taiwan by Chou and Huang (2017), in which 49 children (aged 8–12 years) diagnosed with ADHD were assigned to either a control group (no intervention) (n=25) or a yoga intervention group (n=24). The yoga group involved an eight-week intervention (two 45-minute sessions each week) consisting of physical postures, body and breath awareness, concentration, and relaxation. Children were measured pre- and post-intervention on their physical fitness levels and cognitive performance on the Visual Pursuit Test (measuring selective and sustained attention) and the Determination Test (measuring reaction speed, attention, and reactive stress tolerance). The yoga group showed significant improvement on their response time and accuracy rate post-intervention, whereas the control group showed no improvement. The authors concluded that yoga can increase sustained attention, interference control, and attention shifting among children diagnosed with ADHD.

Jenson and Kenny (2004) recruited nineteen boys (aged 8–13 years) who had a diagnosis of ADHD and were taking medication. They randomly assigned the boys to either a weekly one-hour yoga group (n=11) or a monthly one-hour cooperative games control group (n=8) over five months. The yoga session consisted of breathing practice, asana, relaxation, and meditation. Results on the Conners' Rating Scales (Conners, 1997), a parent- and teacher-rated assessment tool for ADHD and other emotional and behavioral difficulties, suggest that the yoga sessions helped reduce symptoms of hyperactivity and restlessness, particularly at times when medication had worn off or was not being used (evenings and weekends). Anecdotal evidence from parents and participants suggested that the yoga had been helpful, with one boy reporting that he used the relaxation practice to help him sleep. However, the study was limited by its small sample size and differences in contact time between the yoga group and the control group, and that participants were not blinded to the purpose of the study and group assignment. The authors propose that this population may benefit from a more intensive yoga program (i.e., more frequent than one session per week) and recommend further research being conducted.

A controlled pilot study, carried out in Germany by Haffner et al. (2006) randomly assigned nineteen children (twelve boys and seven girls) aged 8–11 with ADHD to practice either yoga or conventional motor exercise (well-known active games). The children who performed yoga improved significantly on test scores on attention tasks and had fewer ADHD symptoms following the intervention (as rated by their parents or caregivers) versus the control group. The authors concluded that yoga may be "an effective complementary or concomitant treatment for attention deficit hyperactivity disorder."

Along with these controlled studies there have also been a small number of noncontrolled studies published on the benefits of yoga-based interventions for children with a diagnosis of ADHD (Grosswald, Stixrud, Travis, & Bateh, 2008; Hariprasad, Arasappa, Varambally, Srinath, & Gangadhar, 2013; Harrison, Manocha, & Rubia, 2004; Lange et al., 2014; Mehta et al., 2011, 2012). These studies report beneficial effects of yoga on clinician/researcher-rated and parent-rated symptoms of ADHD, improved self-esteem, and relationships. Children also self-reported better quality of sleep, reduced anxiety, more ability to focus at school, and fewer relationship problems. One particular project studied the effects of a family yoga intervention (Harrison et al., 2004). Along with the beneficial effects of yoga on the child's ADHD symptoms, this study also showed significant improvements on parent-rated parental stress and an increased ability to handle their child's behavior. Despite their limitations, these studies provide evidence that yoga interventions for children and young people with ADHD are feasible in both clinical and educational settings, and that there have been no adverse effects reported.

These preliminary findings suggest that yoga can provide benefits for children and young people with a diagnosis of ADHD. However, there is a lack of research that specifically investigates the potential mechanisms. Therefore, the following section examines some of the findings from other fields of research which relate to ADHD and its potential effects, and that may be applied to yoga.

Research from other fields related to ADHD

The physical and psychological benefits of structured physical exercise for those with ADHD have been highlighted in the literature (Cerillo-Urbina et al., 2015; Den Heijer et al., 2017; Grassman, Alves, Santos-Galduroz, & Galduroz, 2014). A recent systematic review concluded that physical exercise might be a potential treatment option for children with ADHD and that acute physical exercise has potential benefits above and beyond psychostimulant medication (Halperin, Berwid, & O'Neill, 2014). Cardiovascular exercise has been shown to increase catecholamines and proteins/enzymes that are typically downregulated in ADHD (e.g., dopamine). Complex sensory motor sequences have also been shown to increase connectivity between the two hemispheres of the brain and support the engagement of the PFC and sensory motor areas (including the cerebellum, basal ganglia, and thalamus). The positive effects of exercise on executive functioning skills, attentional networks, and the dorsolateral PFC have also been documented (Chang et al., 2012; Grassman et al., 2014; Smith et al., 2010). These parts of the brain are affected in children and adults with ADHD.

Yoga movement is a form of physical exercise and often involves complex sensory motor sequences, balance, and limited aerobic activity. Yoga asana may therefore bring some of the exercise benefits described earlier. However, yoga is more than just physical exercise. Yoga promotes physical movement along with mental focus, concentration, and mindfulness. Yoga practice involves bringing focused awareness to the body and the breath and developing a deeper awareness of self and our connection to others. Being able to focus the mind on balance and coordination of complex movements, as well as synchronizing movement and breath, requires full concentration and may also enhance attentional networks. Providing a combination of physical movement with attentional training (mindfulness) may provide greater benefits for people with ADHD (Best, 2010; Clark, Schumann, & Mostofsky, 2015).

There is a growing body of literature on the benefits of mindfulness-based interventions for young people and adults living with ADHD (Cairncross & Miller, 2016; Evans et al., 2017; Mitchell, Zylowska, & Kollins, 2015; Zylowska, 2012). In terms of the mechanisms of mindfulness, it has been suggested that meditation and mindfulness could be thought of as a type of attentional or working memory training for children and adults with ADHD (Mrazek, Franklin, Phillips, Baird, & Schooler, 2013). This is supported by past studies of mindfulness and meditation which show that engaging in meditation can activate the ACC and the PFC (Cahn & Polich, 2006; Hölzel et al., 2007), areas of the brain associated with attention and emotion regulation. Studies of short-term and long-term meditators have also found increased connectivity in the brain and a thickening of the corpus callosum, both areas that are affected in ADHD (Luders et al., 2012; Luders et al., 2011; Moyer et al., 2011). In addition, meditation has been found to reduce the activity of the DMN, suggesting that meditation and mindfulness practice may help to support individuals with ADHD to improve sustained attention and focus (Brewer et al., 2011; Garrison et al., 2015).

> There is a growing body of literature on the benefits of mindfulness-based interventions for young people and adults living with ADHD.

A recent meta-analysis concluded that mindfulness-based therapies have been shown to significantly improve attentional capacity (particularly in adults) and hyperactivity/impulsivity (across all ages) in individuals diagnosed with ADHD (Cairncross & Miller, 2016). As yoga practice (including asana, meditation, and yoga nidra) encourages and develops mindfulness of body, breath, emotions, and mental processes, it could be argued that these studies support the use of yoga for ADHD, with yoga offering the enhanced benefit of combining both mindfulness and physical movement (Best, 2010; Clark et al., 2015).

There has also been research investigating the effects of specific yoga practices, which may have implications for ADHD. For instance, research suggests multiple physiological effects of pranayama, including activation of the PFC, increased oxygen supply, and increased parasympathetic drive (Ankad, Herur, Patil, Shashikala, & Chinagudi, 2011; Brown, Gerbarg, & Meunch, 2013; Nivethitha, Mooventhan, & Manjunath, 2016; Sharma et al., 2014; Streeter et al.,

2017). These findings may describe discrete mechanisms that may explain why yoga can be beneficial to ADHD where hypoactivation of the PFC, executive functioning difficulties, and emotional dysregulation (co-occurring with low levels of parasympathetic activity) are prevalent (Bunford, Evans, & Wymbs, 2015).

Although there is no specific research on the effects of pranayama on ADHD symptoms, a few studies may be of relevance to those living with ADHD. In particular, one study looked at the cognitive benefits of *bhramari* (humming bee breath) in healthy male students. *Bhramari* was associated with an improvement in response inhibition when compared to slow breathing, and the authors speculate that *bhramari* may therefore be particularly supportive for individuals affected by ADHD who find it difficult to inhibit their emotional and behavioral responses (Rajesh, Ilavarasu, & Srinivasan, 2014). *Nadi shodhana*, or alternate-nostril breathing (ANB), may also be particularly beneficial in bringing calm and balance to those with ADHD. This practice has been shown to activate both hemispheres of the brain and to increase brain symmetry and connectivity, which is particularly important for ADHD, where brain scans show a reduced volume of the corpus callosum (Curatolo et al., 2010; Emond et al., 2009). Studies have also shown improvements in cognitive functions such as attentiveness and working memory performance with ANB (Garg, Malhotra, Tripathi, & Agarwal, 2016; Telles, Raghuraj, Maharana, & Nagendra, 2007). It may therefore be inferred that ANB would be supportive for those with ADHD.

Children and adults with ADHD report significant benefits from the practice of yoga nidra (translated as "yogic sleep," a practice to promote relaxation and self-inquiry), including a deep sense of rest and rejuvenation. Sleep issues can be a major factor for individuals living with ADHD. Yoga nidra has been shown to positively affect sleep quality in adults with self-reported sleep difficulties (Gutman et al., 2017).

To date there has been no scientific research on the effects of yoga nidra on people with ADHD, and so it is unclear what the benefits or specific neurological mechanisms might be. One study found that yoga nidra increased levels of dopamine in the brains of healthy individuals (Kjaer et al., 2002). So because people affected by ADHD tend to have low levels of dopamine, this may be one of the mechanisms by which yoga nidra could be of benefit. However, further research needs to be carried out in this area.

Rationale for yoga in ADHD treatment

The process of long and arduous assessment, being prescribed medication to change behavior, and the use of diagnostic labels that often identify an individual with their mental health condition (such as "he is ADHD") can seriously impact the social and emotional health of a child or adult. Individuals may develop a deeply held narrative about themselves as disordered, bad, or different, and these beliefs can be detrimental to a person's wellbeing, self-esteem, and confidence. Therefore, changing the relationship a person has to themselves and their behavior can have a dramatic impact, and yoga may support this process. Through yoga philosophy and practice people are encouraged to welcome and accept who they are; their feelings, thoughts, behaviors, and situations. In Yoga Sutra 11.6 (*ekatmata iva asmita*), Patanjali states that false identification can happen easily when we mistake the body, mind, or senses for the true self, and that this leads to suffering. Through yoga and meditation practice, people are encouraged to access the seer (*cit* or *purusa*), the aspect of themselves that is healthy and knowing. The more that people with a diagnosis of ADHD can connect to their true self, the less they may suffer.

Given the potential physical, cognitive, psychological, and functional benefits described earlier, yoga may offer a low-risk complementary treatment option for those living with ADHD. For young people or adults who cannot tolerate—or do not want—medication, yoga may be a viable alternative treatment option (Chou & Huang, 2017). It may be offered flexibly as a group-based intervention, or specific practices may be integrated into one-to-one, family, or group-based therapeutic work (Weintraub, 2012). Yoga can empower an individual to look within for their own healing and provide them with tools to develop self-awareness and self-management of their ADHD symptoms. Collectively, these findings provide a growing evidence base and rationale for anecdotal evidence of yoga's efficacy for people with ADHD.

Considerations when working with people with ADHD

The guidance provided in this section offers general considerations and yoga practices for those living with ADHD. However, every person with a diagnosis of ADHD is unique and will potentially have very different struggles and strengths. If possible, a yoga teacher/therapist should make a thorough assessment of each individual's needs and their personal goals for the yoga sessions. For example, it will be important to take into account if an individual is currently taking medication, if they experience any side effects, and if they find the medication supports them in managing their symptoms. The yoga can then be tailored to specific symptoms or issues (e.g., sleep).

> Every person with a diagnosis of ADHD is unique and will potentially have very different struggles and strengths.

Yoga for ADHD has many components. The practices themselves are helpful, along with the environment provided, and the sensitivity that is offered. The following considerations and yoga practices can be applied to yoga groups/classes or one-to-one yoga therapy sessions. Mental health practitioners with a strong personal yoga practice may wish to integrate yoga into their current therapeutic work. Many of the practices detailed do not require a yoga mat or any special equipment and can be easily woven into individual or group-based therapeutic programs for ADHD.

Environment

Before doing anything else, creating a safe and appropriate space for people with ADHD is essential.

People with a diagnosis of ADHD can be particularly sensitive to visual and auditory stimuli and can become easily distracted and overwhelmed. Therefore, an environment low on stimulation—for example, uplighters rather than overhead lights, clear wall space, and neutral colors—can help to promote calm and focus. In general, it is recommended that props are kept to a minimum. Props can easily become a source of distraction for those with ADHD (particularly children), and can increase excitability and hyperactivity (e.g., props may be thrown around the room). Despite this, certain weighted props like eye pillows, sandbags, and heavy blankets can be very grounding and promote relaxation, and they therefore have a place in class. A few published studies have shown the benefits of deep touch pressure via weighted blankets or weighted vests for children with ADHD (Hvolby & Bilenberg, 2010; Lin, Lee, Chang, & Hong, 2014; Vandenberg, 2001). Eye pillows may support people with ADHD to tune out visual stimuli and come to a resting posture more easily. Bo Forbes (2016) states that weighted eye pillows produce a light pressure on the eyeballs that can lower the heart rate by activating the oculocardiac reflex, a physiological mechanism that reduces the pulse rate in relationship to pressure on the eyeballs, or extraocular pressure.

Routine and ritual versus novelty

Routine, rhythm, and structure are particularly important for those living with ADHD. In general, those with ADHD report that their minds are muddled and that they can find it hard to organize their thoughts and feelings. It is therefore helpful if their environment provides them with some organization, predictability, and structure. Repetition and consistency can also support people to internalize a self-practice. Ritual and repetition is supportive and can build a sense of security and calm (Weintraub, 2012). For example, beginning the session with a particular chant/breathing practice each week, then moving into some asana followed by a yoga nidra practice, and then pranayama and meditation to close.

However, it is equally important for those with ADHD symptoms to maintain their interest and motivation. As previously mentioned, those with attentional difficulties may struggle to focus if they do not have sufficient interest in an activity. Therefore, ritual and routine need to be carefully balanced with novelty and variation throughout the yoga sequence to inspire curiosity and hold their attention.

Sensitivity, nonjudgment, and compassion

Young people and adults with ADHD can experience low self-esteem due to their difficulties and thus be particularly sensitive to criticism. They may believe that they cannot focus or that they cannot relax. It is therefore important to show sensitivity relating to this and to provide messages of acceptance and kindness, such as "It is OK for the mind to wander." People with ADHD are often reprimanded for making mistakes or for being careless and inaccurate. If they experience this with yoga then they will be less likely to engage and experience its benefits. It is important for a yoga teacher/therapist to be aware of this. Rather than focusing on individuals, it may be helpful to address the whole class/group and to adopt a calm voice to gently bring people back to their own experiences; for example, "Just notice any urge to move off the mat."

Being prepared to be responsive and flexible to the needs of your clients or group is vital; for instance,

sitting practices can be extremely hard and on occasion distressing for people with ADHD; keeping practices and sessions short and building them up gradually can offset this distress.

Calm and focus

If students arrive with high energy and are finding it difficult to concentrate, it may be helpful to meet them where they are by matching that energy and then guiding them to a more stable and focused state; for example, introducing a practice such as lively 'Hari Om' chanting and tapping/clapping, or a more vigorous sun salutation sequence, and then moving into more calming, grounding postures. If a group becomes excitable or chatty, sounding a bell (chimes or a singing bowl) or singing a chant can cue people to calm and focus and signal a transition. In particular, the use of a call and response chant or rhythm can capture attention and reengage people and bring them back into the group.

Overstimulation

It is usually best to avoid overstimulating practices such as *kapalabhati*. Novel, fun, and playful approaches may need to be balanced with calming and grounding practices if students become overstimulated and hyperactive.

Group agreements

To help promote safety if working in a group or class format, it may be useful to introduce some group agreements around the qualities and behaviors that the group would like to foster. This can be particularly important for children and teenagers with ADHD, who often need firm external boundaries and clear ground rules to support them in developing self-regulation. These agreements can be discussed together, everyone can contribute, and they can be displayed and reviewed regularly. For example, "Respecting and listening to each other," "Looking after ourselves and one another," and "Keeping ourselves and others safe" are possible agreements. Younger students, particularly those with difficulties related to hyperactivity and impulsivity, may find it difficult to take turns and/or listen to each other in a group setting. The use of a talking piece (Zimmerman & Coyle, 2009) can help to encourage awareness of communication, and support the development of respectful listening, self-regulation, turn taking, and inhibition of responses (e.g., calling out or talking over each other).

> Younger students, particularly those with difficulties related to hyperactivity and impulsivity, may find it difficult to take turns and/or listen to each other in a group setting.

Self-awareness and self-regulation

Yoga provides multiple opportunities for developing self-regulation for people with ADHD. Throughout a yoga session students are invited to move in a deliberate or purposeful fashion. There is often a sequence that is followed in which students are continually asked to focus and maintain their attention (e.g., through focusing on the breath or the sensations in their bodies). This can be enhanced by the many transitions between postures during which the yoga teacher/therapist may have to shift attention and then refocus. With gentle prompting, a student can learn to recognize how restlessness feels, the urge or compulsion to move, and to note impulses but not have to act on each one as it arises. They can then begin to conquer restlessness, seeing it purely as a mental event that they do not have to identify with or act upon. Rather than fighting with this or becoming self-critical, students can be invited to recognize the restlessness and see it as a messenger. By turning toward this experience with kindness, the awareness becomes stronger and the attention span longer. Students can be encouraged to notice how urges may arise (e.g., to roll across each other's yoga mats, singing out loud during relaxation) and how to inhibit these responses and stay on task.

Working on this capacity to self-regulate can be balanced with the development of social skills and awareness of others. This may be encouraged through awareness of social interactions outside the yoga session or can be developed within a group-based yoga class. For example, yoga within a group setting may involve turn taking, listening, and showing sensitivity to others. The yoga teacher/therapist can model attentive, nonjudgmental presence and curiosity about their own experiences and those of others. When offered in this way, yoga can support young people and adults with ADHD to learn how to take care of themselves and others.

Psychoeducation

In order to facilitate self-awareness, to normalize experience, and to encourage self-acceptance, it can be useful to bring in some psychoeducation on ADHD into yoga sessions. This can be particularly powerful when conducted in a group setting, but can also be useful within one-to-one therapy. The psychoeducation component might cover areas such as the diagnostic criteria, considering ADHD from a multidimensional perspective, and the personal impact and individual experiences of ADHD. People can be invited to consider the potential that ADHD offers them, as well as to consider some of the challenges they recognize. Throughout the subsequent yoga sessions the teacher/therapist might mention typical ADHD patterns to increase students' self-awareness and their ability to identify such patterns. It is essential to encourage students with loving kindness and compassion because of how much self-criticism and self-judgment people with ADHD often place on themselves. Yoga professionals are encouraged to offer examples to normalize people's experiences and thus enable them to realize their potential by seeing how others have used yoga to facilitate this. It is helpful to make apparent for students the role of environment and circumstances, because this is often where the greatest level of change occurs, and so it helps the individual not to place all of the challenges within themselves.

It is essential to encourage students with loving kindness and compassion because of how much self-criticism and self-judgment people with ADHD often place on themselves.

Working with families

When working with children and young people, involving their parents, caregivers, and other family members can be beneficial. Van der Oord, Bögels, and Peijnenburg (2012), in their work on mindfulness-based interventions for ADHD, recommend offering separate classes specifically for parents and carers running alongside the young people's groups. Providing parallel yoga classes/groups for parent and carers gives them an opportunity to connect with other parents and carers in a supportive and nonjudgmental environment. Not only can yoga provide parents and carers with deep rest, greater self-awareness, and self-compassion, it can also enhance their connections with their children and can potentially lead to improvements in their children's behavior. Often, if parents and carers are engaging in yoga practice, then this will enhance the children's experience of yoga and support them in developing and sustaining a home practice.

Specific yoga practices for ADHD

Specific yoga practices for ADHD include asana, pranayama, singing and chanting, mudra, yoga nidra, and meditation and mindfulness (see Table 4.1).

Asana

When teaching asana, it can be helpful for people with ADHD to focus on grounding and calming postures. Keeping low to the ground (on all fours) and/or referring to feeling the physical body in connection with the mat/earth over the course of the session can help to build a sense of stability and connectedness. Working slowly, with fewer asana and with a continual

invitation to direct awareness back to the body and breath, can also be helpful for when the mind wanders. Encouraging mindfulness of body sensation during asana practice also helps to provide focus for an overactive mind. Developing the ability to notice when the mind has wandered off and then gently guiding it back without criticism or judgment is an important skill to encourage in this population.

Standing postures

Standing postures can help with developing strength and focus to the scattered and disconnected energy that those with ADHD can experience. Metaphors can be used to support feelings of strength and stability. For example, in *tadasana* (mountain pose), evoking the sense of a mountain, "imagining that the feet are the base of the mountain, with its huge base deeply rooted to the Earth, feeling this stability as you engage with the peak of the mountain—the crown of the head—as it lifts up into the clouds," or, in warrior pose, noticing feelings of strength and stability and/or qualities of the warrior (such as courage) in the body.

Balancing postures

Balancing postures, often used to cultivate concentration, are very effective. Poses such as *vrksasana* (tree) can help students to slow down, find their feet, and center themselves. It may be useful to provide a visual image of the roots of the tree moving down through the earth/feet while breathing out. Finding a *drishti* point (a gazing direction for the eyes to focus attention) for concentration can also support balance and stability. This can be tremendously powerful for people with ADHD who do not believe they have the capacity for stillness.

Forward bends

Forward bends such as child's pose, seated forward bends, and standing forward bends, are believed to have a calming effect on the nervous system; this

Table 4.1

Specific yoga practices for ADHD

Yoga practice	Examples	Potential benefits for ADHD
Asana: Focus on grounding and calming practices Bring mindful awareness to breath and body	Standing postures: Mountain Warrior I Warrior II	Develop strength and focus
	Balancing postures: Tree pose	Promote concentration and balance
	Forward bends: Child's pose Seated forward bend Standing forward bend	Calming and grounding
	Sun salutations Dynamic yoga flow	Support neural networks involved in motor planning, memory, and attention
Pranayama	Education on proper breathing (e.g., three-part breathing)	Develops self-awareness of breathing and how the breath connects to one's mental and emotional state
	Ujjayi (ocean-sounding breath)	Calming breath, promotes mental focus
	Coherent breathing	Supports regulation of the nervous system
	Bhramari (humming bee breath)	Uplifting, promotes calm and mental focus
	Nadi shodhana (alternate-nostril breathing)	Emotional and mental balance and concentration
Sound, chanting, singing	Call-and-response mantra/chanting	Uplifting and calming, promotes connection to self and others
Mudra		Supports intention, concentration, and focus
Yoga nidra		Promotes self-connection, deep rest, and repair
Meditation and mindfulness	Walking meditation	Builds self-awareness, focused attention, and concentration
	Moving body scan	Increases body awareness and self-compassion
	Progressive muscle relaxation	Promotes body awareness and relaxation

effect can be seen when working with individuals with ADHD, and hence it is recommended such poses are included in a yoga sequence, and that they are integrated once a degree of calm is present.

Sun salutations and dynamic yoga flow

If attention is scattered and more dynamic energy is needed to capture attention (as is often the case, especially at the beginning of sessions), sun salutations and dynamic yoga flow sequences are very helpful. Furthermore, series of interlinked movements can support neural networks involved in motor planning, memory and attention, all of which may be otherwise compromised. For some people with ADHD it may be useful to begin with flowing sequences and then move on to more calming and grounding practices. Ultimately, it is most useful to meet a young person, an adult, or a group where they are at any given moment, and offer a balanced asana practice.

Pranayama

Education on proper breathing

The breath is one of the quickest and most reliable indicators of current state. Many people with ADHD have adopted a dysregulated pattern of breathing, such as holding their breath or chest breathing. These breathing patterns can take people away from connecting to themselves and focusing their attention. Therefore, simply supporting children and adults with ADHD to become aware of their breathing, and begin to notice its influence on emotional states, can help them regulate and alter their behavior. Some psychoeducation about proper breathing (three-part breath/belly breathing) is advised. For example, it can be helpful to provide information on how the breath can send and alter messages to the brain, thereby enhancing a desire to practice.

People with ADHD may struggle with sitting still and focusing for long periods and can become restless and agitated. Instead, they may prefer to engage in breathing practices while walking, or moving in asana (at least at the beginning). They may also find it beneficial to count the breath rate silently in their minds (e.g., breathing in for three counts then breathing out for six). This will help to anchor them to the present moment and support them to focus and build concentration. They may also say a simple word or phrase in their mind, to help keep their attention on the breath (e.g., "breathing in, I am aware of breathing in; breathing out, I am aware of breathing out").

The following pranayama practices are recommended for people with ADHD.

Ujjayi (ocean-sounding breath)

Ujjayi is a form of resistance breathing that uses a light contraction of the upper throat muscles. It can be practiced throughout asana and helps to capture attention. The energy needed and the noise created by this breath are particularly helpful in promoting focus.

Coherent breathing

Coherent breathing is a very simple practice that can be used effectively with people of all ages and abilities. This practice, named and described by Stephan Elliott (2005), supports the synchronization (or coherence) between activity of the heart, lungs, and brain. Coherent breathing creates an equal inhale and exhale, gently and slowly for a specific period of time. For adults, the average ideal breath is between 5 and 6 bpm. For children 5–10 years of age, Brown and Gerbarg (2012) recommend 10 bpm. Coherent breathing is often practiced using an audio track that signals a bell at regular intervals at the desired breath rate. The sounding of the bell can be particularly helpful for refocusing the wandering mind.

Bhramari (humming bee breath)

Bhramari is a wonderfully uplifting breath practice since it can be playful, and yet it also requires focus. Humming supports the elongation of the exhalation, thus providing a calming regulatory effect for those with ADHD. Additionally, the blocking out of visual and auditory stimuli, while focusing on the humming sound, can be particularly calming to people with ADHD, who are often struggling to tune out various visual and auditory stimuli.

Nadi shodhana (alternate-nostril breathing)

Alternate-nostril breathing (ANB) may be particularly supportive for people with ADHD. This practice is believed to balance the flow of energy in the *nadis* (described in the literature as energy channels): *ida* (left-sided, passive, feminine) and *pingala* (right-sided, active, male). Alternating the breath between the two sides helps to support emotional and mental balance and harmony. ANB involves coordinating left and right hand movements, while also attending to the breath going in and out. This breath is therefore particularly useful for those with ADHD because it requires full concentration and sustained focus. For younger children this practice can be simplified by using the index fingers of both hands to block each nostril in turn. This can also be done without the use of a mudra by directing the attention to each nostril in turn to increase mental challenge and stimulation.

Singing and chanting

A less direct but very effective way to work with the breath is through the use of sound such as singing and chanting. For those with additional anxiety, being asked to focus specifically on the breath can increase the sense of threat and therefore exacerbate anxiety. Chanting helps to regulate the breath, ensuring deep breathing with longer exhalations. Chanting and singing are fun and engaging and therefore hold attention more easily. They provide the opportunity for expression using soothing, repetitive, methodical patterns, and repetitions, which can support mood and concentration and have a calming and healing effect. Singing has been shown to engage certain brain regions such as the sensorimotor cortex, areas of the PFC, basal ganglia, thalamus, and cerebellum (Loui, 2015). With particular relevance to ADHD, the cognitive benefits of singing may include better verbal working memory, improved information processing and implicit motor control, and goal-directed attention (Kleber, Veit, Birbaumer, Gruzelier, & Lotze, 2010).

Working with different sounds or seed mantras located in different parts of the body is playful, engaging, and helps to bring attention to the body promoting self-regulation. One such chant is Hari Om, in which "ha" vibrates in the abdomen, "ri" in the throat, and "OM" in the crown of the head. A nice way to do this is through call and response, adding hand movements such as tapping the tops of the thighs when singing hari and clapping the hands during OM. This practice requires full concentration as the thigh taps and claps alter. From a neurological perspective, singing while also coordinating complex motor movements such as tapping repetitively engages many areas of the brain that are implicated in ADHD, the PFC, cerebellum and brain stem areas, as well as the frontal, parietal, and temporal lobes (Mavridis & Pyrgelis, 2016). This is a fun way to build the ability to manage sequential tasks, and also to inhibit responses (e.g., turn taking, controlling speed and volume of the voice) even when excited.

Mudra

There are at least 25 major mudras in hatha yoga and many of these can be very helpful for ADHD (Hirschi, 2016). Many people with ADHD will fidget, tap hands, and squirm in their seats. These practices help to focus attention and ground the person in the present moment more easily. Students can be advised to take this learning off the mat, as these mudras can also be done with hands in pockets to prepare for entering a meeting at work or classes at school.

Yoga nidra

Many people with ADHD and their parents and carers feel concerned that people with a diagnosis of ADHD will not be able to lie still or focus enough to meditate and relax. However, guided relaxation and yoga nidra are often cited as the most profound part of a person's yoga session, providing them with an experience of deep rest and stillness through a protocol that engages attention with minimal effort. Participation in a gentle asana practice or sequence (such as *pawan-muktasana*, a slow, steady, joint-freeing series) can be supportive in preparing the body and mind for yoga nidra. Students are allowed to lie down in whatever position works for them (for example, some prefer lying face down or resting in child's pose). Students may also choose eye pillows, sandbags, and heavy blankets, all of which reduce visual distractions and provide a feeling of containment and grounding for some people with ADHD. It is essential that people are given permission to be just as they are. A powerful part of the practice can be the use of affirmations (*sankalpas*) such as "My mind is unwavering and serene." Through all of these practices, students are encouraged to hold a sense of no expectation and observe things the way they are without trying to change them. Paradoxically, change often happens as a consequence.

Meditation and mindfulness

As mentioned in the research section, meditation and mindfulness practice may be particularly beneficial for children and adults with ADHD. However, they will typically find it easier to start with mindfulness of movement (e.g., yoga asana or walking meditation) before engaging in a short sitting meditation. For those who find it difficult to connect to themselves and lack body awareness, practicing a progressive muscle relaxation (tensing and releasing parts of the body in turn) or a moving body scan (gently moving the part of the body being focused on) will be more tolerable than a full, still body scan or a silent *savasana*. The formal meditation and mindfulness practices are often shorter and briefer than in those classes offered to the general population.

Future directions

There is currently very limited access to mind-body therapies within mainstream healthcare for those with a diagnosis of ADHD. Yoga and mindfulness-based interventions may be available in the community, but they aren't regularly recommended or prescribed by medical professionals. The diagnostic rates of ADHD are increasing (Centers for Disease Control and Prevention, 2010), and as healthcare services are squeezed there is greater need for tools and therapies that can support a person with the challenges they face on a daily basis. Some parents of children with ADHD, and adults with ADHD, are wary of reliance on medication and of adverse side effects in particular. As an alternative, they are looking for tools and techniques over which they themselves exert some control.

There is increasing awareness of the benefits of yoga and mindfulness as complementary treatments for ADHD alongside regular medication and psychosocial interventions. Although in its infancy, the evidence base for yoga in supporting those with ADHD is growing. However, there is an urgent need for more robust longitudinal research on the benefits of yoga and meditation for ADHD, assessing the validity and effectiveness of specific practices, and the application of those practices to different age groups across the lifespan. There is a huge opportunity for collaboration between academic, mental health, and yoga communities to better understand how yoga can support this population. The lack of studies looking at the effects of yoga and meditation on the neurophysiology of children and adults with ADHD represents a major gap in current research. Further research into the specific mechanisms of change will support the evidence base for the use of yoga and mindfulness in the treatment of people with ADHD.

There is increasing awareness of the benefits of yoga and mindfulness as complementary treatments for ADHD alongside regular medication and psychosocial interventions.

As well as in mental healthcare, there is a growing interest in yoga and mindfulness in schools and across the education system (Khalsa & Butzer, 2016). Young people with ADHD who are accessing education may be exposed to yoga at an earlier age. These school-based interventions may be extremely supportive, and offer them tools and techniques, which could change their long-term health and education outcomes. Research that evaluates the impact of these school-based yoga interventions may also contribute to the growing body of evidence showing the benefits of yoga for those with ADHD.

Inviting a child or adult who is hyperactive and has attention differences to engage in something slow, peaceful and meditative may at first appear counter-intuitive. However, engaging in relaxing and calming activities can often bring them the much needed rest and repair that they so desperately need. Yoga is a holistic intervention that can support a person with ADHD on a physical, mental, emotional, and spiritual level. It is a low-cost intervention, it connects people to community support, and, unlike mainstream medication therapy, generally has no negative side effects. Finding a *sangha* (community) to practice with can help an individual to remain motivated to practice, decrease social isolation, and increase feelings of wellbeing. Yoga enables people to reveal their true nature and true potential. It supports a coming home, a remembering of the inner peace and the resources they already have within themselves. They are tools for living, for being, and for empowering people to be just who they are.

References

American Academy of Pediatrics: Subcommittee on Attention-Deficit/Hyperactivity Disorder., Steering Committee on Quality Improvement and Management. (2011). ADHD: Clinical Practice Guideline for the Diagnosis, Evaluation, and Treatment of Attention-Deficit/Hyperactivity Disorder in Children and Adolescents. *Pediatrics, 128*(5), 1007–1022. http://doi.org/10.1542/peds.2011-2654

American Psychiatric Association (2013). *Diagnostic and Statistical Manual of Mental Disorders, Fifth Edition*. Arlington, VA: American Psychiatric Publishing.

Ankad, R. B., Herur, A., Patil, S., Shashikala, G. V., & Chinagudi, S. (2011). Effect of short-term pranayama and meditation on cardiovascular functions in healthy individuals. *Heart Views: The Official Journal of the Gulf Heart Association, 12*(2), 58–62. doi:10.4103/1995-705X.86016.

Barkley, R., Murphy, K. R., & Fischer, M. (2007). *ADHD in Adults: What the Science Says.* New York, NY: Guilford Press.

Baughman, F. (2006). *The ADHD Fraud: How Psychiatry Makes Patients of Normal Children.* Trafford Publishing, Victoria: Canada.

Best, J.R. (2010). Effects of physical activity on children's executive function: Contributions of experimental research on aerobic exercise, *Developmental Review, 30*(4), 331–351.

Biederman, J., Milberger, S., Faraone, S. V., Kiely, K., Guite, J., Mick, E., Ablon, S., Warburton, R., & Reed, E. (1995). Family-environment risk factors for attention-deficit hyperactivity disorder: A test of Rutter's indicators of adversity. *Archives of General Psychiatry, 52*, 464–470.

Botting, N., Powls, A., Cooke, R. W., & Marlow, N. (1997). Attention deficit hyperactivity disorders and other psychiatric outcomes in very low birthweight children at 12 years. *Journal of Child Psychology and Psychiatry, 38*, 931–941.

Brewer, J. A., Worhunsky, P. D., Gray, J. R., Tang, Y. Y., Weber, J., & Kober, H. (2011). Meditation experience is associated with differences in default mode network activity and connectivity. *Proceedings of the National Academy of Sciences, 108*(50), 20254–20259. doi:10.1073/pnas.1112029108.

Brown, R. P., & Gerbarg, P.L. (2012). *The Healing Power of the Breath: Simple techniques to reduce stress and anxiety, enhance concentration and balance your emotions.* Boston, MA: Shambhala Publications.

Brown, R. P., Gerbarg, P. L., & Muench, F. (2013). Breathing practices for treatment of psychiatric and stress-related medical conditions. *Psychiatric Clinics of North America, 36*, 121–140.

Bunford, N., Evans, S., W., & Wymbs, F. (2015). ADHD and emotion dysregulation among children and adolescents, *Clinical Child & Family Psychology Review, 18*, 185–217.

Bymaster, F. P., Katner, J. S., Nelson, D. L., Hemrick-Luecke, S. K., Threlkeld, P. G., Heiligenstein, J. H., Morin, S. M., Gehlert, D. R., & Perry, K. W. (2002). Atomoxetine increases extracellular levels of norepinephrine and dopamine in prefrontal cortex of rat: A potential mechanism for efficacy in attention deficit / hyperactivity disorder. *Neuropsychopharmacology, 27*, 699–711.

Cahn, B.R., & Polich, J. (2006). Meditation states and traits: EEG, ERP, and neuroimaging studies. *Psychological Bulletin, 132*, 180–211.

Cairncross, M. & Miller, C. J. (2016). The effectiveness of mindfulness-based therapies for ADHD: A meta-analytic review. *Journal of Attention Disorders,* doi: 10.1177/1087054715625301

Castellanos, F. X., & Proal, E. (2012). Large-scale brain systems in ADHD: Beyond the prefrontal–striatal model. *Trends in Cognitive Sciences, 16*, 17–26.

Centers for Disease Control and Prevention (2010). Increasing prevalence of parent-reported attention deficit/hyperactivity disorder among children: United States, 2003–2007. *Morbidity and Mortality Weekly Report, 59*(44), 1439–1443.

Cerillo-Urbina, A. J., Garcia-Hermoso, A., Sanchez-Lopez, M., Pardo-Guijarro, M. J., Santos Gomez, J. L., & Martinez-Vizcaino, V. (2015). The effects of physical exercise in children with attention–deficit/hyperactivity disorder: A systematic review and meta-analysis of randomized control trials. *Child: Care, Health and Development*, 41(6), 779–788.

Chang, Y. K., Labban, J. D., Gapin, J. I., & Etnier, J. L. (2012) The effects of acute exercise on cognitive performance: A meta-analysis. *Brain Research*, 1453: 87–101.

Chou, C. C., & Huang, C. J. (2017). Effects of an 8-week yoga program on sustained attention and discrimination function in children with attention deficit hyperactivity disorder. *PeerJ*, 5, e2883; doi:10.7717/peerj.2883.

Clark, D., Schumann, F., & Mostofsky, S.H. (2015). Mindful movement and skilled attention. *Frontiers in Human Neuroscience*, 29(9), 297. doi:10.3389/fnhum.2015.00297.

Conners, C. K. (1997). *Conners' Rating Scales–Revised*. Toronto, Canada: Multi-Health Systems.

Cortese, S., & Castellanos, F. X. (2012). Neuroimaging of attention-deficit/hyperactivity disorder: Current neuroscience-informed perspectives for clinicians. *Current Psychiatry Reports*, 14, 5.

doi:10.1007/s11920-012-0310-y.

Curatolo, P., D'Agati, E., & Moavero, R. P. (2010). The neurological basis of ADHD. *Italian Journal of Pediatrics*, 36, 79.

Den Heijer, A. E., Groen, Y., Tucha, L., Fuermaier, A. B. M., Koerts, J., Lange, K. W., Thome, J., & Tucha, O. (2017). Sweat it out? The effects of physical exercise on cognition and behavior in children and adults with ADHD: A systematic literature review. *Journal of Neural Transmission*, 124 (Suppl 1), S3–S26. doi:10.1007/s00702-016-1593-7.

Easton, N., Steward, C., Marshall, F., Fone, K., & Marsden, C. (2007). Effects of amphetamine isomers, methylphenidate and atomoxetine on synaptosomal and synaptic vesicle accumulation and release of dopamine and noradrenaline in vitro in the rat brain. *Neuropharmacology, 52*, 405–414.

Elliott, S. (2005). *The new science of breath: Coherent breathing for autonomic nervous system balance, health and wellbeing*. Texas: Coherent Press.

Ellison-Wright, I., Ellison-Wright, Z., & Bullmore, E. (2008). Structural brain change in Attention Deficit Hyperactivity Disorder identified by meta-analysis. *BMC Psychiatry*, 30(8), 51. doi:10.1186/1471-244X-8-51.

Emond, V., Joyal, C., & Poissant, H. (2009). Structural and functional neuroanatomy of attention-deficit hyperactivity disorder (ADHD). *Encephale*, 35(2), 107–14. doi:10.1016/j.encep.2008.01.005.

Evans, S., Ling, M., Hill, B., Rinehart, N., Austin, D., & Sciberras, E. (2017). Systematic review of meditation-based interventions for children with ADHD. *European Child & Adolescent Psychiatry*, online publication, doi:10.1007/s00787-017-1008-9

Faraone, S. V., Sergeant, J., Gillberg, C., & Biederman, J. (2003). The worldwide prevalence of ADHD: is it an American condition? *World Psychiatry*, 2(2), 104–113.

Fayyad, J., De Graaf, R., Kessler, R., Alonso, J., Angermeyer, M., Demyttenaere, K., De Girolamo, G., Haro, J. M., Karam, E. G., Lara, C., Lépine, J. P., Ormel, J., Posada-Villa, J., Zaslavsky, A. M., & Jin, R. (2007). Cross-national prevalence and correlates of adult attention-deficit hyperactivity disorder. *British Journal of Psychiatry*, 190(5),402–409. doi:org/10.1192/bjp.bp.106.034389.

Forbes, B. (2016). Happiness Toolkit: Why an eye pillow is your stress Rx. Retrieved from: https://www.yogajournal.com/yoga-101/happiness-toolkit-eye-pillow-stress-rx

Garg, R., Malhotra, V., Tripathi, Y., & Agarwal, R. (2016). Effect of left, right, and alternate nostril breathing on verbal and spatial memory. *Journal of Clinical and Diagnostic Research*, 10(2), CC01–CC03.

Getahun, D., Rhoads, G. G., Dimissie, K., Lu, S., Quinn, V. P., Fassett, M. J., Wing, D. A., & Jacobsen, S. J. (2013). In utero exposure to ischemic-hypoxic conditions and attention-deficit/hyperactivity disorder. *pediatrics*, 131, e53–e61.

Garrison, K. A., Zeffiro, T. A., Scheinost, D., Constable, R. T., & Brewer, J. A. (2015). Meditation leads to reduced default mode network activity beyond an active task. *Cognitive Affective & Behavioural Neuroscience,* 15(3): 712–720. doi: 10.3758/s13415-015-0358-3

Gouldarins, J. B., Marques, J. C. B., & De Oliveira, J. A. (2017). Attention deficit hyperactivity disorder and motor impairment: A critical review. *Perceptual Motor Skills, 124*(2), 425–440. doi:org/10.1177/0031512517690607.

Grassmann, V., Alves, M. V., Santos-Galduroz, R. F., & Galduroz, J. C. (2014). Possible cognitive benefits of acute physical exercise in children with ADHD: A systematic review. *Journal of Attention Disorders*, 21(5), 367–371. doi:10.1177/1087054714526041.

Grosswald, S. J., Stixrud, W. R., Travis, F., & Bateh, M. A. (2008). Use of transcendental meditation technique to reduce symptoms of attention deficit-hyperactivity disorder (ADHD) by reducing stress and anxiety: An exploratory study. *Current Issues in Education*, 10, 1–16.

Gutman, S. A., Gregory, K. A., Sadlier-Brown, M. M., Schlissel, M. A., Schubert, A. M., Westover, L. A., & Miller, R. C. (2017). Comparative effectiveness of three occupational therapy sleep interventions: A randomized controlled study. *OTJR: Occupation, Participation & Health,* 37(1), 5–13.

Haffner, J., Roos, J., Goldstein, N., Parzer, P., & Resch, F. (2006). The effectiveness of body-oriented methods of therapy in the treatment of attention-deficit hyperactivity disorder (ADHD): Results of a controlled pilot study. *Zeitschrift Fur Kinder - Und Jugendpsychiatrie Und Psychotherapie*, 34, 37–47.

Halperin, J. M., Berwid, O. G., & O'Neill, S. O. (2014). Healthy body, healthy mind? The effectiveness of physical activity to treat ADHD in children. *Child & Adolescent Psychiatric Clinics*, 23(4), 899–936. doi:10.1016/j.chc.2014.05.005.

Hariprasad, V. R., Arasappa, R., Varambally, S., Srinath, S., & Gangadhar, B. N. (2013). Feasibility and efficacy of yoga as an add-on intervention in attention deficit-hyperactivity disorder: An exploratory study. *Indian Journal of Psychiatry*, 55, S379–S384.

Harrison, L., Manocha R., & Rubia, K. (2004). Sahaja Yoga Meditation as a family treatment programme for children with attention-deficit hyperactivity disorder. *Clinical Child Psychology and Psychiatry*, 9(4), 479–497.

Hartmann, T. (2003). *The Edison Gene: ADHD and the Gift of the Hunter Child*. Rochester, VT: Park Street Press.

Hirschi, G. (2016). *Mudras: yoga in your Hands*. Newburyport, MA: Weiser.

Hjern, A., Weitoft, G. R., & Lindblad, F. (2010). Social adversity predicts ADHD-medication in school children–a national cohort study. *Acta Paediatrica*, 99(6), 920–924. doi:10.1111/j.1651-227.2009.01638.x.

Hölzel, B. K., Ott, U., Hempel, H., Hackl, A., Wolf, K., Stark, R., & Vaitl, D. (2007). Differential engagement of anterior cingulate cortex and adjacent medial frontal cortex in adept meditators and nonmeditators. *Neuroscience Letters, 421*, 16–21.

Hoza, B. (2007). Peer functioning in children with ADHD. *Journal of Pediatric Psychology, 32*(6), 655–663.

Huntley, Z., & Young, S. (2012). Alcohol and substance use history among ADHD adults: The relationship with persistent and remitting symptoms, personality, employment and history of service use. *Journal of Attention Disorders, 18*(1), 82–90.

Hvolby, A. (2015). Associations of sleep disturbance with ADHD: Implications for treatment. *Attention Deficit Hyperactivity Disorder, 7*(1), 1–18.

Hvolby, A., & Bilenberg, N. (2010). Use of ball blanket in attention-deficit hyperactivity disorder sleeping problems. *Nordic Journal of Psychiatry, 65*, 89–94.

Jensen, P. S., & Kenny, D.T. (2004). The effects of yoga on the attention and behavior of boys with attention deficit/hyperactivity disorder. *Journal of Attention Disorders, 7*, 205–216.

Jensen, P. S., Shervette, R. E., Xenakis, S. N., & Richters, J. (1993). Anxiety and depressive disorders in attention deficit with hyperactivity: New findings. *American Journal of Psychiatry, 150*(8), 1203–1209.

Kessler, R. C, Adler, L., Barkley, R., Biederman, J., Conners, C. K., Demler, O., Faraone, S. V., Greenhill, L. L., Howes, M. J., Secnik, K., Spencer, T., Ustun, T. B., Walters, E. E., & Zaslavsky, A. M. (2006). The prevalence and correlates of adult ADHD in the United States: Results from the National Comorbidity Survey Replication. *American Journal of Psychiatry, 163*, 716–723.

Khalsa, S. B. S., & Butzer, B. (2016). Yoga in school settings: A research review. *Annals of the New York Academy of Sciences, 1373*, 45–55.

Kjaer, T. W., Bertelsen, C., Piccini, P., Brooks, D., Alving, J., & Lou, H. C. (2002). Increased dopamine tone during meditation-induced change of consciousness. *Brain Research. Cognitive Brain Research, 13*(2), 255–259.

Kleber, B., Veit, R., Birbaumer, N., Gruzelier, J., & Lotze, M. (2010). The brain of opera singers: Experience-dependent changes in functional activation. *Cerebral cortex, 5*(1), 1144–1152.

Kuo, F. E., & Faber Taylor, A. (2004). A potential natural treatment for attention-deficit/hyperactivity disorder: Evidence from a national study. *American Journal of Public Health, 94*(9), 1580–1586.

Lange, K. M., Makulska-Gertruda, E., Hauser, J., Reissmann, A., Kaunzinger, I., Tucha, L., Tucha, O., & Lange, K. W. (2014). Yoga and the therapy of children with attention deficit hyperactivity disorder. *Journal of Yoga and Physical Therapy, 4*, 168. doi:10.4172/2157-7595.1000168.

Lin, H. Y., Lee, P., Chang, W., & Hong, F. Y. (2014). Effects of weighted vests on attention, impulse control, and on-task behavior in children with attention deficit hyperactivity disorder. *American Journal of Occupational Therapy, 68*(2), 149–158. doi:10.5014/ajot.2014.009365.

Linnet, K. M., Dalsgaard, S., Obel, C., Wisborg, K., Henriksen, T. B., Rodriguez, A., Kotimaa, A., Moilanen, I., Thomsen, P. H., Olsen, J., & Jarvelin, M. R. (2003). Maternal lifestyle factors in pregnancy risk of attention deficit hyperactivity disorder and associated behaviors: Review of the current evidence. *American Journal of Psychiatry, 160*(6), 1028–1040.

Loui, P. (2015). A Dual-Stream Neuroanatomy of Singing. *Music Perception, 32*(3), 232–241. doi:10.1525/mp.2015.32.3.232.

Luders, E., Clark, K., Narr, K. L., & Toga, A. W. (2011). Enhanced brain connectivity in long-term meditation practitioners. *Neuroimage, 57*(4), 1308–1316.

Luders, E., Phillips, O. R., Clark, K., Kurth, F., Toga, A. W., & Narr, K. L. (2012). Bridging the hemispheres in meditation: Thicker callosal regions and enhanced fractional anisotropy (FA) in long-term practitioners. *Neuroimage, 61*(1), 181–187.

Mavridis, I. N., & Pyrgelis, E. S. (2016), Brain activation during singing: "Clef de Sol Activation" is the "concert" of the human brain. *Journal of Medical Problems in Performing Artists, 31*(1), 45–50.

McCann, D., Barrett, A., Cooper, A., Crumpler, D., Dalen, L., Grimshaw, K., Kitchin, E., Lok, K., Porteous, L., Prince, E., Songuga-Barke, E., OWarner, J., & Stevenson, J. (2007). Food additives and hyperactive behaviour in 3-year-old and 8/9-year-old children in the community: A randomised, double-blinded, placebo-controlled trial. *The Lancet, 370*(9598), 1560–1567.

Mehta, S., Mehta, V., Mehta, S., Shah, D., Motiwala, A., Vardhan, J., Mehta, N., & Mehta, D. (2011). Multimodal behavior program for ADHD incorporating yoga and implemented by high school volunteers: A pilot study. *ISRN Pediatrics*. Article publication online. doi:10.5402/2011/780745.

Mehta, S., Shah, D., Shah, K., Mehta, S., Mehta, N., Mehta, V., Mehta, V., Mehta, V., Motiwala, S., Mehta, N., & Mehta, D. (2012) Peer-mediated multimodal intervention program for the treatment of children with ADHD in India: One-year follow up. *ISRN Pediatrics*. Article publication online. doi:10.5402/2012/419168.

Metin, B., Krebs, R. M., Wiersema, J. R., Verguts, T., Gasthuys, R., Van der Meere, J. J., Achten, E., Roeyers, H., & Sonuga-Barke, E. (2015). Dysfunctional modulation of the default mode network activity in attention-deficit hyperactivity disorder. *Journal of Abnormal Psychology, 124*(1), 208–214.

Mick, E., Biederman, J., Faraone, S. V., Sayer, J., & Kleinman, S. (2002). Case-control study of attention deficit hyperactivity disorder and maternal smoking, alcohol use and drug use during pregnancy. *American Journal of Child and Adolescent Psychiatry*, 41, 378–385.

Millichap, G.J., & Yee, M. M. (2012). The diet factor in attention-deficit hyperactivity disorder. *Paediatrics*, *129*(2), 330–337.

Mitchell, J. T., Zylowska, L., & Kollins, S. H. (2015). Mindfulness meditation training for attention-deficit/hyperactivity disorder in adulthood: Current empirical support, treatment overview, and future directions. *Cognitive Behavioural Practice*, *22*(2), 172–191. doi:10.1016/j.cbpra.2014.10.002.

Moyer, C. A., Donnelly, M. P, Anderson, J. C., Valek, K. C., Huckaby, S. J., Wiederholt, D. A., Doty, R. L., Rehlinger, A. S., & Rice, B. L. (2011). Frontal electroencephalographic asymmetry associated with positive emotion is produced by very brief meditation training, *Psychological Science*, *22*(10), 1277–1279.

Mrazek, M. D., Franklin, M. S., Phillips, D. T., Baird, B., & Schooler, J. W. (2013). Mindfulness training improves working memory capacity and GRE performance while reducing mind wandering. *Psychological Science*. Article publication online. doi:10.1177/0956797612459659.

National Institute of Health and Clinical Excellence (2018, March). *Attention deficit hyperactivity disorder: diagnosis and management* (NICE Guideline NG87). Retrieved from: https://www.nice.org.uk/guidance/ng87.

Nivethitha, L., Mooventhan, A., & Manjunath, N. (2016). Effects of various *prāṇāyāma* on cardiovascular and autonomic variables. *Ancient Science of Life*, *36*(2), 72–77. doi:10.4103/asl.ASL_178_16.

Piek, J. P., Pitcher, T. M., & Hay, D. A. (1999). Motor coordination and kinaesthesia in boys with attention deficit-hyperactivity disorder. *Developmental Medicine & Child Neurology*, *41*, 159–165.

Pliszka, S. R. (2005). The neuropsychopharmacology of attention-deficit/hyperactivity disorder. *Biological Psychiatry*, *57*, 1385–1390.

Polanczyk, G., de Lima, M. S., Horta, B. L., Biederman, J., & Rohde, L. A. (2007). The worldwide prevalence of ADHD: A systematic review and metaregression analysis. *American Journal of Psychiatry*, *164*, 942–948.

Rajesh, S. K., Ilavarasu, J. V., & Srinivasan, T. M. (2014). Effect of bhramari pranayama on the response inhibition: Evidence from the stop signal task. *International Journal of Yoga*, *7*(2), 138–141. doi:10.4103/0973-6131.133896.

Remschmidt, H. (2005). Global consensus on ADHD/HKD. *European Child & Adolescent Psychiatry*, 14, 127–137.

Rucklidge, J. J., Brown, D. L., Crawford, S., & Kaplan, B. J. (2006). Retrospective reports of childhood trauma in adults with ADHD. *Journal of Attention Disorders*, *9*(4), 631–641.

Sharma, V. K., Rajajeyakumar, M., Velkumary, S., Subramanian, S. K., Bhavanani, A. B., Madanmohan, Sahai, A., & Thangavel, D. (2014). Effect of fast and slow pranayama practice on cognitive functions in healthy volunteers. *Journal of Clinical and Diagnostic Research*, *8*(1), 10–13. doi:10.7860/JCDR/2014/7256.3668.

Shifrin, J. G., Proctor, B. E., & Prevatt, F. F. (2010). Work performance differences between college students with and without ADHD. *Journal of Attention Disorders*, 13, 489–496.

Shum, S. B. M, & Pang, M. Y. C. (2009). Children with attention deficit hyperactivity disorder have impaired balance function: Involvement of somatosensory, visual, and vestibular systems. *Journal of Pediatrics*, *155*(2), 245–249.

Sibley, M. H., Swanson, J., Arnold, E., Hechtman, L. T., Owens, E. B., Stehli, A., Abikoff, H., Hinshaw, S. P., Molina, B. S. G., Mitchell, J. T., Jensen, P. S., Howard, A. L., Lakes, K. D., & Pelham, W. E. (2017). Defining ADHD symptom persistence in adulthood: Optimizing sensitivity and specificity. *Journal of Child Psychology and Psychiatry and Allied Disciplines*, *58*(6), 655–662. doi:10.1111/jcpp.12620.

Siegfried, C. B., Blackshear, K., & National Child Traumatic Stress Network, with assistance from the National Resource Center on ADHD: A Program of Children and Adults with Attention-Deficit/Hyperactivity Disorder (CHADD) (2016). *Is it ADHD or child traumatic stress? A guide for Clinicians*. Los Angeles, CA & Durham, NC: National Center for Child Traumatic Stress.

Smith, P. J., Blumenthal, J. A., Hoffman, B. M., Cooper, H., Strauman, T. A., Welsh-Bohmer, K., Browndyke, J. N., & Sherwood, A. (2010). Aerobic exercise and neurocognitive performance: A meta-analytic review of randomized controlled trials. *Psychosomatic Medicine*, *72*(3), 239–252.

Streeter, C. C., Gerbarg, P. L., Whitfield, T. H., Owen, L., Johnston, J., Silveri, M. M., Gensler, M., Faulkner, C. L., Mann, C., Wixted, M., Hernon, A. M., Nyer, M. B., Brown, E. R., & Jensen, J. E. (2017). Treatment of major depressive disorder with Iyengar yoga and coherent breathing: A randomized controlled dosing study. *Journal of Alternative and Complementary Medicine*, *23*(3), 201–207. doi:10.1089/acm.2016.0140.

Swing, E. L., Gentile, D. A., Anderson, C. A., & Walsh, D. A. (2010). Television and video game exposure and the development of attention problems. *Pediatrics*, *126*(2), 214–221.

Telles, S., Raghuraj, P., Maharana, S., & Nagendra, H. R. (2007). Immediate effect of three yoga breathing techniques on performance on a letter-cancellation task. *Perceptual and Motor Skills*, 104(3 Pt 2), 1289–1296.

Thomas, R., Sanders, S., Doust, J., Beller, E., & Glasziou, P. (2015). Prevalence of attention-deficit/hyperactivity disorder: A systematic review and meta-analysis. *Pediatrics*, 135(4), e994–e1001.

Vaidya, C. J., & Stollstorff, M. (2008). Cognitive neuroscience of attention deficit hyperactivity disorder: Current status and working hypotheses. *Developmental Disabilities Research Reviews*, *14*(4), 261–267.

Van der Oord, S., Bögels, S. M., & Peijnenburg, D. (2012). The effectiveness of mindfulness training for children with adhd and mindful parenting for their parents. *Journal of Child and Family Studies*, 21(1), 139–147. doi:10.1007/s10826-011-9457-0.

Vandenberg, N. L. (2001). The use of a weighted vest to increase on-task behavior in children with attention difficulties. *American Journal of Occupational Therapy*, 55, 621–628.

Voigt, R. G., Katusic, S. K., Colligan, R. C., Killian, J. M., Weaver, A. L., & Barbaresi, W. J. (2017). Academic achievement in adults with a history of childhood attention-deficit/hyperactivity disorder: A population-based prospective study. *Journal of Developmental Behavioural Pediatrics*, *38*(1), 1–11. doi:10.1097/DBP.0000000000000358.

Volkow, N. D., Wang, G. J., Kollins, S. H., Wigal, T. L., Newcorn, J. H., Telang, F., Fowler, J. S., Zhu, W., Logan, J., Ma, Y., Pradhan, K., Wong, C., & Swanson, J. M. (2009). Evaluating dopamine reward pathway in ADHD: Clinical implications. *JAMA*, *302*, 1084–1091.

Volkow, N. D., Wang, G.-J., Newcorn, J. H., Kollins, S. H., Wigal, T. L., Telang, F., Fowler, J. S., Goldstein, R. Z., Klein, N., Logan, J., Wong, C., & Swanson, J. M. (2011). Motivation deficit in ADHD is associated with dysfunction of the dopamine reward pathway. *Molecular Psychiatry*, *16*(11), 1147–1154. doi:10.1038/mp.2010.97.

Weinstein, D., Staffelbach, D., & Biaggio, M. (2000). attention-deficit hyperactivity disorder and posttraumatic stress disorder: Differential diagnosis in childhood sexual abuse. *Clinical Psychology Review, 20*, 359–378.

Weintraub, A. (2012). *Yoga Skills for Therapists: Effective Practices for Mood Management*. New York: W.W. Norton & Company.

Willcutt, E.G. (2012). The prevalence of DSM-IV attention-deficit/hyperactivity disorder: A meta-analytic review. *Neurotherapeutics, 9*, 490–499.

World Health Organization (2012). Pharmacological and nonpharmacological interventions for children with attention deficit hyperactivity disorder (ADHD). Retrieved from: http://www.who.int/mental_health/mhgap/evidence/child/q7/en/

Yoon, S. Y. R., Jain, U., & Shapiro, C. (2012). Sleep in attention-deficit/hyperactivity disorder in children and adults: Past, present, and future. *Sleep Medicine Reviews*, 16, 371–388.

Zimmerman, J., & Coyle, V. (2009). *The Way of Council* (2nd ed.). USA: Bramble Books.

Zylowska, L. (2012). *The Mindfulness Prescription for Adult ADHD*. Boston, MA: Trumpeter Books.

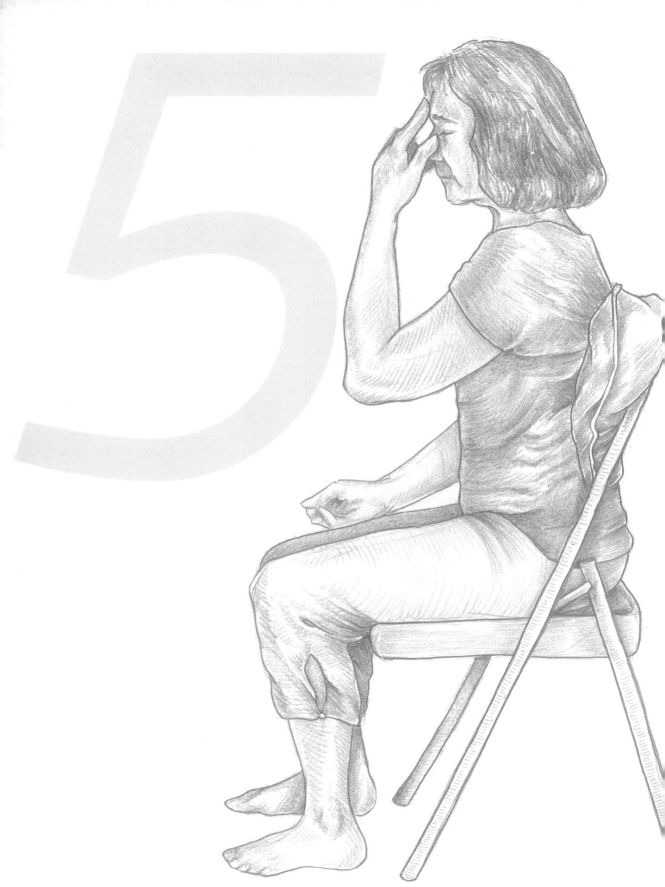

Insomnia

Sat Bir Singh Khalsa and Lisa Sanfilippo

5

Overview

Insomnia is highly prevalent, affecting 10% to 20% of the general population, with approximately 50% having a chronic course (Buysse, 2013). A large U.S. survey indicated that overall prevalence estimate of broadly defined insomnia is as high as 23.6% (Roth *et al.*, 2011); and, although there is high variability globally, similar estimates of prevalence have been recorded for Japan, Australia, the UK and Germany (Havens, Grandner, Youngstedt, Pandey, & Parthasarathy, 2017). The presence of insomnia is a known risk factor for impaired functioning and the occurrence of both medical and psychological conditions, as well as increased healthcare utilization and costs.

Broadly defined, insomnia is experienced as a difficulty initiating sleep at the beginning of the night, difficulty maintaining sleep throughout the night, waking up too early, or a complaint of light, non-restorative, or unsatisfying sleep quality. Sleep maintenance insomnia is currently the most common manifestation, although it is not unusual for individuals to experience a combination of some or all of these symptoms. Insomnia is considered clinically significant if it meets a certain threshold of severity, and there are several clinical guidelines for this diagnosis. A common set of criteria requires the persistence of the aforementioned symptoms for at least three months (thus distinguishing chronic insomnia from more commonly experienced short-term episodes) occurring with a frequency of at least three times per week despite there being adequate opportunities for sleep, accompanied by daytime symptoms of clinically significant distress such as fatigue or mood disturbance and/or an impairment in social, occupational, or cognitive functioning. Chronic insomnia

can also be divided into primary insomnia, in which the insomnia appears to exist on its own, or secondary insomnia, in which there is a clearly defined underlying cause for the insomnia such as a psychological or medical condition, medication side effects, or drug misuse (Buysse, 2013; Medalie & Cifu, 2017; Morin & Benca, 2012).

The etiology and maintenance of insomnia involves genetic, environmental, behavioral, psychological, and physiological factors, all of which contribute to an underlying psychophysiological hyperarousal (Buysse, 2013). There are predisposing factors that increase the risk of developing insomnia, which include a family history of, and a lifelong propensity for, stress-related low quality sleep. Precipitating factors involved in etiology can include medical, environmental, or psychosocial stressful life circumstances that initiate a pattern of poor sleep.

> Chronic insomnia can be divided into primary insomnia, in which the insomnia appears to exist on its own, or secondary insomnia, in which there is a clearly defined underlying cause for the insomnia such as a psychological or medical condition, medication side effects, or drug misuse.

There are also perpetuating factors. It is not uncommon that the original precipitant for insomnia has been a life circumstance causing a sleep disturbance (e.g., a stressful life event or situation, a bout of jet lag, a prescription medication known to interfere with sleep quality) resulting in acute insomnia, which then progressed to chronic insomnia despite the resolution or removal of the precipitating factor. Those with insomnia may engage in behaviors and develop other psychological factors (e.g., conditioned behaviors and associations) that lead to a counterproductive repeating cycle of continued sleep disturbance. For example, many spend excessive time in bed trying to "catch up" on sleep, despite the fact that increased time in bed at night and increased attention and effort to "try to sleep" exacerbates psychophysiological hyperarousal and perpetuates insomnia. Another example of a counterproductive behavior is conducting business in the bedroom or in the evening just before bed without allowing sufficient wind-down time before sleep initiation. An additional perpetuating psychological factor is mental rumination, that is, allowing counterproductive and/or catastrophic thinking about sleep (such as worrying about the negative effects of sleep deprivation and the impending inability to function well the next day) to proliferate during sleep onset or during mid-sleep awakenings. Physiological perpetuating factors include evidence of chronically elevated activation of the stress system, manifesting as elevated levels of both stress hormones and metabolic and sympathetic activity.

It has been argued that insomnia is not strictly a sleep disorder, but rather a disorder of elevated psychophysiological hyperarousal, characterized by cognitive, emotional and physiological hyperarousal. However, although hyperarousal is a strong component underlying insomnia, it is likely that both neurophysiological hyperarousal and psychological and behavioral processes contribute (Levenson, Kay, & Buysse, 2015).

Medication

Because the field of sleep disorders is neither well represented in medical school education nor familiar to the general population, many healthcare providers and individuals with chronic insomnia are unaware of the characteristics and consequences of this disorder and the currently available treatments, and many sufferers are therefore largely untreated.

The most common conventional approach to treatment is pharmacological. Over-the-counter medications include antihistamines and various herbal preparations, which have mild sedative effects (and may linger, causing fatigue during the subsequent day). However, these medications are often insufficient to treat chronic insomnia over the long term, since they are unlikely to be strong enough in their sleep-inducing or sleep-maintaining role to have any

> Patients who withdraw from hypnotic medication may often experience a complete resumption of insomnia symptoms, suggesting the significant criticism that this approach does not address the underlying causes of insomnia and its persistence.

significant effect on chronic established insomnia. Physicians widely prescribe hypnotic medications, mostly benzodiazepine-related drugs, that come in a variety of forms and half-lives. Although these are more effective than over-the-counter medications, their side effects can include aberrant night-time behaviors (e.g., confusional arousals, sleepwalking) or cognitive impairments (e.g., memory loss), and it is not uncommon for patients to develop tolerance to these medications, with their efficacy waning over several weeks to reach a point of minimal benefit (Medalie & Cifu, 2017; Reynolds & Ebben, 2017). Furthermore, patients who withdraw from hypnotic medication may often experience a complete resumption of insomnia symptoms, suggesting the significant criticism that this approach does not address the underlying causes of insomnia and its persistence. On the other hand, behavioral treatments for insomnia do address these underlying factors (Reynolds & Ebben, 2017).

Behavioral treatments

Cognitive behavioral therapy for insomnia (CBTI)

Research on the efficacy of behavioral treatments for chronic insomnia is extensive and has a long history, justifying the contention that this should be the first-line approach in the treatment of insomnia (Qaseem et al., 2016). These treatments represent a number of discrete behavioral and psychological approaches to insomnia care generally referred to as cognitive behavioral therapy for insomnia (CBTI); these treatments are often offered together as individual or group sessions lasting up to eight weeks involving patient education and behavioral practices. Reviews of CBTI for the treatment of insomnia reveal robust effect sizes that are maintained at long-term follow-up (van Straten et al., 2018) and good efficacy in comparison with pharmacotherapy (Mitchell, Gehrman, Perlis, & Umscheid, 2012). Unfortunately, despite the fact that CBTI is likely also more cost-effective than pharmacotherapy, due to socioeconomic factors and the lack of knowledge and education in sleep medicine, these treatments are not generally known to either healthcare providers or the general public. In addition, there are very few qualified therapists, to whom access is limited due to the sparse number of sleep clinics where they work (Reynolds & Ebben, 2017).

Conventional CBTI

There are five somewhat discrete approaches within conventional CBTI (Buysse, 2013; Morin & Benca, 2012).

1. Sleep hygiene focuses on addressing common-sense behavioral and environmental issues that can contribute to insomnia, including adjusting caffeine intake, allowing for a wind-down time before bed, adopting a regular exercise program (but avoiding vigorous exercise just before bed), avoiding alcohol as a sleep aid, and maintaining an appropriate sleeping environment with respect to noise, light, temperature, and the quality of the bed.

2. Stimulus control addresses conditioning factors in the maintenance of insomnia. The bedroom is reconfigured to reserve it for only either sex or sleep. Patients are advised not to lie in bed at night for prolonged periods of time trying to fall asleep, but to leave the bedroom after 15–20 minutes if unable to fall asleep and to adopt a quiet, restful waking activity until drowsiness occurs, at which time sleep can be initiated again. The aim is to re-associate the bedroom and the experience of drowsiness with successful sleep onset and maintenance. Regular sleep and wake times are encouraged to recondition the mind and body to a regular sleep pattern.

3. CBT is the most widely used form of psychotherapy for psychological conditions and is also very useful in insomnia (as CBTI). Patients learn to identify dysfunctional and catastrophic ruminative thoughts and how to replace these with more realistic thought patterns that are more conducive to sleep. Cognitive restructuring assists in reframing dysfunctional beliefs and attitudes toward sleep and insomnia to prevent their negative impact on sleep.

4. Sleep restriction therapy utilizes the sleep drive—the accumulated propensity for sleep or sleepiness—in an attempt to use sleep deprivation to consolidate the sleep episode. Patients may be advised to adopt relatively short night sleep opportunities for a period of weeks so that the resulting cumulative sleep deprivation will consolidate the sleep episode. Once this is achieved, the sleep episode can be slowly lengthened to normal duration. It is likely that this strategy also reconditions the mind and body to experience a consolidated sleep episode. Another key recommendation for individuals with insomnia is to avoid daytime napping, which takes away from the sleep drive available for night-time sleep.

5. Relaxation treatments have been aimed at reducing the well-known cognitive and

psychophysiological arousal associated with insomnia, including elevated SNS activity and stress hormone levels. Muscle relaxation and guided imagery-related strategies have been most studied in connection with CBTI. However, there is now significant implementation of, and research on, mind-body medicine strategies such as meditation, yoga, and tai chi for insomnia.

Rationale for meditation in the treatment of insomnia

Meditation works on both cognitive and physiological levels, reducing mind wandering and rumination while also eliciting the relaxation response, a coordinated endogenous behavior in the mind and body that is effectively opposite to the stress response. Importantly, meditation practice also leads to the development of metacognition, a key underlying principle in CBT, in which the relationship and reactivity to thoughts and thought patterns is changed. Mind-body practices such as yoga, tai chi and qi gong include the additional strategies of breath regulation and body movement and exercise, augmenting the effects of reducing psychophysiological arousal by affecting physiology directly (Schmalz, Streeter, & Khalsa, 2016).

Studies on meditation dating back to the 1970s clearly demonstrate some degree of efficacy in insomnia treatment. Most of the early studies used so-called single-point, concentrative or closed-focus meditation in which attention is held on a single target such as a word, sound, or the breath (Carr-Kaffashan & Woolfolk, 1979; Schoicket, Bertelson, & Lack, 1988; Woolfolk, Carr-Kaffashan, & McNulty, 1976). More recent studies have evaluated open-focus meditation practices such as mindfulness or *vipassana*, in which attention is focused on the flow of thought and sensation. The scientific clinical rationale for this form of meditation for insomnia has been discussed by

Jason Ong and others (Garland, Zhou, Gonzalez, & Rodriguez, 2016; Larouche, Cote, Belisle, & Lorrain, 2014; Ong, Ulmer, & Manber, 2012) with respect to its effects on metacognition and psychophysiological arousal, leading to balanced appraisals, cognitive flexibility, equanimity, and commitment to values as important characteristics for improving sleep. There are now insomnia treatment studies of mindfulness meditation alone (Black, O'Reilly, Olmstead, Breen, & Irwin, 2015) as well as others reviewing studies using the formalized Mindfulness-Based Stress Reduction program (Garland et al., 2014; Gross et al., 2011; Ong et al., 2014) and the Mindfulness-Based Cognitive Therapy program (Heidenreich, Tuin, Pflug, Michal, & Michalak, 2006). A recent meta-analysis has revealed that mindfulness meditation demonstrated significant beneficial effects in total wake time, sleep onset latency, sleep quality, and sleep efficiency, as compared with controls, suggesting that it may mildly improve some sleep characteristics in patients with insomnia, and could serve as an adjunct treatment to medication for sleep complaints (Gong et al., 2016).

In general, there is no medical or psychophysiological reason prohibiting the use of meditative strategies in combination with conventional behavioral strategies in the treatment of insomnia, except perhaps in cases of trauma (discussed later). There are published studies of interventions that have incorporated meditation together within a CBTI intervention with significant success (Jacobs, Benson & Friedman, 1993, 1996; Jacobs et al., 1993; Ong, Shapiro & Manber, 2009).

Research review of yoga therapy for insomnia

There has been less research conducted on the efficacy of yoga for insomnia, although it is likely to have greater treatment potential than meditation alone given the added practices of breath regulation and physical postures and exercises. Indeed, there are a few studies suggesting the efficacy of breath regulation on its own for insomnia (Choliz, 1995; Tsai, Kuo, Lee, & Yang, 2015). The earliest study to evaluate yoga for insomnia was a single-group trial conducted on a small sample in India (Joshi, 1992). Subsequently, this author's laboratory (Khalsa, 2004) conducted a single-group trial of an eight-week Kundalini yoga–based self-care intervention on a mixed population of patients with primary and secondary chronic insomnia. Subjects were instructed to practice for at least 30 minutes per day on their own with the same sequence of practices that included the breathing meditation Shabad Kriya (a specific practice within the tradition of Kundalini yoga as taught by Yogi Bhajan), a slow breathing practice that includes both a segmented inhaling and exhaling pattern together with a prolonged breath retention in the breath cycle in coordination with meditation on a mentally repeated mantra. Statistically significant improvements were observed on sleep-wake diaries in sleep efficiency, total sleep time, total wake time, sleep onset latency, and time spent awake at night after sleep onset. A subsequent RCT on subjects with chronic primary sleep onset insomnia using the same intervention showed similar improvements (Khalsa, 2010). Kozasa et al. (2010) published a review of studies of mind-body therapies for insomnia, concluding that "…self-reported sleep was improved by all mind-body treatments, among them yoga, relaxation, Tai Chi, and music." A more recent review of meditative movement intervention trials on insomnia reported that seventeen high quality RCTs showed beneficial effects for various populations on a range of sleep measures (Wang et al., 2016). Studies of the efficacy of yoga for insomnia secondary to other conditions, including osteoarthritis (Buchanan, Vitiello, & Bennett, 2017; Taibi & Vitiello, 2011), menopause (Afonso et al., 2012; Buchanan et al., 2017), and cancer (Cohen, Warneke, Fouladi, Rodriguez, & Chaoul-Reich, 2004; Mustian, 2013; Mustian, Janelsins, Peppone, & Kamen, 2014), have also shown benefit. Given the higher propensity for insomnia in the elderly, it is encouraging to find that trials of yoga for insomnia in Israel (Halpern et al., 2014) and in India (Manjunath & Telles, 2005) on geriatric populations have shown positive results. A current weakness of this evidence base relates to the variety of intervention characteristics across relatively few studies, including content of the yoga intervention (although most trials incorporate the fundamental components of traditional yoga including postures/exercises, pranayama, relaxation and meditation/mindfulness), the style/school of yoga practice, overall intervention duration,

It is clear that yoga has significant potential for the successful treatment of both primary and secondary chronic insomnia.

frequency of practice, session practice length, as well as poor reporting of the exact content. The evidence is also insufficient to allow any conclusion regarding the most effective components of yoga practice, or whether specific yoga practices are more efficacious than a simple general yoga practice.

It is clear that yoga has significant potential for the successful treatment of both primary and secondary chronic insomnia. However, there are relatively few studies in this area and there is significant need for additional RCTs of yoga for chronic insomnia to further establish its efficacy and to elucidate dose-response characteristics (that is, how the individual responds to different levels of yogic activity). Future studies should also evaluate a modified CBTI program that incorporates a significant yoga therapy component.

Integrative and yoga therapy approaches

Both individual yoga traditions and integrative approaches have been directed toward the task of improving sleep and overcoming insomnia.

The first mention of yoga asana specifically for insomnia may have been B. K. S. Iyengar's recommendations in *Light on Yoga* (1966). Iyengar notes the following poses in the appendix entitled *Curative Asanas for Various Diseases*: (1) inversions, that is, shoulder stand and cycle, including *halasana* (plow pose) and headstand; (2) *uttanasana* (standing forward bend); and (3) breath practices (*bhastrika, nadi sodhana, suryabhedana pranayama*, and *sanmukhi mudra*). Iyengar recommends these practices be adapted according to ability and by observing the reactions of the body.

Disordered sleep is addressed in Kundalini yoga through *shabad kriya* (see earlier) and bridge pose and table pose, as taught by Yogi Bhajan (Khalsa, 1996). The practice of *shabad kriya* has demonstrated beneficial effects for alleviating primary and secondary insomnia (Khalsa, 2004).

Judith Lasater (2011) offers a sequence of insomnia-focused supported poses (using props such as blankets, blocks, and belts) entitled *Elusive Dreams* to induce the relaxation response in preparation for sleep and to overcome insomnia. The sequence features chest and hip openers, an inversion, a seated wide-legged forward bend, and a version of *savasana*, complemented by modern lifestyle habits.

Yoga nidra (yoga sleep) is a guided relaxation practice that leads practitioners into the hypnagogic state, the threshold between alpha and theta brainwaves, as cited in popular yoga and wellbeing literature (Brody, 2017; Hill, 2017). The effects of yoga nidra are often cited in relationship to the benefits of meditation for treating insomnia. In particular, yoga nidra is theorized to treat insomnia by inducing and reinforcing the brainwave patterns associated with transitioning into and maintaining deep sleep.

Guidelines for yoga teachers/therapists

Although yoga practice in general may be of benefit for insomnia, the following guidelines for a therapeutic approach address specific concerns (Sanfilippo, 2019).

1. **Sleep onset.** Yoga asana and pranayama can be used prior to bedtime to induce relaxation, which facilitates sleep onset and promotes sleeps maintenance. Yoga and pranayama are believed to be particularly effective in conjunction with behavioral and lifestyle changes (e.g., sleep hygiene and resetting set sleep and wake times). Two sleep-preparation asana sequences devised by Lisa Sanfilippo, the Simple Sleep Sequence (see Figure 5.1) and Deeper Sleep Sequence (Sanfilippo, 2019), may be offered to alleviate muscle tension and induce relaxation for sleep readiness based on common tension hotspots. These include lengthened exhale breathing in the cat/cow pose, lower body stretches (thigh, hip, and hamstring) and twists to alleviate tension in the diaphragm, gentle backbends, and forward bends. Pranayama includes a gentle form of *ujjayii* (an extended breath that produces a gentle sighing sound in the throat associated with the toning of the glottis) with lengthened exhalation, modified *dirga pranayama* (a three-part breath into the low belly, middle ribcage, and upper chest, then all three sequentially), and *chandra bhedana* (breathing in and out through the left nostril) or *shabad kriya*. This method aligns practices with appropriate times of day to support the functioning of circadian rhythms as well as addressing the hyperarousal that underpins insomnia.

2. **Daytime relaxation to promote night-time sleep.** Relaxing practices can be conducted during daytime to support sleep at night by

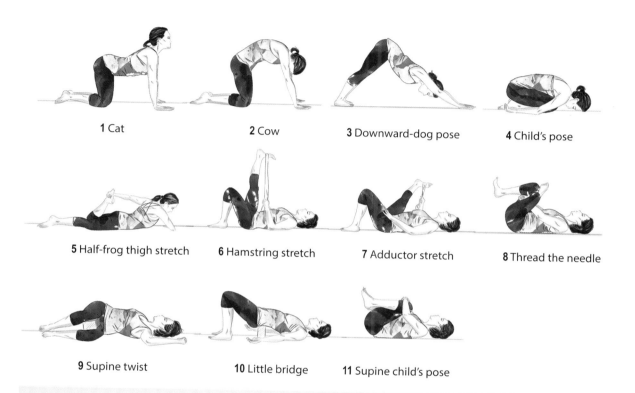

1 Cat **2** Cow **3** Downward-dog pose **4** Child's pose

5 Half-frog thigh stretch **6** Hamstring stretch **7** Adductor stretch **8** Thread the needle

9 Supine twist **10** Little bridge **11** Supine child's pose

Figure 5.1

Simple Sleep Sequence. This sequence can be practiced on the floor, on a yoga mat, or in bed (in which case, omit Pose 3). Each pose is to be held for five breaths (preferably with a lengthened exhalation) or until the practitioner experiences a release in the muscle(s) being stretched. Pose 5 should be done on each side before progressing to Poses 6–8, which are completed in sequence first on one side of the body, and then repeated on the other side. Continue to Pose 9 on each side, then include Pose 10 on either a brick or firm pillow under the sacrum for up to three minutes. Finish with Pose 11. © Lisa Sanfilippo / Illustrations by Masha Pimas establishing the habits and states of consciousness that decrease the nervous system hyper-arousal underlying insomnia for many people. It is beneficial to practice yoga in the afternoon between 2 pm and 5 pm, during which many people experience a dip in energy, rather than turning to caffeine or other stimulants. Napping should also be avoided because this decreases the sleep drive needed to build up tiredness at bedtime. Relaxing or restorative practices may include a modified *viparita karani* (legs-up-the-wall or legs-on-the-chair pose), restorative/supported *supta baddha konasana* (cobbler or goddess pose), or simple open-focus meditation practices, which can enable the practitioner to achieve restful and restorative states.

3. **Promoting daytime wakefulness.** Practices that stimulate the SNS and raise the heart rate in a sustained way should be practiced at times of day in which wakefulness is desirable. The contrasting practices, relaxing versus stimulating, can help the client/student to align with circadian rhythms to support good sleep. Vigorous practices, for example, holding an intense asana such as a warrior pose or handstand, or doing a stimulating breath practice such as *kapalabhati* (the vigorous abdomen-pumping pranayama known as shining-skull breath) or breath of joy (a three-part sharp inhalation with vigorous arm movements followed by a vigorous exhalation on a forward bend), will generally increase heart rate, and when practiced regularly can also increase a person's capacity to shift from a state of high excitation to a resting state. This may increase the capacity to adapt to stress, which is often a significant underlying factor in insomnia. However, it is recommended to avoid intense aerobic activity or yoga known to stimulate the SNS response late in the evening.

4. **Reducing anxiety related to lack of sleep.** In the earlier section describing psychological perpetuating factors for insomnia, it was noted that catastrophic thinking about sleeplessness (e.g., panic about being able to function during the day) is a key perpetuating factor of insomnia. Yoga, pranayama, and meditation may help to address these negative thought patterns, and explicitly thought-focused practices such as journaling, thought labeling, cognitive reframing (as used in CBT), and some mindfulness practices may help to interrupt the ruminations and develop alternate thoughts or patterns of thinking. In addition, using yoga practices that manage morning grogginess or a dip in energy in the afternoon may help to alleviate anxiety about not being able to function due to lack of sleep. In addition to practicing in the afternoon, restorative postures, meditation, or yoga nidra (yogic sleep) practiced in the morning can help regain some deep rest after sleeping poorly, and enable starting the day with better physical and psychological resilience. Providing practices to restore energy sustainably without actually sleeping can help a person to decrease or prevent the use of stimulants in order to remain wakeful.

5. **Timing of practice.** Time of day is important in undertaking yoga practices geared toward alleviating insomnia, particularly when they are new to the practitioner. For more experienced practitioners who are genuinely easeful in these poses, headstand and shoulder stand can have a relaxing effect and facilitate sleep even when practiced late in the day. However, for a newer practitioner, these poses may be too stimulating before bed due to the intense effort involved, and possibly due to some of the inversion effects as well. In these cases, modifications like *setubandhasana* (little bridge pose) or *viparita*

karani (legs up the wall pose) may substitute for shoulder stand, and a similarly relaxing effect to that created by headstand may be achieved by a wide-legged forward bend with head down, resting on a block. There is debate about backbends such as *urdhva dhanurasana/chakrasana* (full wheel/bow pose), which may activate the thoracic nerve plexus by pulling the shoulders back and pressing against gravity, which can activate the SNS, thus preventing some people from sleeping. For teachers and students alike, noting the effects on the individual is essential.

6. **Regular practice creates more durable effects.** Yoga for insomnia works cumulatively, building over time and decreasing levels of hyperarousal, as well as reducing anxiety about sleep; also, those who practice yoga in general may experience benefits for their sleep.

Guidelines for yoga classes

In general yoga classes, integrating several guidelines can help to avoid triggering insomnia, alleviate it, and promote better sleep in general (Sanfilippo, 2019). First, students can learn to tolerate longer durations of time in a relaxed state when the yoga teacher/therapist integrates restorative poses into general classes, beginning with deep stretching to alleviate tension in the musculature. To help students with alternatives to caffeine and other stimulants for dealing with fatigue, yoga teachers can highlight postures such as *viparita karani* and *supta baddha konasana*, as well as simple poses like child's pose with the belly supported by a bolster. Utilizing pre-bedtime breath and meditation practices such as *ujjayi* with extended exhalation, three-part breath, *chandra bhedana* or *shabad kriya*, reinforces a student's capacity to enter the nonwaking brainwave states associated with dropping off to sleep and maintaining sleep, thus helping to build a sense of safety and familiarity in the relaxed state that is necessary to recover from problems with sleep.

Tailoring interventions in a yoga therapy approach

A yoga therapy approach to insomnia tailors interventions to the individual's needs, offering both yogic practices and lifestyle changes. As with all yoga therapy practices, individual screening is necessary to separate primary from secondary insomnia; it is also recommended that the client complete a sleep log (indicating their sleep habits) listing factors affecting sleep for one week (or more) to help the yoga teacher/therapist assess the causes of the disordered sleep (although they do not perform a mental health diagnosis). The yoga teacher/therapist will then devise an individual program for the client, incorporating the yoga interventions into a practical routine. For example, the yoga teacher/therapist may give a set of bedtime asana practices first, enabling the client to establish a routine, and then where appropriate add daytime breath and anti-stress practices that support the downregulation of the sympathetic nervous system (SNS) required for sleep onset and maintenance. Through managing states of wakefulness, stress, and tiredness throughout the day, a client can learn how to self-regulate sleep and wake states.

> Through managing states of wakefulness, stress, and tiredness throughout the day, a client can learn how to self-regulate sleep and wake states.

Depending upon the initial causes, perpetuating factors and the physical, mental, and emotional make-up of the individual, certain postures and practices may be more or less effective. Yoga therapy fits the practice to the person. For example, the type of insomnia that accompanies depressive symptoms can be different to that which accompanies an anxious presentation. For instance, for a client with co-occurring depression, some stimulating morning and daytime practices may be used to activate the SNS. Breath of joy (three inhalations with arms moving up, then out to a

Chapter 5

T-shape, and then up again on the inhalation, followed by a forward bend on the exhale) may also be helpful in this regard (Weintraub, 2004). However, adopting a similar practice could be overactivating for a person with co-occurring anxiety. For the anxious client, daytime practices may include standing grounding postures such as warrior poses, which are activating but have less of a direct stimulating effect on the SNS. Khalsa's research (2010), as noted earlier, has shown *shabad kriya* to be effective in alleviating insomnia. However, where trauma or breathing difficulties are present, care should be taken in prescribing the use of this method, because for some clients the breath retentions and breath count may induce panic rather than relaxation. Indeed, for clients with co-occurring PTSD or complex trauma, it is essential to approach yoga practices for insomnia with sensitivity to avoid possible unintended and/or paradoxical effects. For example, a closed-eyes meditation may be deeply relaxing for some, but could induce panic or terror in those who are still experiencing the effects of trauma.

> For clients with co-occurring PTSD or complex trauma, it is essential to approach yoga practices for insomnia with sensitivity to avoid possible unintended and/or paradoxical effects.

Guidelines for therapists in other modalities

Therapists employing other mental health modalities can bring knowledge of yoga therapy principles into their work with clients suffering from insomnia, or they may refer clients to a qualified yoga therapist for more in-depth treatment. For those who have the requisite training, yogic therapeutic principles can be integrated into other practices by

- encouraging good daily sleep hygiene and providing basic psychoeducation about the impact of habits on sleep will empower clients, helping them to decrease their anxiety about sleep. Establishing a yoga practice to calm them down before bed will provide relaxation;

- promoting good daily sleep hygiene, particularly the aspect of insomnia that relates to self-restricted sleep arising from anxiety, depression, or lack of awareness about circadian rhythms;

- encouraging clients to integrate habits and practices at home: while complementary and holistic therapies such as psychotherapy, massage therapy, and acupuncture sessions may provide important ingredients in reestablishing healthy sleep patterns, the best outcomes occur when the positive habits and integration of practices that promote the ability to relax into sleep are continued at home;

- learning and advocating the use of simple yoga and breath techniques to induce relaxation within a session can help clients to integrate helpful physical practices that help restore sleep. Therapists should undertake to learn simple practices themselves, so that they are more capable of imparting these to their clients. Simple breath techniques such as *ujjayii* with lengthened exhale or three-part breathing (*dirga pranayama*) may be used after therapeutic consultation. This can provide a way into yoga practices and give encouragement to the client, and are generally safe enough to impart without formal yoga teacher training; and

- building internal resources for sleep: it may be useful to help clients wean themselves off the use of external sleep aids, unless medically necessary (e.g., breathing/CPAP machines for sleep apnea). Those suffering from insomnia often develop anxiety around sleep and rely on external props or aids such as recordings, specific scents, pillows, and herbs. In the longer term, however, these may encourage dependency; the risk here is that unavailability of such props can induce panic or cause distress, thereby delaying or preventing sleep. In the case of dependency on insomnia medications, through yoga a client may become able to decrease or stop taking sleep medications—always, of course, with the assistance of their doctor. Furthermore, the use of electronic apps is discouraged: as well as the risk of dependence, evidence suggests that the blue-light emissions from the use of electronic devices prior to sleep may shift circadian rhythms (by affecting the conversion of serotonin to melatonin) and diminish the onset of sleep over time. Some newer devices may offer a night-time mode that emits red-spectrum light, but many devices do not.

Precautions

There are a few additional precautions to the recommended guidelines pertaining to particular conditions.

Trauma

If insomnia is due to posttraumatic stress, some postures and body positions may initially induce a negative response, and may continue do so in the long term, especially those that expose vulnerable parts of the body or cause a person to feel overly restricted. Sitting or lying immobile (whether in meditation or restorative poses) with the eyes closed may be uncomfortable or distressing for someone who has experienced trauma. Similarly, the ability to sit or release into a supported pose may only be possible after significant release in muscle tension through active asana, or the capacity may need to be built through other supportive practices, including psychotherapy.

Physical limitations and pain

Some of the more complex yoga postures, such as shoulder stand, although indicated as useful for insomnia, are not appropriate for new practitioners and/or those with injuries. More gentle alternatives may include *setu bhandasana* (bridge pose) or *viparita karani* (legs-up-the-wall pose) because they are also beneficial for sleep and may achieve some of the same inversion functions. In addition, where insomnia is due to chronic physical pain, very limited asana or non-asana based approaches may be best.

> Where insomnia is due to chronic physical pain, very limited asana or non-asana based approaches may be best.

Future directions

Future directions for yoga therapy for insomnia are expected to include developments in both research and practice. As the incidence of insomnia rises to almost epidemic levels, it is of growing importance for yoga teachers and mental health providers to integrate a working knowledge of the potential of yoga to ameliorate sleep problems and promote better sleep in the general population. A yoga teacher/therapist may seek further training to include a holistic approach, offering a range of interventions, or to focus solely on providing asana and pranayama solutions tailored to individual client needs and capacities.

Both mainstream and specialist medicine will benefit from a research base that documents the specific effects of different practices on treating and alleviating insomnia, including contraindications and effective dosage. Broadening the qualitative and quantitative research about both individual practices and combination yoga therapy approaches will add to the general knowledge of this holistic approach, as well as research investigating yoga practices alone and in combination with other treatments such as psychotherapy and therapeutic exercise. Yoga teachers/therapists may undertake studies or join with academic or medical research programmes to conduct trials of various practices as mentioned in this chapter. Better or more extensive research may be of benefit to include physical practices of asana and pranayama into CBTI approaches, with the potential to bring these two approaches together through public health and private insurance systems. Better research may help the yoga teaching and therapy community make the case for offering, and securing funds to provide, insomnia interventions in schools and workplaces, in addition to what they may currently offer in yoga studios and holistic wellbeing centers.

References

Afonso, R. F., Hachul, H., Kozasa, E. H., Oliveira Dde, S., Goto, V., Rodrigues, D., Tufik, S., & Leite, J. R. (2012). Yoga decreases insomnia in postmenopausal women: A randomized clinical trial. *Menopause, 19*(2), 186–193.

Black, D. S., O'Reilly, G. A., Olmstead, R., Breen, E. C., & Irwin, M. R. (2015). Mindfulness meditation and improvement in sleep quality and daytime impairment among older adults with sleep disturbances: A randomized clinical trial. *Journal of the American Medical Association Internal Medicine, 175*(4), 494–501.

Buchanan, D. T., Landis, C. A., Hohensee, C., Guthrie, K. A., Otte, J. L., Paudel, M., Anderson, G. L., Caan, B., Freeman, E. W., Joffe, H., LaCroix, A. Z., Newton, K M., Reed, S., & Ensrud, K. E. (2017). Effects of yoga and aerobic exercise on actigraphic sleep parameters in menopausal women with hot flashes. *Journal of Clinical Sleep Medicine, 13*(1), 11-18.

Buchanan, D. T., Vitiello, M. V., & Bennett, K. (2017). Feasibility and efficacy of a shared yoga intervention for sleep disturbance in older adults with osteoarthritis. *Journal of Gerontological Nursing,* 11:1-10.

Brody, K. (2017) *Your brain on yoga nidra,* accessed from https://www.yogajournal.com/meditation/your-brain-on-yoga-nidra.

Buysse, D. J. (2013). Insomnia. *Journal of the American Medical Association, 309*(7), 706-716.

Carr-Kaffashan, L., & Woolfolk, R. L. (1979). Active and placebo effects in treatment of moderate and severe insomnia. *Journal of Consulting and Clinical Psychology, 47*(6), 1072-1080.

Choliz, M. (1995). A breathing-retraining procedure in treatment of sleep-onset insomnia: Theoretical basis and experimental findings. *Perceptual and Motor Skills, 80*(2), 507-513.

Cohen, L., Warneke, C., Fouladi, R. T., Rodriguez, M. A., & Chaoul-Reich, A. (2004). Psychological adjustment and sleep quality in a randomized trial of the effects of a Tibetan yoga intervention in patients with lymphoma. *Cancer, 100*(10), 2253-2260.

Garland, S. N., Carlson, L. E., Stephens, A. J., Antle, M. C., Samuels, C., & Campbell, T. S. (2014). Mindfulness-based stress reduction compared with cognitive behavioral therapy for the treatment of insomnia comorbid with cancer: A randomized, partially blinded, noninferiority trial. *Journal of Clinical Oncology, 32*(5), 449-457.

Garland, S. N., Zhou, E. S., Gonzalez, B. D., & Rodriguez, N. (2016). The quest for mindful sleep: A critical synthesis of the impact of mindfulness-based interventions for insomnia. *Current Sleep Medicine Reports, 2*(3), 142-151.

Gong, H., Ni, C. X., Liu, Y. Z., Zhang, Y., Su, W. J., Lian, Y. J., Peng, W., & Jiang, C. L. (2016). Mindfulness meditation for insomnia: A meta-analysis of randomized controlled trials. *Journal of Psychosomatic Research, 89*, 1-6.

Gross, C. R., Kreitzer, M. J., Reilly-Spong, M., Wall, M., Winbush, N. Y., Patterson, R., Mahowald, M., & Cramer-Bornemann, M. (2011). Mindfulness-based stress reduction versus pharmacotherapy for chronic primary insomnia: A randomized controlled clinical trial. *Explore, 7*(2), 76-87.

Halpern, J., Cohen, M., Kennedy, G., Reece, J., Cahan, C., & Baharav, A. (2014). Yoga for improving sleep quality and quality of life for older adults. *Alternative Therapies in Health and Medicine, 20*(3), 37–46.

Havens, C. M., Grandner, M. A., Youngstedt, S. D., Pandey, A., & Parthasarathy, S. (2017) International variability in the prevalence of insomnia and use of sleep-promoting medications, supplements and other substances. *Sleep, 40*(Suppl 1), A117–A118.

Heidenreich, T., Tuin, I., Pflug, B., Michal, M., & Michalak, J. (2006). Mindfulness-based cognitive therapy for persistent insomnia: A pilot study. *Psychotherapy and Psychosomatics, 75*(3), 188–189.

Hill, E. (2017) *How yoga nidra works,* accessed from https://www.huffingtonpost.com/entry/how-yoga-nidra-works_us_58efcea5e4b048372700d692

Iyengar, B. K. (1968). *Light on yoga; yoga dīpikā.* London: G. Allen & Unwin.

Jacobs, G. D., Benson, H., & Friedman, R. (1993). Home-based central nervous system assessment of a multifactor behavioral intervention for chronic sleep-onset insomnia. *Behavior Therapy, 24*, 159–174.

Jacobs, G. D., Benson, H., & Friedman, R. (1996). Perceived benefits in a behavioral-medicine insomnia program: A clinical report. *The American Journal of Medicine, 100*(2), 212–216.

Jacobs, G. D., Rosenberg, P. A., Friedman, R., Matheson, J., Peavy, G. M., Domar, A. D., & Benson, H. (1993). Multifactor behavioral treatment of chronic sleep-onset insomnia using stimulus control and the relaxation response. A preliminary study. *Behavior Modification, 17*(4), 498–509.

Joshi, K. S. (1992). Yoga treatment of insomnia: An experimental study. *Yoga Mimamsa, 33*(4), 24–26.

Khalsa, S. B. S. (2004). Treatment of chronic insomnia with yoga: A preliminary study with sleep-wake diaries. *Applied Psychophysiology and Biofeedback*, 29(4), 269–278.

Khalsa, S. B. S. (2010). A randomized controlled trial of a yoga treatment for chronic insomnia [Abstract]. *Applied Psychophysiology and Biofeedback, 35*, 179.

Khalsa, S. P. K. (1996), *Kundalini Yoga: The Flow of Eternal Power: A Simple Guide to the Yoga of Awareness as taught by Yogi Bhajan, Ph.D.* The Berkley Publishing Group, New York, NY. (pg. 263–265).

Kozasa, E. H., Hachul, H., Monson, C., Pinto Jr, L., Garcia, M. C., Mello, L. E., & Tufik, S. (2010). Mind-body interventions for the treatment of insomnia: A review. *Revista Brasileira De Psiquiatria, 32*(4), 437–443.

Larouche, M., Cote, G., Belisle, D., & Lorrain, D. (2014). Kind attention and non-judgment in mindfulness-based cognitive therapy applied to the treatment of insomnia: State of knowledge. *Pathologie-Biologie, 62*(5), 284–291.

Lasater, J. H. (2011). *Relax and renew: restful yoga for stressful times.* Berkeley, CA: Rodmell.

Levenson, J. C., Kay, D. B., & Buysse, D. J. (2015). The pathophysiology of insomnia. *Chest, 147*(4), 1179–1192.

Manjunath, N. K., & Telles, S. (2005). Influence of yoga and ayurveda on self-rated sleep in a geriatric population. *The Indian Journal of Medical Research, 121*(5), 683–690.

Medalie, L., & Cifu, A. S. (2017). Management of chronic insomnia disorder in adults. *Journal of the American Medical Association, 317*(7), 762–763.

Mitchell, M. D., Gehrman, P., Perlis, M., & Umscheid, C. A. (2012). Comparative effectiveness of cognitive behavioral therapy for insomnia: A systematic review. *BMC Family Practice, 13*, 40–2296–13–40.

Morin, C. M., & Benca, R. (2012). Chronic insomnia. *Lancet, 379*(9821), 1129–1141.

Mustian, K. M. (2013). Yoga as treatment for insomnia among cancer patients and survivors: A systematic review. *European Medical Journal Oncology, 1*, 106–115.

Mustian, K. M., Janelsins, M., Peppone, L. J., & Kamen, C. (2014). Yoga for the treatment of insomnia among cancer patients: Evidence, mechanisms of action, and clinical recommendations. *Oncology & Hematology Review, 10*(2), 164–168.

Ong, J. C., Manber, R., Segal, Z., Xia, Y., Shapiro, S., & Wyatt, J. K. (2014). A randomized controlled trial of mindfulness meditation for chronic insomnia. *Sleep, 37*(9), 1553–1563.

Ong, J., & Sholtes, D. (2010). A mindfulness-based approach to the treatment of insomnia. *Journal of Clinical Psychology, 66*(11), 1175–1184.

Ong, J. C., Shapiro, S. L., & Manber, R. (2008). Combining mindfulness meditation with cognitive-behavior therapy for insomnia: A treatment-development study. *Behavior Therapy, 39*(2), 171–182.

Ong, J. C., Shapiro, S. L., & Manber, R. (2009). Mindfulness meditation and cognitive behavioral therapy for insomnia: A naturalistic 12-month follow-up. *Explore, 5*(1), 30–36.

Ong, J. C., Ulmer, C. S., & Manber, R. (2012). Improving sleep with mindfulness and acceptance: A metacognitive model of insomnia. *Behaviour Research and Therapy, 50*(11), 651–660.

Qaseem, A., Kansagara, D., Forciea, M. A., Cooke, M., Denberg, T. D., & Clinical Guidelines Committee of the American College of Physicians (2016). Management of chronic insomnia disorder in adults: A clinical practice guideline from the American College of Physicians. *Annals of Internal Medicine, 165*(2), 125–133.

Reynolds, S. A., & Ebben, M. R. (2017). The cost of insomnia and the benefit of increased access to evidence-based treatment: Cognitive behavioral therapy for insomnia. *Sleep Medicine Clinics, 12*(1), 39–46.

Roth, T., Coulouvrat, C., Hajak, G., Lakoma, M. D., Sampson, N. A., Shahly, V., Shillington, A. C., Stephenson, J. J., Walsh, J. K., & Kessler, R. C. (2011). Prevalence and perceived health associated with insomnia based on DSM-IV-TR; international statistical classification of diseases and related health problems, tenth revision; and research diagnostic criteria/international classification of sleep disorders, second edition criteria: Results from the America insomnia survey. *Biological Psychiatry, 69*(6), 592–600.

Schmalzl, L., Streeter, C. C., & Khalsa, S. B. S. (2016). Research on the psychophysiology of yoga. In S. B. S. Khalsa, L. Cohen, T. McCall, & S. Telles (Eds.), *The Principles and Practice of Yoga in Health Care* (pp. 49–69). Pencaitland, UK: Handspring Publishing Limited.

Schoicket, S., Bertelson, A. D., & Lack, P. (1988). Is sleep hygiene a sufficient treatment for sleep-maintenance insomnia? *Behavior Therapy, 19*, 183–190.

Sanfilippo, L. (2019). *Yoga Therapy for Insomnia and Sleep Recovery.* Singing Dragon, London.

Taibi, D. M., & Vitiello, M. V. (2011). A pilot study of gentle yoga for sleep disturbance in women with osteoarthritis. *Sleep Medicine, 12*(5), 512–517.

Tsai, H. J., Kuo, T. B., Lee, G. S., & Yang, C. C. (2015). Efficacy of paced breathing for insomnia: Enhances vagal activity and improves sleep quality. *Psychophysiology, 52*(3), 388–396.

van Straten, A., van der Zweerde, T., Kleiboer, A., Cuijpers, P., Morin, C. M., & Lancee, J. (2018). Cognitive and behavioral therapies in the treatment of insomnia: A meta-analysis. *Sleep Medicine Reviews, 38*:3–16.

Wang, F., Eun-Kyoung Lee, O., Feng, F., Vitiello, M. V., Wang, W., Benson, H., Fricchione, G. L., & Denninger, J. W. (2016). The effect of meditative movement on sleep quality: A systematic review. *Sleep Medicine Reviews, 30*, 43–52.

Weintraub, A. (2004) *Yoga for Depression: A Compassionate Guide to Relieve Suffering through Yoga.* Broadway Books.

Woolfolk, R. L., Carr-Kaffashan, L., & McNulty, T. F. (1976). Meditation training as a treatment for insomnia. *Behavior Therapy, 7*, 359–365.

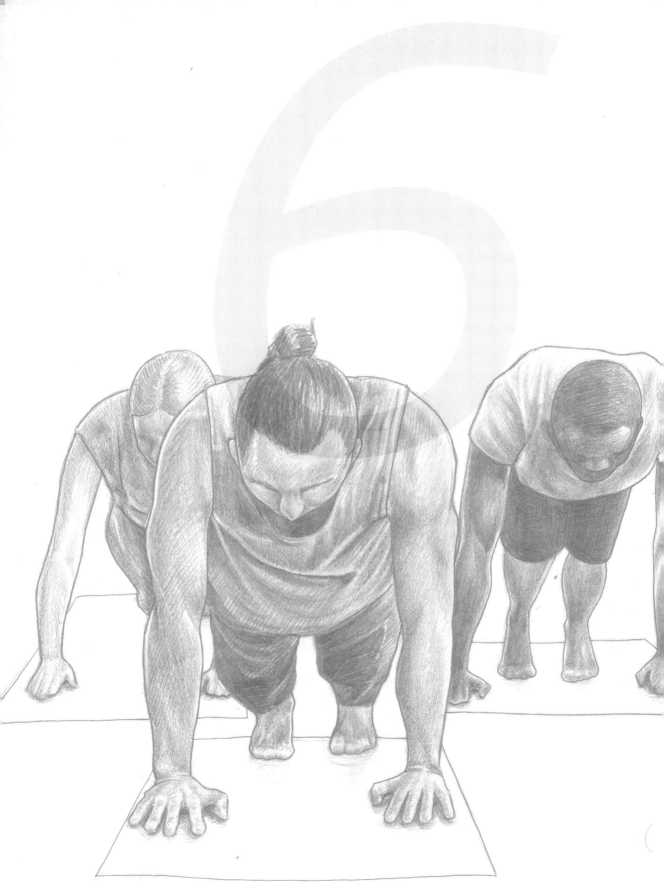

Trauma

Dana Moore and Daniel J. Libby

6

Overview

Trauma is the general term used to describe the negative consequences of the direct or indirect experience of an overwhelmingly distressing event such as an accident, assault, or natural disaster that involved actual or threatened death, serious injury, or sexual violence. The results of trauma include disabling symptoms across biological, cognitive, emotional, and spiritual domains. For many people, traumatic experiences adversely change their sense of who they are and how they relate to the world around them.

Studies estimate the rate of exposure to traumatic events as high as 90% in the general population (Breslau, 2002; Kilpatrick et al., 2013). Only a small proportion develop symptoms of posttraumatic stress disorder (PTSD), estimated to be around 6.8% to 7.8% of the US adult population (Kessler, Chiu, Demler, Merikangas, & Walters, 2005; Kilpatrick et al., 2013). Exposure to trauma is most closely associated with the development of PTSD, but it has also been linked to the development of other mental health conditions including depressive disorders, anxiety disorders, and addiction (Galea et al., 2002). The number, duration, and intensity of symptoms varies among individuals and depends on pretrauma factors (e.g., poor premorbid psychiatric functioning, previous traumatic events, poor social support, and low socioeconomic status), peritrauma factors (e.g., intensity and duration of the traumatic event, unpredictable and uncontrollable emotional response to the event, and perceived social support), and posttrauma factors (e.g., avoidant coping style and perceived social support) (Heron-Delaney, Quinn, Lee, Slater, & Pascalis, 2013; Ozer, Best, Lipsey, & Weiss, 2003).

Studies estimate the rate of exposure to traumatic events as high as 90% in the general population.

Although there is debate within the scientific community (Kamens, Elkins, & Robbins, 2017) about how best to represent the varied clinical presentations and experiences resulting from traumatic events, most of them fall into one of the four clusters of PTSD symptoms outlined by the *Diagnostic and Statistical Manual of Mental Disorders, Fifth Edition* (DSM-5) (American Psychiatric Association, 2013):

1. **Re-experiencing.** Trauma is associated with the experience of repeated intrusive memories, thoughts, and feelings related to the traumatic event(s). The intensity of these intrusions varies from being a repeated annoying distraction to a full re-experiencing of the trauma as if it were happening in the present moment (dissociative flashbacks). These symptoms often occur at night in the form of nightmares. Individuals often experience intensely distressing physiological and psychological reactions to these intrusive memories.

2. **Avoidance.** Trauma survivors engage in both conscious and unconscious avoidance of internal reminders (thoughts, feelings, and physical sensations) and external reminders (people, places, conversations, activities, objects, and situations) that might trigger the re-experiencing symptoms. This avoidance often becomes generalized so that fear responses related to the traumatic event are transferred to other non-related situations, resulting in increased withdrawal and isolation from the external world of

Chapter 6

people and places, as well as greater disconnection from the internal world of self and body.

3. **Alterations in arousal and reactivity**. The common link underlying many of the symptoms and co-occurrences of trauma is a fundamental inability to appropriately regulate physiological responses to incoming sensory stimuli. Individuals recovering from trauma often have difficulty maintaining physiological energy levels in a way that is context-appropriate and which supports goal-directed behavior, and instead alternates between states of hyperarousal and hypoarousal. This physiological dysregulation results in a smaller range of potential psychological or behavioral responses, those that are generally focused on defense, escape, avoidance, and retaliation. Common behavioral manifestations include irritable or aggressive behavior, reckless or self-destructive behavior, hypervigilance, exaggerated startle response, problems with concentration, and sleep disturbances.

4. **Negative changes in thought and mood**. Trauma symptoms also include persistent and exaggerated negative expectations about the self, others, and the world; persistent, distorted blaming of oneself or others about the cause(s) or consequences of the trauma; pervasive difficult emotions including fear, horror, anger, guilt, and shame; decreased interest and engagement in life activities; feeling detached and estranged from others; and a persistent inability to experience positive emotions. In addition, dissociative amnesia—an inability to remember parts or all of the traumatic event—is common, and ongoing dissociative symptoms are a defining feature in many individuals with PTSD (Lanius, Brand, Vermetten, Frewen, & Spiegel, 2012).

The experience of symptoms among trauma survivors is heterogeneous, and the four-symptom cluster model does not reflect the full range of experiences that people can have after trauma (van der Kolk, 2014). For example, the terms *complex trauma* and *complex PTSD* have been used to describe the experiences of individuals who have undergone prolonged, repeated, or inescapable trauma, often perpetrated by a caregiver or another trusted authority figure (Cook et al., 2017; Herman, 1992). Survivors of interpersonal trauma often experience more debilitation, including dissociative symptoms, and may require more intensive and different treatment approaches than those whose trauma was not interpersonal in nature (Forbes et al., 2014; Gershuny & Thayer, 1999). Up to 30% of individuals with PTSD meet the criteria for a dissociative subtype marked by states of depersonalization and derealization. These individuals tend to have greater functional impairment and are at a greater risk of suicide.

Childhood trauma

Although the DSM-5 includes a developmental subtype of PTSD called posttraumatic stress disorder in preschool children (American Psychiatric Association, 2013), the term *developmental trauma disorder* is increasingly being used to more accurately describe the clinical presentation of those who have survived adverse childhood events (van der Kolk, 2010). Individuals who experience trauma early in life often develop in a way that their lives and nervous systems become organized around the trauma, resulting in severe emotional and physiological dysregulation, attentional and behavioral dysregulation, and self- and relational dysregulation (van der Kolk, 2010). These children are likely to have lifelong challenges to their very basic sense of self, often leading to a range of psychological, emotional, and behavioral habits that evolve into personality disorders, eating disorders, and other psychiatric disorders (Ball & Links, 2009; Gershuny & Thayer, 1999). Results from the landmark ACE study (Felitti et al., 1998) of over 17,000 patient volunteers showed that trauma during childhood is associated with problems including learning and behavioral problems that persist into adulthood, resulting in higher rates of mental health disorders including chronic depression, high-risk health behaviors such as addiction, and suicidal behavior, as well as chronic medical diseases including chronic obstructive pulmonary disease (COPD), heart disease, cancer, and emphysema (Felliti et al., 1998).

Trauma and adult health

Regardless of age, trauma is associated with higher rates of medical and physical health problems (Byers, Covinsky, Neylan, & Yaffe, 2014; Pacella, Hruska, & Delahanty, 2013; Sareen et al., 2007; Schnurr & Jankowski, 1999) including pain (Lew, Tun, & Cifu, 2009), poor body awareness (van der Kolk, Pelcovitz, Roth, Mandel, McFarlane, & Herman, 1996), and digestive issues (Pacella, Hruska, & Delahanty, 2013). In addition, trauma is also associated with higher rates of affective, anxiety, and substance-use disorders (Brown, Campbell, Lehman, Crisham, & Mancill, 2001; Jacobsen, Southwick, & Kosten, 2001; Shalev et al., 2014), as well as decreased quality of life (Zatzick et al., 1997) and disability (Byers et al., 2014; Smith, Schnurr, & Rosenheck, 2005). These co-occurrences exacerbate symptoms and complicate treatment (Back, Sonne, Killeen, Danksy, & Brady, 2003; Brady & Clary, 2003; Cloitre & Koenen, 2001; Zlotnick, Mattia, & Zimmerman, 1999).

These common co-occurrences, combined with an inability to regulate the body's and/or mind's reactions to events and circumstances, often result in significant psychosocial challenges, including unemployment (Smith et al., 2005), legal troubles (Donley et al., 2012; Kubiak, 2004; Wilson & Zigelbaum, 1983), divorce (Kulka et al., 1990), and homelessness (O'Connell, Kasprow, & Rosenheck, 2008; Washington et al., 2010). For individuals who do not get help,

trauma increases the risk of suicide (Krysinska & Lester, 2010).

Development of symptoms

The path that leads from a traumatic event to the development of posttraumatic symptoms begins with an event that is perceived as unsafe, unpredictable, and uncontrollable. The nervous system then activates a defensive biobehavioral response marked by fight/flight behaviors or immobilization shutdown behaviors. If the event and the individual's own physical and mental responses to the event are overwhelming, they become unable to integrate the memories of the thoughts, images, sensations, and emotions experienced during the event into their existing view of the world and their relationship to it. These memories persist as implicit, behavioral, and somatic memories, dissociated from normal conscious experience, and are subsequently relived in the form of intrusive re-experiencing symptoms accompanied by ongoing defensive biobehavioral responses. The loss of control over physical and mental processes and the resulting emotional and behavioral responses are an intricate part of the traumatic experience. Consequently, people develop stress reactions not only to the event, but to their emotional, physical, and behavioral responses to the event, which may have been similarly experienced as being unsafe, unpredictable, and uncontrollable.

> The loss of control over physical and mental processes and the resulting emotional and behavioral responses are an intricate part of the traumatic experience.

The individual's continued efforts to understand the experience or to keep recollections of the experience outside of awareness leads to fragmented, incomplete, and disorganized personal narratives; increased allostatic load (Cicchetti, 2011); and increasingly negative changes in thought and mood. The continued automatic activation of defensive biobehavioral responses is interwoven with a continued perception of a threat in both the external environment (e.g., people, places and things) and in the internal environment (e.g., sensations, emotions, and thoughts).

Trauma and self-regulation

Traumatic events typically arouse one of two types of defensive biobehavioral response: fight/flight or behavioral shutdown/freeze. The fight/flight system involves activation of the sympathetic nervous system (SNS) in order to prepare the body for action—fleeing the threat or fighting back against it. The behavioral shutdown/freeze system involves the activation of the evolutionarily older (dorsal) branch of the vagus nerve, preparing the body to reduce metabolic activity for stillness to avoid detection or for dissociation. The type of defensive system that is engaged depends on many factors, including the individual's history of taking effective action.

PTSD is characterized by a perpetuation of this defensive and often disorganized biobehavior even in response to objectively unthreatening circumstances. The polyvagal theory, proposed by Stephen Porges (1995, 2011), explains these biobehavioral responses to stress and trauma as a means to understanding the ongoing dysregulation of physiological, cognitive, emotional, and behavioral processes we may observe in trauma survivors, and how yoga may help.

At any particular time, and in response to threat, the autonomic nervous system (ANS) coordinates all of the body's systems supporting distinct goal-directed behavior. The bimodal view of the ANS as consisting of an SNS and a peripheral nervous system (PNS) has evolved into an understanding that behaviors arise from various combinations of activation of one of the three divisions of the ANS. A number of global states (Porges, 2011) or preparatory sets (Payne & Crane-Godreau, 2015), with distinct patterns of autonomic, sensorimotor, affective, attentional, and cog-

nitive activity, can result from various combinations of activation of these three ANS branches. These coordinated processes are unconscious, largely automatic responses. Trauma survivors may display maladaptive behaviors due to a disorganized response among the various divisions of the ANS.

According to the polyvagal theory, the mammalian ANS functions hierarchically, such that more evolutionarily advanced systems regulate the phylogenetically older systems. The most evolutionarily advanced division of the ANS from which behavior can arise is the social engagement system. Mediated by activity in the ventral branch of the vagus nerve, the social engagement system brings human physiological arousal levels into a range that allows us to be present during social interaction and to engage in affiliative behaviors. During a potentially threatening event, the social engagement system supports "tend and befriend" behaviors such as protecting offspring and seeking social support (Taylor et al., 2000). In the absence of threat, this system recruits the physiological resources and neurological circuits that not only support social behavior but also support health, growth, and restoration. Activation of the social engagement system is associated with improved cognitive performance, adaptation, and health (Thayer et al., 2009).

At baseline levels of functioning, and in response to everyday challenges, many trauma survivors become unable to activate the social engagement neural network and instead experience a chronic activation of the fight/flight response. This involves activation of the SNS, supporting escape, defense, and retaliation behaviors; such hyperarousal is associated with hyperactivity of the amygdala, the part of the brain that mediates fear and anger. Over time the amygdala becomes hyperresponsive to both trauma-related and unrelated cues (Garfinkle & Liberzon, 2009), reflecting a generalization of the fear response. In addition to hyperreactivity in the circuits involved in the fear response, there is a relative deactivation in those areas of the brain responsible for inhibiting and extinguishing the fear response and preventing its generalization. For example, studies show functional hypoactivity in the hippocampus, ventromedial prefrontal cortex (vmPFC), ventral anterior cingulate cortex (vACC) and dorsal anterior cingulate cortex (dACC) (Etkin, Prater, Schatzberg, Menon, & Greicius, 2009; Garfinkle & Liberzon, 2009; Sherin & Nemeroff, 2011) and variations in neurotransmission, including decreases in the neurotransmitter GABA, which inhibits fear networks (e.g., Vaiva et al., 2004). In addition to manifesting directly as hyperarousal symptoms such as hypervigilance and exaggerated startle response, these biobehavioral responses contribute to the experience of the other clusters of symptoms, and inhibit internal regulatory and homeostatic mechanisms (Thayer et al., 2009).

> Yoga in particular may be an ideal practice for engaging the social engagement system and for reregulating the defensive biobehavioral responses that are at the root of posttraumatic stress.

Often when an event is life-threatening, especially when there is no opportunity for escape, the evolutionarily oldest branch of the ANS is activated, which is mediated by the dorsal vagal complex (DVC). This activation decreases physiological activity to support immobilization behaviors, including disengagement, freezing, and feigning death. For many trauma survivors, this branch of the ANS is dominant and manifests in symptoms such as anhedonia, flattened affect, and dissociation (Frewen & Lanius, 2006). Up to a third of people with PTSD exhibit decreased arousal in response to traumatic reminders, and individuals with the dissociative subtype of PTSD show increased activation of the rostral ACC and medial prefrontal cortex (mPFC), representing a hyperinhibition of active defensive responses (van der Kolk, 2004; Lanius et al., 2010).

Posttraumatic stress is marked by fundamentally dysregulated coordination of the systems people use to engage in goal-directed behaviors while managing environmental demands. Trauma survivors chronically respond to both ordinary and extraordinary challenges with defensive behaviors that interrupt the functioning of the cortical and subcortical circuits responsible for self-regulation, maintaining a coherent sense of self, and connecting with others (Damasio, 1999; Hayes, van Elzakker, & Shin, 2012; Porges, 2003; Sherin & Nemeroff, 2011). Recovery from trauma requires the reregulation of these response networks so that the appropriate neural resources are recruited to fit goal-directed behavior at the appropriate time. Yoga in particular may be an ideal practice for engaging the social engagement system and for reregulating the defensive biobehavioral responses that are at the root of posttraumatic stress.

Trauma recovery

The phase-oriented approach

The phase-oriented approach is the standard of care when it comes to the treatment of trauma (Figure 6.1) (Chu, 2011; van der Hart, Brown, & van der Kolk, 1989; van der Kolk, McFarlane, & van der Hart, 1996). This approach posits that recovery from trauma is most effectively achieved when recovery progresses in steps. Phase 1 goals are focused on safety, stabilization, self-regulation, and symptom reduction. Research suggests that the ability to regulate arousal is a prerequisite to recovery from trauma (Cloitre et al., 2010; Ford, Steinberg, & Zhang, 2011), and professional guidelines advocate an initial phase focused on somatic experience, affect regulation, and distress tolerance to improve outcomes (Cloitre et al., 2012). Phase 2 involves processing of the trauma—the purposeful remembering and re-understanding of the trauma, its circumstances, and its consequences—with the assistance of a licensed, trained professional. Phase 3 is focused on the evolution from posttraumatic stress to

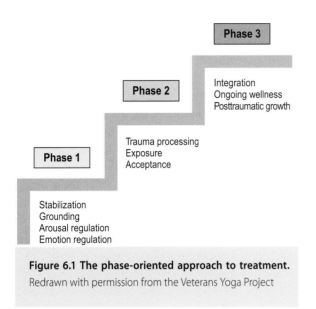

Figure 6.1 The phase-oriented approach to treatment.
Redrawn with permission from the Veterans Yoga Project

posttraumatic growth via the development of mission and purpose, focus on ongoing health and wellness, and reintegration into a day-to-day existence with resilient responses to the ordinary and extraordinary challenges life presents.

The limitations of psychotherapy

There are many psychotherapeutic treatments for trauma. The therapies with the most research support, prolonged exposure (PE) (Foa, Hembree, & Rothbaum, 2007), cognitive processing therapy (CPT) (Resick & Schnicke, 1993), trauma-focused cognitive behavioral therapy (TF-CBT) (Foa, Keane, & Friedman, 2000), and eye-movement desensitization and reprocessing (EMDR) (Shapiro & Forrest, 2001) are all evidence-based therapies, with meta-analyses showing very large effect sizes in clinical trials (Benish, Imel, & Wampold, 2008; Bradley, Greene, Russ, Dutra, & Westen, 2005). PE, CPT and TF-CBT are all trauma-focused interventions involving the processing of the traumatic memory or its meaning. They are cognitive-behavioral in nature and involve talking

about, writing about, or thinking about the memories to help extinguish the fear response that was learned during the traumatic event, in exchange for more effective and adaptive responses. Although not all treatment approaches involve direct focus on extinguishing the learned fear response (e.g., CBT without exposure; EMDR), these treatments are intended to allow the patient to process and integrate the memories of the thoughts, images, sensations, and emotions that had become cut off from conscious awareness.

Unfortunately, these treatments, and the research supporting their use, are limited (Olatunji, Deacon, & Abramowitz, 2009; Steenkamp, 2016; Yehuda & Hoge, 2016) in that they do not successfully treat all patients (Bradley et al., 2005). In fact, a majority of people who begin evidence-based psychotherapeutic therapies for PTSD drop out of treatment (Schottenbauer, Glass, Arnkoff, Tendick, & Gray, 2008). For those who do complete treatment, many are left with clinically significant residual symptoms even if they no longer meet the full criteria for PTSD. For example, up to half of all veterans who receive PE and CPT do not achieve clinically meaningful improvement (Steenkamp, Litz, Hoge, & Marmar, 2015).

In addition, there is scant evidence that these treatments are effective in treating complex trauma, developmental trauma disorder, or even PTSD in individuals who are also suffering from co-occurring psychiatric, medical, and substance-use disorders (Steenkamp, 2016). Furthermore, some patients have adverse reactions to exposure-based treatment, including worsening of symptoms, hospitalization, and drop-out from treatment (Steenkamp et al., 2015; Yehuda & Hoge, 2016).

The lack of attention to Phase 1 goals may be at the root of the limitations of evidence-based treatments for trauma. In practice, these psychotherapeutic treatments may not focus enough on the Phase 1 goals of self-regulation, grounding, interoceptive awareness, and development of coping skills that set the foundation for managing the overwhelming experience of trauma processing that is the goal of Phase 2, which is the crux of these treatments. Therefore, when survivors engage in Phase 2 purposeful exposure to trauma-related stimuli, they may lack the internal physiological, cognitive, and emotional resources required to stay grounded in the present moment, understand the effects of the trigger, and successfully integrate them into a cohesive sense of self with a past, present, and future.

Rationale for yoga in trauma recovery
A holistic approach

In her seminal work, *Trauma and Recovery*, Judith Herman (1992) writes, "To understand trauma you have to think like a theologian, a philosopher and a jurist." Now, thanks to the pioneering work on the psychobiology of trauma done by Bessel van der Kolk (2006, 2014), we know that we also have to think like a yoga teacher/therapist. Just as trauma has adverse effects across physiological, emotional, and cognitive domains, yoga has demonstrated healing and self-regulatory effects across those same domains (Gard, Noggle, Park, Vago, & Wilson, 2014). Several excellent comprehensive frameworks have been proposed to explain the ways that yoga may improve psychological wellness in the face of stress and trauma (Gard, Noggle et al., 2014; Payne & Crane-Godreau, 2015; Schmalzl, Powers, & Blom, 2015).

> Many individuals suffering from the symptoms of trauma turn to mind-body practices to treat their self-reported emotional and mental problems.

Many individuals suffering from the symptoms of trauma turn to mind-body practices to treat their self-reported emotional and mental problems (Libby, Pilver, & Desai, 2013). There has been an increase in the use of yoga in Veterans Administration (VA) PTSD treatment nationally, which appears to be propelled primarily by veteran preferences for CAM treatments (Libby, Pilver, & Desai, 2012; McPherson & Schwenka, 2004). In addition, yoga is attractive to those with avoidance symptoms because a self-administered CAM practice provides a greater sense of safety, predictability, and control than treatments that require regular contact with a treatment provider (Chaitow, 2013; Eisenberg et al., 1998; Libby, 2018; Libby et al., 2012). Even in yoga classes with other students, unlike in group therapy, individuals are able to navigate social interactions at a more natural pace. In other words, a trauma survivor can go to a yoga class and gain some of the benefit of social support without having to feel pressured to engage in social interactions with others.

Yoga and arousal regulation

The inability to regulate physiological arousal is a primary functional deficit among trauma survivors. The value of yoga in trauma treatment may largely be in its ability to help patients achieve Phase 1 goals of stabilization and self-regulation. Self-regulation includes ANS regulation and has been associated with psychological wellbeing (Chaitow, 2013; Gard, Noggle et al., 2014). Yoga practices lead to a more adaptive use of ANS states, and in particular a shift to activation of the VVC-social engagement system. This shift occurs during and immediately after the yoga practice, and with regular practice there is greater propensity toward remaining in that preparatory set as a baseline level of physiological regulation.

Yoga practice may also provide tools for speeding up recovery from a defensive response; for example, coming back to baseline more quickly after a triggered distressing memory. It is thought that yoga practice trains the ANS to be more dynamically adaptive to stressors, supporting coordinated responses of the body during stress to return to homeostasis (Streeter,

Gerbarg, Saper, Ciraulo, & Brown, 2012; Thayer and Sternberg, 2006). Many components of yoga, including conscious breathing, meditation, physical activity and relaxation, chanting, and social interaction, are associated with direct positive effects on physiological arousal via regulation of the ANS (Bernardi, Valle, Coco, Calciati, & Sleight, 1996; Delgado-Pastor, Perakakis, Subramanya, Telles, & Vila, 2013; Jerath, Edry, Barnes, & Jerath, 2006; Yackle et al., 2017). Over time, these yoga practices may lead to changes in neural functioning, including areas associated with the fear response and its inhibition. For example, a reduction in the size of the amygdala was found after eight weeks of daily mindfulness meditation (Holzel et al., 2010), and reduced activity of the amygdala was shown after twelve weeks of Iyengar yoga (Cohen et al., 2009). Similarly, mindfulness meditation has been associated with increases in hippocampal volume and activity (Gotink et al., 2016; Holzel, 2011; Luders et al., 2009; Pickut et al., 2013).

Top-down and bottom-up mechanisms

Emotions are processed by the nervous system via both top-down and bottom-up mechanisms. Thoughts and beliefs can generate and influence emotions, associated sensorimotor activity, and autonomic functioning (top-down) as when we mindfully return our attention to the breath after noticing the mind wandering during meditation. Conversely, autonomic functioning and sensorimotor activity can generate and influence emotions and associated cognitive activity (bottom-up), as when we extend our exhalation and experience the expanded thought–behavior repertoire that accompanies increased ventral–vagal parasympathetic activity. Trauma involves overwhelming experience in sensorimotor, emotional, and cognitive realms that often become fragmented when laid down in memory. Traumatic experiences are largely processed as a felt experience of sensations and perceptions in the body involving bottom-up sensory-based fear responses, rather than

cognitive constructs or coherent memories that can be verbally recalled. Similarly, ongoing posttraumatic symptoms are often experienced as bottom-up sensory-based emotional responses. Therefore, the use of cognitive top-down approaches may be less effective against triggered trauma-related sensorimotor experiences than approaches that integrate sensorimotor bottom-up processes.

Yoga practice develops coordination between top-down and bottom-up processes by facilitating improved integration of cortical executive control networks and subcortical autonomic functioning, which in turn leads to coordinated responses among musculoskeletal, autonomic, emotional/motivational, attentional, and cognitive/appraisal processes (Gard, Noggle et al., 2014; Payne & Crane-Godreau, 2015; Wells, Lang, Schmalzl, Groessl, & Strauss, 2016). Repeated use of VVC-enhancing practices creates implicit and procedural memories that can then operate unconsciously from a subcortical level (Roediger, 1990) as internal resources and capacities supporting goal-directed behavior and resilience to stress.

Yoga and avoidance

Avoidance is one of the primary symptom clusters of PTSD, and addressing avoidance is one of the first goals in the phase-oriented approach to treatment. Yoga practices may directly address the symptoms of avoidance by encouraging non-reactive awareness of the impulse to divert attention away from unpleasant internal or external stimuli. It then follows that not acting on the impulse toward avoidance can increase the ability to accept and experience thoughts, feelings, and sensations as they occur; they then become less overwhelming and the individual feels more in control (Dick et al., 2014).

The dissociative symptoms of trauma have been characterized as a type of avoidance coping strategy. A lack of body awareness and stunted movement patterns—forms of avoidance of feelings and sensations—are common among trauma survivors. The loss of a sense of integrated self may be a result of this lack of body awareness and movement (Damasio, 1999; Haselager et al., 2011). Mindfulness has been associated with activation of the midline structures of the brain associated with greater body awareness, further suggesting that yoga practices which decrease avoidance may lead to a greater sense of self (Brewer et al., 2011; Damasio, 1999).

Yoga and re-experiencing symptoms

The skills learned in yoga are important for coping with the defensive biobehavioral responses and impulses toward avoidance that accompany re-experiencing symptoms. This is especially important for the survivor who experiences an increase in those symptoms that accompany Phase 2: trauma-processing and integration. For the person in trauma recovery, the difficult work of cognitive/verbal processing of trauma memories with their mental health clinician is made easier by having the support of self-regulation skills. In other words, as bottom-up self-regulation resources are developed, top-down processes are freed up to perform the higher-order executive functions necessary for skillful, intentional responses, especially in stressful situations. These assist the patient in allowing contact with conditioned stimuli and in managing the discomfort that arises from that exposure. The ability to self-regulate may also lead to greater feelings of self-efficacy, propelling the treatment process and decreasing the likelihood of treatment dropout. Yoga practice may also provide those recovering from trauma time to integrate the therapeutic insights and changes that arise in psychotherapy or counseling.

Yoga may also support Phase 2 goals, with or without concurrent psychotherapeutic treatment, by extinguishing the neural associations between interoceptive and proprioceptive cues and the overwhelming sensorimotor, emotional, and cognitive

> Yoga practice may also provide those recovering from trauma time to integrate the therapeutic insights and changes that arise in psychotherapy or counseling.

experiences associated with the trauma. Yoga can be viewed as a type of cognitive-behavioral therapy that inherently affords opportunities for exposure-based extinction of fear responses to sensorimotor stimuli. Whereas trauma-focused treatment purposefully exposes the patient to stimuli that trigger reminders of the trauma, yoga practice allows traumatic triggers to arise in real time, in the natural flow of that person's moment-to-moment experience. When a yoga class or yoga therapy session is appropriately taught, the individual's experience unfolds in such a way that the nervous system can remain nondefensive while the teacher/therapist is helping to gently support the contextualization of experience. When anxiety-provoking stimuli (e.g., traumatic memories, unconscious proprioceptive cues) arise, they do so in an internal and external environment that encourages nonreactive mindful awareness. The learned association between the stimuli and trauma reaction may then be extinguished and the person experiences a state of openness and curiosity about their environment. Greater accurate interoception may be one bottom-up mechanism by which yoga facilitates the integration of traumatic experiences and subsequent reduction of intrusive symptoms (Mitchell et al., 2014; Payne, Levine, & Crane-Godreau, 2015). In other words, implicit sensory processes are conditioned to inhibit reactivity and promote calm active engagement.

Yoga and negative changes in thought and mood

Trauma changes the way we interpret perceptions of our most basic and often unconscious sensory experiences, including neuroceptive cues that help us to distinguish between safety and threat, which fundamentally changes our relationship to physical reality. After trauma, the brain manages perceptions so that they are interpreted through a more defensive lens. Recovery begins to occur when the brain re-organizes that relationship to sensations/perceptions via both top-down and bottom-up processes. Yoga practices including mindfulness are associated with increases in positive affect and decreases in negative affect (Engen & Singer, 2015; Killingsworth & Gilbert, 2010; Narasimhan, Nagarathna, & Nagendra, 2011; Pascoe & Bauer, 2015), which may be mediated in part by changes in neuroendocrine functioning (Carney, Cuddy, & Yap, 2010; Streeter et al., 2010, 2012). Yoga is also associated with improvements in cognitive functioning including attention, memory, and executive functioning (Froeliger, Garland, & McClernon, 2012; Gard, Taquet et al., 2014; Rocha et al., 2012).

In addition to providing the self-regulation skills necessary to support Phase 1 stabilization and Phase 2 processing, the practice of yoga can also support Phase 3 goals of integration, finding meaning and purpose, and post-traumatic growth, as well as ongoing health and wellness. Indeed, qualitative studies have found that yoga interventions go beyond the focus on symptoms to include the development of aspects of personal growth such as compassion toward the self, a greater awareness of the mind-body connection, a sense of empowerment, greater mental clarity, and acceptance of the self and others (Jindani & Khalsa, 2015; West, Liang, & Spinazzola, 2017).

Research overview

Research into the effects of yoga on trauma is in its infancy. There is solid evidence about the basic mechanisms of yoga and its ability to regulate the physiological dysfunctions that underlie trauma symptoms, as well as coherent models of how yoga may improve trauma symptoms (Gard, Noggle et al., 2014; Payne & Crane-Godreau, 2015; Schmalzl et al., 2015; Wells et al., 2016). However, there is less solid evidence from clinical trials demonstrating the ability of yoga to facilitate recovery from PTSD symptoms. Unfortunately, many studies examining the effectiveness of yoga do not meet the rigorous criteria that are required for inclusion in reviews and meta-analyses (e.g., West et al., 2002; Balasubramaniam, Telles, & Doraiswamy, 2013). In general, studies have shown that yoga is a promising intervention, but one that requires much more study.

There are many challenges to studying yoga as an intervention. There are many potential active ingredients in any particular yoga intervention and studies examining yoga and trauma use a wide variety of interventions and approaches, arising from the many different lineages of yoga.

In addition to the heterogeneity among treatment protocols, the study designs and methodologies in clinical trials vary greatly. For example, a major consideration for research and practice is that yoga may be an excellent complementary but insufficient alternative treatment for PTSD (c.f., Price et al., 2017). As suggested by the phase-oriented approach to recovery, yoga may be more suited to support more standard psychological treatments for PTSD, rather than replace them. Ultimately, this is an empirical question. The studies, both RCTs and uncontrolled trials, that have examined yoga as a treatment for trauma have used yoga as an alternative treatment (e.g., Streeter et al., 2010) or a complementary therapy (e.g., Price et al., 2017; van der Kolk et al., 2014) or they didn't describe or control for the effect of concurrent psychosocial treatments (e.g., Jindani, Turner, & Khalsa, 2015; Mitchell et al., 2014; Reinhardt et al., 2018; Thordardottir, Gudmundsdottir, Zoëga, Valdimarsdottir, & Gudmundsdottir, 2014).

In the field of yoga and yoga therapy, there is general agreement that yoga interventions for individuals with PTSD should be made trauma-sensitive (Emerson & Hopper, 2011; Emerson, Sharma, Chaudhry, & Turner, 2009; Libby, 2018; Wells et al., 2016; Horton, 2016). However, the extent to which yoga interventions are made trauma-sensitive in research trials has not been adequately measured. While some studies report adherence to trauma-sensitive principles, the extent to which this generally occurs is unknown. Future research should determine how to best assess the perceived sense of safety, predictability, and control on the part of the student during the yoga intervention, and the extent to which that influences outcomes.

Yoga is not traditionally seen as a short-term intervention. Most of the studies examining the effects of yoga on symptoms of PTSD have interventions that are twelve sessions or fewer. Longer term interventions may have a greater effect on outcomes. For example, Price et al. (2017) studied the effect of a 20-week trauma-sensitive yoga protocol for a small sample of female trauma survivors and found effect sizes comparable to evidence-based treatments for PTSD. Other studies indicate that symptoms improve over time with regular practice (e.g., Reinhardt et al., 2018).

In most of the RCTs that have found symptom improvement from yoga, that improvement has been modest, and it has not been greater than the active control group. Several uncontrolled studies have found clinically and statistically significant results (e.g., Price et al., 2017), but other studies have not (e.g., Staples, Hamilton, & Uddo, 2013). Descriptions of the results from several RCTs follow.

Van der Kolk et al. (2014) compared a trauma-sensitive yoga intervention consisting of ten weekly 60-minute trauma-sensitive yoga classes (n=31 of the 32 participants assigned to the yoga group completed the treatment and assessment) with a supportive talk therapy group (n=29/32) for a sample of women with chronic, treatment-resistant PTSD. Results showed that the yoga intervention led to significantly greater decreases in PTSD than the control group, both in terms of mean PTSD symptom severity and the percentage of participants no longer meeting diagnostic criteria for PTSD. Participants were required to be engaged in ongoing supportive therapy and continuing with whatever medications they were taking. A breakdown of symptom change by symptom cluster was not provided.

Mitchell et al. (2014) compared a Kripalu yoga intervention consisting of twelve weekly or six twice-weekly 75-minute classes adhering to trauma-sensitive principles (n=14/20) to an assessment control group of women with PTSD or subthreshold PTSD (n=12/18). The researchers found clinically significant decreases in symptoms in both groups, which were maintained at follow-ups after one month. Results show that the yoga group reported coping significantly better with their PTSD than those in the control group. The authors did not report whether participants were concurrently engaged in other therapies, or whether they were encouraged to practice yoga at home.

Jindani, Turner, and Khalsa (2015), in the largest RCT to examine yoga for PTSD, found greater decreases in PTSD symptoms in the yoga group (n=29/59) than in a wait-list control group (n=21/21) using a trauma-informed protocol that included eight weekly 90-minute Kundalini yoga classes and recommended home practice. In addition, 39% of the yoga group were involved in undescribed "other therapies." The authors did not report changes in symptoms by symptom cluster, although participants in the yoga condition did show positive changes in measures of sleep, positive affect, and perceived stress.

Another study (Thordardottir et al., 2014) compared a hatha yoga intervention consisting of twice-weekly 60-minute classes for six weeks (n=26/31) with a wait-list control (n=32/35) for a group of earthquake survivors in Iceland. Both groups showed significant reductions in symptoms. They did not report whether participants were engaged in other treatments, or if the yoga classes were trauma-informed.

Reinhardt et al. (2018) examined an intervention consisting of ten classes of weekly Kripalu yoga (n=14/20) compared with a no-treatment assessment control (n=12/18) in a sample of military veterans and active duty personnel. Results revealed decreases in PTSD symptoms in both groups that were not clinically or statistically significant.

Overall, evidence for the efficacy of yoga over active control groups is sparse. Most of the RCTs described earlier resulted in symptom improvement for both the yoga group and the active control group. The small sample sizes, in addition to the limitations described earlier, may underplay yoga's ability to support healing from posttraumatic stress.

In addition, a number of other studies have examined meditation or breathwork alone, or in conjunction with other psychosocial interventions for PTSD (e.g., Bormann et al., 2006; Seppälä et al., 2014; Simpson et al., 2007; Stankovic, 2011). These interventions share some commonalities with the various yoga styles that have been examined, in that they often have predictable beneficial effects for trauma recovery. Future dismantling research may help us understand how the various aspects of these mind-body programs, such as the relaxation effect and improvements in self-regulation, increased body awareness, and the capacity for mindfulness, may each influence recovery from trauma-related challenges.

Recommendations for practice

Just over a decade ago, David Emerson, Dana Moore, and Jody Carey developed Trauma-Sensitive Yoga at Bessel van der Kolk's Trauma Center in Boston. Since then many other yoga teachers and mental health professionals have followed their lead and developed trauma-sensitive yoga classes, protocols, and programs. There are trauma-sensitive yoga programs for specific populations such as veterans, prisoners, mental health hospital patients, and survivors of interpersonal violence and natural disasters. These programs are staffed by industry-leading practitioners and trainers who are highly specialized in teaching trauma-sensitive yoga to special populations. They have their own best practices, teaching principles, and theoretical guidelines (e.g., Emerson & Hopper, 2014; Libby, 2014; Miller, 2015; Horton, 2016). What they have in common is their dedication to using various yoga practices such as movement, meditation, and breathing to help individuals heal from trauma.

These programs fall into one of three types of trauma-sensitive yoga programs that range from an implicit to an explicit focus on trauma. The three types of trauma-sensitive yoga are (1) trauma-sensitive yoga teaching, (2) trauma-sensitive yoga classes, and (3) trauma-focused yoga therapy.

Understanding these three types of trauma-sensitive yoga will serve the field in at least three ways. First, this perspective will help instructors find the best teaching match for their training, aspirations, and what is required of them for more in-depth work with trauma and yoga. Second, referral sources like physicians, social workers, and mental health professionals can make better informed referrals for clients who would benefit from trauma-sensitive yoga. Third, this perspective will help people seeking trauma-sensitive yoga by themselves find the most appropriate type of experience.

> The three types of trauma-sensitive yoga are (1) trauma-sensitive yoga teaching, (2) trauma-sensitive yoga classes, and (3) trauma-focused yoga therapy.

Recommendations for practice that apply across the spectrum from general yoga classes taught in an implicit trauma-sensitive way to the most explicit trauma-focused yoga therapy can be captured by the cardinal therapeutic principle of all trauma healing: to help the survivor feel connected and empowered (Herman, 1992). Everything in a trauma-oriented yoga class/session should serve this principle. A trauma-informed yoga teacher makes decisions in each of the following dimensions during a yoga class to help the students feel connected and empowered: the teacher's language; their method of providing assists; the ways in which they support students to perform each yoga exercise; the class size/dynamics; how the teacher takes into account skill level, yoga experience, and physical health issues; the class environment; and the teacher's level of training. Each of these aspects of teaching yoga is made according to the spectrum of implicit to explicit focus on trauma (see Table 6.1).

Three types of trauma-oriented yoga

Trauma-oriented yoga can be taught along a spectrum from implicit to explicit trauma focus. At the implicit end of the spectrum, regular yoga classes are taught in a trauma-sensitive manner, but the teacher does not address trauma directly or ask for trauma history disclosure. At the explicit end, the teacher or health professional offers trauma-focused yoga therapy to individuals who self-identify as having a trauma history and who wish to use yoga to help heal themselves from trauma.

Trauma-sensitive yoga teaching

At the implicit end of the spectrum yoga classes are taught using trauma-sensitive guidelines: that is, given the prevalence of trauma in contemporary culture, the teacher assumes that one or more students in their class has a trauma history that could be exacerbated by experiences in the yoga class. By avoiding common trauma-symptom triggers, trauma-sensitive yoga teaching reduces the chances of traumatic memories arising during class. The teacher maintains focus on teaching a general yoga class and does not provide exercises intended to release trauma, process trauma, discharge energy, or in any other way attempt to facilitate trauma healing. The instructor presents a broad spectrum of movement, breathing, and meditative exercises to improve general health and wellbeing.

Teaching yoga with sensitivity to the potential trauma histories of students is best practice for any yoga teacher, and involves choices in eight domains of a trauma-sensitive yoga class:

(1) environment, (2) language, (3) student characteristics, (4) teacher characteristics, (5) class dynamics, (6) yoga practices, (7) assists, and (8) intention/purpose of the class.

Recommendations for trauma-sensitive yoga teaching

To make a regular yoga class trauma-sensitive, the teacher practices the following principles and guidelines:

- Maintains professional boundaries inside and outside of class.

- Avoids language that contains sexual innuendo and direct or indirect reference to sex, erogenous zones, or close associations to sex.

- Empowers students to learn from their own experiences rather than using a controlling

Table 6.1

Comparison of trauma-oriented yoga ranging from implicit to explicit focus

	Implicit ⟶ Explicit		
	General yoga classes taught with trauma-sensitivity	**Trauma-sensitive yoga classes/sessions offered to special populations with trauma histories**	**Trauma-focused yoga therapy**
Recommendations for teacher training	Basic yoga teacher certification Trauma-sensitive yoga teaching training	Basic yoga teacher certification Trauma-sensitive yoga teaching training Trauma-sensitive yoga class training	Basic yoga teacher certification and trauma-focused yoga therapy training and traumatic stress training. Examples include Traumatic Stress studies at The Trauma Center at JRI, Somatic Experiencing®, or commensurate training in traumatology Graduate degree and license in counseling, social work, psychology, and training in trauma-focused yoga therapy Supervision by a licensed mental health clinician
Venue	Yoga studios, YMCAs, corporate locations, private homes, parks, community centers	Prisons, shelters, clinics, yoga therapy studios, healthcare settings (e.g., recreational therapy)	Prisons, shelters, clinics, yoga therapy studios, healthcare settings (e.g., mental health treatment)
Participants' characteristics	General yoga population	Individuals with known or suspected trauma histories Students may be experiencing acute symptoms and may be working with other helping agencies	Individuals with known or suspected trauma histories. Students are likely to be experiencing acute symptoms and may be working with other helping agencies
Purpose of the class/session	General health and wellbeing	General health and wellbeing Improvement in the management of symptoms throughout daily activities	Contribute to trauma recovery in all three phases
Exercises	Beginner to advanced levels Comprehensive for complete physical conditioning Modified as necessary for each student Supported by props Follow a three-phase arc: warm-up, work-out, cool-down	Beginner level As comprehensive as possible for complete physical conditioning Modified as necessary for each student Supported by props Follow a three-phase arc: warm-up, work-out, cool-down	Beginner level Focused on trauma healing objectives, the establishment of Phase 1 goals including safety, predictability, and control in internal and external realms Modified as necessary for each student Supported by props Follow a three-phase arc: warm-up, work-out, cool-down

Table 6.1 Continued

Assists	The use of touch with trauma survivors should be thought about with great care and attention. Insensitive use of physical assists can induce hyperarousal symptoms, dissociative symptoms, feelings of anger or paranoia, or other adverse reactions. While physical assists have the potential for therapeutic value in the form of improving alignment, reducing risk of injury, and assisting in opening, stretching, and strengthening, this may only be possible when a trusting therapeutic alliance has been established between the teacher and student, and the student has given explicit consent. Modeling the practice and using verbal assists can limit the need to offer physical assists. Depending on the type of class and the location, it is often most appropriate to have a no-touch policy		
	Ask permission at the beginning of class and, if needed, before each physical assist	Announce to the class whether physical assists will be used, and if so, how	Announce to the class whether physical assists will be used, and if so, how
	Use visual and verbal assists first	Use visual and verbal assists first	Use visual and verbal assists first
	Use the press-point method regularly and the manipulative assist method sparingly	Ask permission before each physical assist	Ask permission before each physical assist
		Use the press-point method regularly and the manipulative assist method more sparingly	Use the press-point method regularly but never the manipulative assist method
	Provide safety assists as needed, deepening and feel-good assists sparingly	Provide safety assists as needed, only provide deepening and feel-good assists if there is strong rapport with the student	Provide safety assists as needed, only provide deepening and feel-good assists if there is strong rapport with the student
Class dynamics	Arrange space between mats so touching a neighbor is difficult and rare	Same as in a general class with these additions:	Same as in a general class and a trauma-sensitive class with these additions:
	Teacher avoids walking around extensively, especially during postures that expose the pelvis, chest, buttocks	Consider mat arrangement where no one is directly behind someone else, and the exits are visible	Consider mat arrangement where no one is directly behind someone else, and the exits are visible
	Students move together in synchronized breathing and moving	Teacher walks around minimally and intentionally	Teacher walks around minimally and intentionally
	Students have time to perform self-selected exercises	Small to medium class size	Teacher walks around only to provide assists or other support
		Institution staff might be present	Small-to-medium class size
			Primary treatment provider could be the yoga teacher
Language	Teacher uses trauma-sensitive language	Teacher uses trauma-sensitive language	Teacher uses trauma-sensitive language
		Teacher may use nature images and metaphor	Teacher may use nature images and metaphor
		Intentional use of silence to support the practice	Intentional use of silence to support the practice
			Yoga therapists may verbalize how the practice can be used to improve symptoms

teaching style that requires students to follow instructions and perform for the teacher.

- Treats each student with equal respect and provides the same teaching service to every student.

- Uses physical assists only for safety and to empower students to maintain control of their bodies.

- Cultivates connection and rapport with students by precisely fulfilling the many mini-contracts they present to students throughout class, for example "Take five more breaths," "Focus your attention on sensations in your body," and "We will be in this posture for three minutes." When the teacher makes such a contract and then fails to fulfill it, there is a break in rapport between teacher and students. A traumatized student could lose connection with the teacher and may not return to class.

- Provides a lightly guided *savasana* (resting pose) to support relaxation and minimize rumination and agitation.

Trauma-sensitive yoga classes

Whereas trauma-sensitive yoga teaching is used in open classes, trauma-sensitive yoga classes are provided explicitly for those suffering from posttraumatic (and current) stress. Such classes occur in places where teachers can receive support, such as prisons, hospitals, clinics, shelters, refugee camps, and post-disaster areas. Although the class is for those with trauma, the yoga teacher does not focus the class on alleviating or coping with symptoms.

Recommendations for trauma-sensitive yoga classes

The teacher

- presents fewer exercises than a general yoga class, making the assumption is that it is often

harder for those with trauma to follow complex yoga instructions because it takes time to forge connection with the body

- supports students to perform each exercise by offering efficient, clear, and predictable verbal guidance

- prioritizes exercises that synchronize breathing and movement, to promote awareness of the mind-body connection

- teaches yogic techniques that specifically promote ANS flexibility as understood from a neuroscientific perspective

- provides opportunities for students to make choices about how they perform the exercises, for example, choosing the right level of challenge or modification option, changing speed or intensity, improving the quality of their movement: this serves as an inroad to developing greater personal agency

- encourages students to explore the challenges and benefits of practicing a variety of exercises with their eyes open and closed: closing the eyes presupposes a feeling of safety within the surroundings

- reserves pelvis-exposing exercises such as the happy baby pose for later stages of trauma healing, when students demonstrate comfort with their bodies in various ways

- maintains calm energy in the class and keeps pace with students' abilities

- cultivates qualities of therapeutic alliance, for instance empathy for the burden of suffering many traumatized people experience, unconditional positive regard for each student equally, and authenticity, presenting themselves as a genuine person rather than projecting an image of a perfect person or yoga teacher

- maintains professional boundaries to avoid confusion for students and to support a safe space, limits periods of silence—the teacher's voice is often an anchor that prevents overwhelming traumatic memories from arising

- announces to the class when they will be moving around the room

- monitors the room often by walking around slowly to see if students are calm or at the edge of being triggered

- provides competent support for a student in distress (see later).

Trauma-focused yoga therapy classes

These classes are specifically designed for students seeking healing from trauma through yoga. The rationale is that the practices may help to transform both psychological and physiological responses in a targeted way. Class size is limited so that the teacher can focus on individual needs and will conduct a brief intake interview with each student prior to class. Due to the level of expertise required to safely and effectively teach this way, more training is needed. Accordingly, classes can be taught by a licensed mental healthcare provider who is either also a certified yoga instructor with training in yoga for trauma or by a trained yoga therapist who also has extra training in yoga for trauma. This type of class directly addresses broad trauma therapy objectives such as self-care, self-regulation, and self-awareness. Students are offered psychoeducation regarding the efficacy of practices and taught how to use them on and off the mat toward their healing. Breathing practices, moving and meditative exercises that have specific effects on the nervous system, psychological systems, and states of consciousness may be taught. Students in these classes must complement the deep work done in such classes with additional psychotherapeutic support, to help them process material that will arise in or as a result of class.

Trauma-informed yoga therapy sessions

In addition to trauma-focused yoga therapy classes, certified yoga therapists with additional training in trauma studies may offer one-to-one sessions to trauma survivors as part of a more extensive treatment plan. This allows for more personalized work, conducted with the support and insight of a comprehensive mental health team. Working in such ways without external support would usually be outside the scope of practice of a yoga therapist, but here they can align their yoga therapeutic approach with Phase 1 trauma-healing goals: safety, stability, and ultimately connection and empowerment.

The ability to effectively guide a trauma survivor through the process of accessing, discharging, and integrating previously dissociated traumatic content requires a special set of competencies. Yoga therapists without adequate training and support from mental health professionals should refrain from venturing into Phase 2 trauma-treatment territory. After a strong rapport has been established and with the necessary groundwork in place, a specially trained yoga therapist may enter this terrain with caution, and ideally with the support from a mental health treatment team.

> The ability to effectively guide a trauma survivor through the process of accessing, discharging, and integrating previously dissociated traumatic content requires a special set of competencies.

If through this process a client experiences a strong traumatic memory, the yoga therapist should normalize the experience as a common trauma reaction and support the student in a way that is uniquely suited to that individual. Furthermore, the well-trained yoga therapist has a set of potent skills to help regulate a client in distress and to help them through the process. If, however, in the rare event that they become a danger to themselves, to another person or to property, then the teacher informs the client that they are obliged to call their local emergency agency.

In summary, we recommend that yoga therapists who work with trauma

- acquire training in traumatic stress

- follow the recommendations for practice for teaching trauma-sensitive yoga classes as defined above

- be familiar with the different interpersonal dynamics of teaching trauma-sensitive to a group and offering yoga therapy to a single individual

- consult with a supervisor or peer-supervision group regularly

- remain within their scope of practice and training.

Trauma-informed yoga therapy in an individual psychotherapy session

As holistic perspectives continue to settle into modern culture, increasing numbers of mental health professionals who provide treatment to traumatized clients include yoga practices such as movement, meditation, and breathing exercises in their sessions. Four ways that mental health therapists with clinical yoga training provide yoga exercises during an individual psychotherapy session are (1) at the beginning of a session

to help the client transition from previous activities to be more present for the session; (2) at the end of a session to help the client transition from the therapy session to their next activity; (3) as the primary theme of a psychotherapy session focusing on, for example, a yoga practice for self-care; and (4) as an intervention during a psychotherapy session to help the client modulate ANS balance.

Mental health professionals who are trained in somatically oriented therapies for trauma such as Somatic Experiencing® (Levine, 1997) and Sensorimotor Psychotherapy (Ogden & Minton, 2000) will find many areas that overlap with trauma-informed yoga. These are forms of therapy utilizing, in part, the natural, biological processes that animals possess when responding to traumatic stress. When the natural processes within an individual are allowed to follow their course they help return the organism to a more neutral state. A central aspect of both of these therapies is enabling the client to track sensation in their body and allowing the sensation to inform a behavioral response.

Although a mental health practitioner without yoga teacher training should not teach complex yoga asanas, helping patients utilize their bodies within their normal range of motion can be very useful. Basic yoga postures are ways of holding our bodies. For example, simple yoga postures like seated or standing mountain pose can be very effective for grounding and self-regulation. Mental health professionals can also teach some basic breathing practices, such as elongating the exhalation or abdominal breathing to help support regulation in the ANS.

Recommendations for practice in trauma-focused psychotherapy

Mental health professionals should

- clearly explain the clinical rationale for including yoga in a treatment plan;

- follow the same recommendations for practice that apply to teaching a trauma-sensitive yoga class; and

- develop sources of professional support from peers and supervisors, as well as yoga therapists.

Students in distress

Key principles:

1. **Prevention**. Teachers provide students with choice-making opportunities throughout the class to keep the students connected and empowered. A student is less likely to become distressed when they feel in control of their experience without pressure to perform to the teacher's standard. Teachers scan the class continuously and track each person in the class so they can notice as early as possible a student becoming distressed. The earlier the teacher intervenes then the less likely it is that the student will become so distressed that they cannot continue the class.

2. **Less-to-more intervention**. The best intervention is often no intervention. Holding the space by allowing students to have their own experiences without interruption can be valuable and empowering. In other cases, the teacher might first make comments to the entire class hoping the student in distress will hear what is said and self-regulate. Making eye contact and continuing to teach the class is one way to communicate to the student that you are there to provide support, but that you are also maintaining your responsibility to the rest of the class. Making direct interpersonal contact with the individual in distress can be used when less direct methods have been insufficient.

3. **Protection**. The teacher does all they can to keep the class going while attending to the student in distress, who is at risk of experiencing intense shame if their distress becomes the focus of the group, particularly so if the class is impacted by their experience.

4. **Help the student regain control**. A student in a dysregulated state is feeling unsafe and is sometimes unpredictable and out of control. The role of the teacher is to help the student re-establish those qualities inside themselves and gain a measure of equilibrium.

Absolute contraindications for all trauma-sensitive yoga settings

Important precautions have been included in the preceding sections. However, if any of the following contraindications are present, the teacher must refuse the student participation in class, refer them to a healthcare provider, or call their local emergency medical system:

- alcohol or illicit drug intoxication

- active psychosis

- derealization/depersonalization

- intense physical pain

- actively suicidal, self-harming, or threatening to harm others

- unmedicated schizophrenia with active symptoms.

Supporting recovery from trauma

Recovering from trauma is a personal journey for each individual. As a result of trauma, a person may lose their basic sense of self, their ability to connect with others, and the knowledge of their place in the world. No one else can fix that. The best that providers can do is be present and available to assist each individual in their journey. As described in this chapter, generally, that means something different for a yoga teacher, a yoga therapist, and a mental health clinician. Nevertheless, the accepted understanding of recovery from trauma requires providers to hold the space and to share the practice. Any particular symptom may arise due to a combination of functional deficits in autonomic, cognitive, or emotional donations. A balanced yoga practice that focuses on whole-person health, wellness, recovery, and resilience will likely more effective than a yoga practice designed to target a specific symptom or cluster of symptoms. This can be achieved by helping students and clients learn the various tools they might find helpful for particular symptoms and empowering them to discover for themselves which tools best meet their needs in any given situation.

> A balanced yoga practice that focuses on whole-person health, wellness, recovery, and resilience will likely more effective than a yoga practice designed to target a specific symptom or cluster of symptoms.

Future directions

The modern field of yoga for trauma is in its infancy, but is growing rapidly. The basis of providing yoga for trauma is to create the conditions for healing to occur. Through all aspects of the yoga encounter, we empower our students to connect with their own thoughts, feelings, and sensations in a way that fosters the body's and the mind's innate homeostatic and healing abilities.

Increasingly, yoga is being integrated into mental healthcare settings. In the field of yoga, teachers and yoga therapists can best prepare themselves by obtaining adequate training. This training should include an understanding of trauma and posttraumatic stress, the mechanisms by which yoga facilitates recovery, the specific practices that have been found to be helpful, and the particular approaches that make yoga safer and more effective for those recovering from trauma. The emergence of yoga therapy as a field will bring important questions about the scope of practice and the limits of yoga for the treatment of mental health disorders. In addition, the field will advance because there is an increasing awareness of the different types of trauma-sensitive yoga being applied in a variety of settings, ranging from yoga studios, to prisons, to healthcare settings. The field will also advance with the inclusion of mental health professionals educating themselves on the value of yoga in trauma recovery and incorporating basic principles into their clinical practice or collaborating with a yoga teacher/therapist.

There is an increasing amount of quality research examining the use of yoga for trauma, including biological studies to understand the neural and physiological mechanisms underlying yoga practices. There will also be attempts to understand which practices are most effective for particular symptoms. As the research accumulates on which aspects of yoga may be more important for trauma recovery, it will be important not to lose sight of the holistic nature of a practice that has integrated European traditions of calisthenics, gymnastics, and military training with the medieval Indian tradition of hatha yoga (Singleton, 2010).

Each of our students and clients has a unique story, presentation, and path to health and wellness. When we are providing yoga for trauma, it is important to remember that we are really providing yoga for this individual or a group of individuals. If we focus on their experience and maintain open communication from a place of unconditional positive regard, our students will guide us in our efforts to support their recovery.

References

American Psychiatric Association (2013). *Diagnostic and Statistical Manual of Mental Disorders, Fifth Edition*. Arlington, VA: American Psychiatric Publishing.

Back, S. E., Sonne, S. C., Killeen, T., Dansky, B. S., & Brady, K. T. (2003). Comparative profiles of women with PTSD and comorbid cocaine or alcohol dependence. *The American Journal of Drug and Alcohol Abuse*, *29*(1), 169–189.

Balasubramaniam, M., Telles, S., & Doraiswamy, P. M. (2013). Yoga on our minds: a systematic review of yoga for neuropsychiatric disorders. *Frontiers in Psychiatry*, *3*, 117.

Ball, J. S., & Links, P. S. (2009). Borderline personality disorder and childhood trauma: Evidence for a causal relationship. *Current Psychiatry Reports*, *11*(1), 63–68.

Benish, S. G., Imel, Z. E., & Wampold, B. E. (2008). The relative efficacy of bona fide psychotherapies for treating post-traumatic stress disorder: A meta-analysis of direct comparisons. *Clinical Psychology Review*, *28*(5), 746–758.

Bernardi, L., Valle, F., Coco, M., Calciati, A., & Sleight, P. (1996). Physical activity influences heart rate variability and very-low-frequency components in Holter electrocardiograms. *Cardiovascular Research*, *32*(2), 234–237.

Bormann, J. E., Gifford, A. L., Shively, M., Smith, T. L., Redwine, L., Kelly, A., Becker, S., Gershwin, M., Bone, P., & Belding, W. (2006). Effects of spiritual mantram repetition on HIV outcomes: A randomized controlled trial. *Journal of Behavioral Medicine*, *29*(4), 359–376.

Bradley, R., Greene, J., Russ, E., Dutra, L., & Westen, D. (2005). A multidimensional meta-analysis of psychotherapy for PTSD. *American Journal of Psychiatry*, *162*(2), 214–227.

Brady, K. T., & Clary, C. M. (2003). Affective and anxiety comorbidity in post-traumatic stress disorder treatment trials of sertraline. *Comprehensive Psychiatry*, *44*(5), 360–369.

Breslau, N. (2002). Epidemiologic studies of trauma, posttraumatic stress disorder, and other psychiatric disorders. *The Canadian Journal of Psychiatry*, *47*(10), 923–929.

Brewer, J. A., Worhunsky, P. D., Gray, J. R., Tang, Y. Y., Weber, J., & Kober, H. (2011). Meditation experience is associated with differences in default mode network activity and connectivity. *Proceedings of the National Academy of Sciences*, *108*(50), 20254–20259.

Brown, T. A., Campbell, L. A., Lehman, C. L., Grisham, J. R., & Mancill, R. B. (2001). Current and lifetime comorbidity of the DSM-IV anxiety and mood disorders in a large clinical sample. *Journal of Abnormal Psychology*, *110*(4), 585.

Byers, A. L., Covinsky, K. E., Neylan, T. C., & Yaffe, K. (2014). Chronicity of posttraumatic stress disorder and risk of disability in older persons. *JAMA Psychiatry*, *71*(5), 540–546.

Carney, D. R., Cuddy, A. J., & Yap, A. J. (2010). Power posing: Brief nonverbal displays affect neuroendocrine levels and risk tolerance. *Psychological Science*, *21*(10), 1363–1368.

Chaitow, L. (2013). *Muscle Energy Techniques*. London, UK: Churchill Livingstone.

Chu, J. A. (2011). *Rebuilding Shattered Lives: Treating Complex PTSD and Dissociative Disorders*. Hoboken, NJ: John Wiley & Sons.

Cicchetti, D. (2011). Allostatic load. *Development and Psychopathology*, *23*(3), 723.

Cloitre, M., Courtois, C. A., Ford, J. D., Green, B. L., Alexander, P., Briere, J., & Van der Hart, O. (2012, November 5). *The ISTSS expert consensus treatment guidelines for complex PTSD in adults*. Retrieved from https://www.istss.org/ISTSS_Main/media/Documents/ISTSS-Expert-Concesnsus-Guidelines-for-Complex-PTSD-Updated-060315.pdf.

Cloitre, M., & Koenen, K. C. (2001). The impact of borderline personality disorder on process group outcome among women with posttraumatic stress disorder related to childhood abuse. *International Journal of Group Psychotherapy*, *51*(3), 379–398.

Cloitre, M., Stovall-McClough, K. C., Nooner, K., Zorbas, P., Cherry, S., Jackson, C. L., Gan, W., & Petkova, E. (2010). Treatment for PTSD related to childhood abuse: A randomized controlled trial. *American Journal of Psychiatry*, *167*(8), 915–924.

Cohen, D. L., Wintering, N., Tolles, V., Townsend, R. R., Farrar, J. T., Galantino, M. L., & Newberg, A. B. (2009). Cerebral blood flow effects of yoga training: Preliminary evaluation of 4 cases. *The Journal of Alternative and Complementary Medicine*, *15*(1), 9–14.

Cook, A., Spinazzola, J., Ford, J., Lanktree, C., Blaustein, M., Cloitre, M., DeRosa, R., Hubbard, R., Kagan, R., Liautaud, J., & Mallah, K. (2017). Complex trauma in children and adolescents. *Psychiatric Annals*, *35*(5), 390–398.

Damasio, A. R. (1999). *The Feeling of What Happens: Body and Emotion in the Making of Consciousness*. New York: Harcourt Brace.

Delgado-Pastor, L. C., Perakakis, P., Subramanya, P., Telles, S., & Vila, J. (2013). Mindfulness (Vipassana) meditation: Effects on P3b event-related potential and heart rate variability. *International Journal of Psychophysiology*, *90*(2), 207–214.

Dick, A. M., Niles, B. L., Street, A. E., DiMartino, D. M., & Mitchell, K. S. (2014). Examining mechanisms of change in a yoga intervention for women: The influence of mindfulness, psychological flexibility, and emotion regulation on PTSD symptoms. *Journal of Clinical Psychology*, *70*(12), 1170–1182.

Donley, S., Habib, L., Jovanovic, T., Kamkwalala, A., Evces, M., Egan, G., Bradley, B., & Ressler, K. J. (2012). Civilian PTSD symptoms and risk for involvement in the criminal justice system. *The Journal of the American Academy of Psychiatry and the Law*, *40*(4), 522.

Eisenberg, D. M., Davis, R. B., Ettner, S. L., Appel, S., Wilkey, S., Van Rompay, M., & Kessler, R. C. (1998). Trends in alternative medicine use in the United States, 1990–1997: Results of a follow-up national survey. *JAMA*, *280*(18), 1569–1575.

Emerson, D., & Hopper, E. (2011). *Overcoming trauma through yoga: Reclaiming your body*. Berkeley, CA: North Atlantic Books.

Emerson, D., Sharma, R., Chaudhry, S., & Turner, J. (2009). Trauma-sensitive yoga: Principles, practice, and research. *International Journal of Yoga Therapy*, 19(1), 123–128.

Engen, H. G., & Singer, T. (2015). Compassion-based emotion regulation up-regulates experienced positive affect and associated neural networks. *Social Cognitive and Affective Neuroscience*, 10(9), 1291–1301.

Etkin, A., Prater, K. E., Schatzberg, A. F., Menon, V., & Greicius, M. D. (2009). Disrupted amygdalar subregion functional connectivity and evidence of a compensatory network in generalized anxiety disorder. *Archives of General Psychiatry*, 66(12), 1361–1372.

Felitti, V. J., Anda, R. F., Nordenberg, D., Williamson, D. F., Spitz, A. M., Edwards, V., Koss, M. P., & Marks, J. S. (1998). Relationship of childhood abuse and household dysfunction to many of the leading causes of death in adults. The Adverse Childhood Experiences (ACE) Study. *American Journal of Preventive Medicine*, 14(4), 245–258.

Foa, E. B., Hembree, E. A., & Rothbaum, B. O. (2007). *Prolonged exposure therapy for PTSD: Emotional processing of traumatic experiences. Therapist guide.* New York: Oxford University Press.

Foa, E. B., Keane, T. M., & Friedman, M. J. (2000). Guidelines for treatment of PTSD. *Journal of traumatic stress*, 13(4), 539–588.

Forbes, D., Lockwood, E., Phelps, A., Wade, D., Creamer, M., Bryant, R. A., McFarlane, A., Silove, D., Rees, S., Chapman, C., Slade, T., Mills, K., Teesson, M., & O'Donnell M. (2014). Trauma at the hands of another: Distinguishing PTSD patterns following intimate and nonintimate interpersonal and noninterpersonal trauma in a nationally representative sample. *The Journal of Clinical Psychiatry*, 75(2), 147–153.

Ford, J. D., Steinberg, K. L., & Zhang, W. (2011). A randomized clinical trial comparing affect regulation and social problem-solving psychotherapies for mothers with victimization-related PTSD. *Behavior Therapy*, 42(4), 560–578.

Frewen, P. A., & Lanius, R. A. (2006). Toward a psychobiology of posttraumatic self-dysregulation. *Annals of the New York Academy of Sciences*, 1071(1), 110–124.

Froeliger, B., Garland, E. L., & McClernon, F. J. (2012). Yoga meditation practitioners exhibit greater gray matter volume and fewer reported cognitive failures: Results of a preliminary voxel-based morphometric analysis. *Evidence-Based Complementary and Alternative Medicine*. Advance online publication.

Galea, S., Ahern, J., Resnick, H., Kilpatrick, D., Bucuvalas, M., Gold, J., & Vlahov, D. (2002). Psychological sequelae of the September 11 terrorist attacks in New York City. *New England Journal of Medicine*, 346(13), 982–987.

Gard, T., Noggle, J. J., Park, C. L., Vago, D. R., & Wilson, A. (2014). Potential self-regulatory mechanisms of yoga for psychological health. *Frontiers in Human Neuroscience*, 8, 770.

Gard, T., Taquet, M., Dixit, R., Hölzel, B. K., de Montjoye, Y. A., Brach, N., Salat, D. H., Dickerson, B. C., Gray, J. R., & Lazar, S. W. (2014). Fluid intelligence and brain functional organization in aging yoga and meditation practitioners. *Frontiers in Aging Neuroscience*, 6, 76.

Garfinkle, S. N., & Liberzon, I. (2009). Neurobiology of PTSD: A review of neuroimaging findings. *Psychiatric Annals*, 39(6), 370.

Gershuny, B. S., & Thayer, J. F. (1999). Relations among psychological trauma, dissociative phenomena, and trauma-related distress: A review and integration. *Clinical Psychology Review*, 19(5), 631–657.

Gotink, R. A., Meijboom, R., Vernooij, M. W., Smits, M., & Hunink, M. M. (2016). 8-week mindfulness based stress reduction induces brain changes similar to traditional long-term meditation practice–a systematic review. *Brain and Cognition*, 108, 32–41.

Haselager, W. F. G., Broens, M. C., & Gonzalez, M. E. Q. (2012). The importance of sensing one's movement in the world for the sense of personal identity. *Rivista internazionale di Filosofia e Psicologia*, 1–11.

Hayes, J. P., van Elzakker, M. B., & Shin, L. M. (2012). Emotion and cognition interactions in PTSD: a review of neurocognitive and neuroimaging studies. *Frontiers in Integrative Neuroscience*, 6, 89.

Herman, J. L. (1992). *Trauma and Recovery* (pp. 34–35). New York: Basic Books.

Heron-Delaney, M., Quinn, P. C., Lee, K., Slater, A. M., & Pascalis, O. (2013). Nine-month-old infants prefer unattractive bodies over attractive bodies. *Journal of Experimental Child Psychology*, 115(1), 30–41.

Hölzel, B. K., Carmody, J., Vangel, M., Congleton, C., Yerramsetti, S. M., Gard, T., & Lazar, S. W. (2011). Mindfulness practice leads to increases in regional brain gray matter density. *Psychiatry Research: Neuroimaging*, 191(1), 36–43.

Horton, C. (Ed.) (2016). *Best Practices for Yoga with Veterans.* Atlanta, GA: YSC-Omega Publications.

Jacobsen, L. K., Southwick, S. M., & Kosten, T. R. (2001). Substance use disorders in patients with posttraumatic stress disorder: a review of the literature. *American Journal of Psychiatry*, 158(8), 1184–1190.

Jerath, R., Edry, J. W., Barnes, V. A., & Jerath, V. (2006). Physiology of long pranayamic breathing: neural respiratory elements may provide a mechanism that explains how slow deep breathing shifts the autonomic nervous system. *Medical Hypotheses*, 67(3), 566–571.

Jindani, F. A., & Khalsa, G. F. S. (2015). A yoga intervention program for patients suffering from symptoms of posttraumatic stress disorder: A qualitative descriptive study. *The Journal of Alternative and Complementary Medicine*, 21(7), 401–408.

Jindani, F., Turner, N., & Khalsa, S. B. S. (2015). A yoga intervention for posttraumatic stress: A preliminary randomized control trial. *Evidence-Based Complementary and Alternative Medicine*.

Kamens, S. N., Elkins, D. N. & Robbins, B. D. (2017). Open Letter to the DSM-5. *Journal of Humanistic Psychology*. 57(6).

Kessler, R. C., Chiu, W. T., Demler, O., Walters, E. E., & Merikangas, K. R. (2005). Prevalence, Severity, and Comorbidity of 12-Month DSM-IV Disorders in the National Comorbidity Survey Replication. *Archives of General Psychiatry*, 62(6), 617–627.

Killingsworth, M. A., & Gilbert, D. T. (2010). A wandering mind is an unhappy mind. *Science*, 330(6006), 932.

Kilpatrick, D. G., Resnick, H. S., Milanak, M. E., Miller, M. W., Keyes, K. M., & Friedman, M. J. (2013). National Estimates of Exposure to Traumatic Events and PTSD Prevalence Using DSM-IV and DSM-5Criteria. *Journal of Traumatic Stress, 26*(5), 537–547.

Krysinska, K., & Lester, D. (2010). Post-traumatic stress disorder and suicide risk: a systematic review. *Archives of Suicide Research, 14*(1), 1–23.

Kubiak, S. P. (2004). The effects of PTSD on treatment adherence, drug relapse, and criminal recidivism in a sample of incarcerated men and women. *Research on Social Work Practice, 14*(6), 424–433.

Kulka, R. A., Schlenger, W. E., Fairbank, J. A., Hough, R. L., Jordan, B. K., Marmar, C. R., Weiss, D. S., & Grady, D. A. (1990). *Trauma and the Vietnam War generation: Report of findings from the National Vietnam Veterans Readjustment Study.* New York: Brunner/Mazel.

Lanius, R. A., Brand, B., Vermetten, E., Frewen, P. A., & Spiegel, D. (2012). The dissociative subtype of posttraumatic stress disorder: Rationale, clinical and neurobiological evidence, and implications. *Depression and Anxiety, 29*, 1–8.

Lanius, R. A., Vermetten, E., Loewenstein, R. J., Brand, B., Schmahl, C., Bremner, J. D., & Spiegel, D. (2010). Emotion modulation in PTSD: Clinical and neurobiological evidence for a dissociative subtype. *American Journal of Psychiatry, 167*, 640–647.

Levine, P. A. (1997). *Waking the tiger: Healing trauma: The innate capacity to transform overwhelming experiences* (Vol. 17). North Atlantic Books.

Lew, H. L., Tun, C., & Cifu, D. X. (2009). Prevalence of chronic pain, posttraumatic stress disorder, and persistent postconcussive symptoms in OIF/OEF veterans: Polytrauma clinical triad. *Journal of Rehabilitation Research and Development, 46*(6), 697.

Libby, D. J. (2014) *Mindful Resilience Yoga for Veterans Coping With Trauma: A Practice Guide.* Alameda, CA: Veterans Yoga Project. Retrieved from www.veteransyogaproject.org/practice.

Libby, D. J. (2018). A Safe, Predictable, and Controllable Environment: Creating SPACE for recovery and resilience. *Yoga Therapy Today*, 32–34.

Libby, D. J., Pilver, C. E., & Desai, R. (2012). Complementary and alternative medicine in VA specialized PTSD treatment programs. *Psychiatric Services, 63*(11), 1134–1136.

Libby, D. J., Pilver, C. E., & Desai, R. (2013). Complementary and alternative medicine use among individuals with posttraumatic stress disorder. *Psychological Trauma: Theory, Research, Practice, and Policy, 5*(3), 277.

Luders, E., Toga, A. W., Lepore, N., & Gaser, C. (2009). The underlying anatomical correlates of long-term meditation: Larger hippocampal and frontal volumes of gray matter. *Neuroimage, 45*(3), 672–678.

McPherson, F., & Schwenka, M. A. (2004). Use of complementary and alternative therapies among active duty soldiers, military retirees, and family members at a military hospital. *Military Medicine, 169*(5), 354.

Miller, R. C. (2015). *The iRest program for healing PTSD: A proven-effective approach to using Yoga Nidra meditation and deep relaxation techniques to overcome trauma.* Oakland, CA: New Harbinger Publications.

Mitchell, K. S., Dick, A. M., DiMartino, D. M., Smith, B. N., Niles, B., Koenen, K. C., & Street, A. (2014). A pilot study of a randomized controlled trial of yoga as an intervention for PTSD symptoms in women. *Journal of Traumatic Stress, 27*(2), 121–128.

Narasimhan, L., Nagarathna, R., & Nagendra, H. (2011). Effect of integrated yogic practices on positive and negative emotions in healthy adults. *International Journal of Yoga, 4*(1), 13–19.

O'Connell, M. J., Kasprow, W., & Rosenheck, R. A. (2008). Rates and risk factors for homelessness after successful housing in a sample of formerly homeless veterans. *Psychiatric Services, 59*(3), 268–275.

Ogden, P., & Minton, K. (2000). Sensorimotor psychotherapy: One method for processing traumatic memory. *Traumatology, 6*(3), 149.

Olatunji, B. O., Deacon, B. J., & Abramowitz, J. S. (2009). The cruelest cure? Ethical issues in the implementation of exposure-based treatments. *Cognitive and Behavioral Practice, 16*(2), 172–180.

Ozer, E. J., Best, S. R., Lipsey, T. L., & Weiss, D. S. (2003). Predictors of posttraumatic stress disorder and symptoms in adults: A meta-analysis. *Psychological Bulletin, 129*(1), 52–73.

Pacella, M. L., Hruska, B., & Delahanty, D. L. (2013). The physical health consequences of PTSD and PTSD symptoms: A meta-analytic review. *Journal of Anxiety Disorders, 27*(1), 33–46.

Pascoe, M. C., & Bauer, I. E. (2015). A systematic review of randomised control trials on the effects of yoga on stress measures and mood. *Journal of Psychiatric Research, 68*, 270–282.

Payne, P., & Crane-Godreau, M. A. (2015). The preparatory set: A novel approach to understanding stress, trauma, and the bodymind therapies. *Frontiers in Human Neuroscience, 9*, 178.

Payne, P., Levine, P. A., & Crane-Godreau, M. A. (2015). Somatic experiencing: Using interoception and proprioception as core elements of trauma therapy. *Frontiers in Psychology, 6*, 93.

Pickut, B. A., Van Hecke, W., Kerckhofs, E., Mariën, P., Vanneste, S., Cras, P., & Parizel, P. M. (2013). Mindfulness based intervention in Parkinson's disease leads to structural brain changes on MRI: A randomized controlled longitudinal trial. *Clinical Neurology and Neurosurgery, 115*(12), 2419–2425.

Porges, S. W. (1995). Orienting in a defensive world: Mammilian modifications of our evolutionary heritage. A Polyvagal Theory. *Psychophysiology, 32*, 301–318.

Porges, S. W. (2003). The polyvagal theory: Phylogenetic contributions to social behavior. *Physiology & Behavior, 79*(3), 503–513.

Porges, S. W. (2011). *The Polyvagal Theory: Neurophysiological Foundations of Emotions, Attachment, Communication, and Self-regulation* (Norton Series on Interpersonal Neurobiology). New York: WW Norton & Company.

Price, M., Spinazzola, J., Musicaro, R., Turner, J., Suvak, M., Emerson, D., & van der Kolk, B. (2017). Effectiveness of an extended yoga treatment for women with chronic posttraumatic stress disorder. *The Journal of Alternative and Complementary Medicine, 23*(4), 300–309.

Reinhardt, K. M., Noggle Taylor, J. J., Johnston, J., Zameer, A., Cheema, S., & Khalsa, S. B. S. (2018). Kripalu yoga for military veterans with PTSD: A randomized trial. *Journal of Clinical Psychology, 74*(1), 93–108.

Resick, P. A., & Schnicke, M. K. (1993). Cognitive processing therapy for rape victims: A treatment manual. Newbury Park, CA: Sage.

Rocha, K. K. F., Ribeiro, A. M., Rocha, K. C. F., Sousa, M. B. C., Albuquerque, F. S., Ribeiro, S., & Silva, R. H. (2012). Improvement in physiological and psychological parameters after 6 months of yoga practice. *Consciousness and Cognition, 21*(2), 843–850.

Roediger, H. L. (1990). Implicit memory: Retention without remembering. *American Psychologist, 45*(9), 1043.

Sareen, J., Cox, B. J., Stein, M. B., Afifi, T. O., Fleet, C., & Asmundson, G. J. (2007). Physical and mental comorbidity, disability, and suicidal behavior associated with posttraumatic stress disorder in a large community sample. *Psychosomatic Medicine, 69*(3), 242–248.

Schmalzl, L., Powers, C., & Blom, E. H. (2015). Neurophysiological and neurocognitive mechanisms underlying the effects of yoga-based practices: Toward a comprehensive theoretical framework. *Frontiers in Human Neuroscience, 9*, 235.

Schnurr, P. P., & Jankowski, M. K. (1999). Physical health and post-traumatic stress disorder: Review and synthesis. *Seminars in clinical neuropsychiatry, 4*(4), 295–304.

Schottenbauer, M. A., Glass, C. R., Arnkoff, D. B., Tendick, V., & Gray, S. H. (2008). Nonresponse and dropout rates in outcome studies on PTSD: Review and methodological considerations. *Psychiatry: Interpersonal and Biological Processes, 71*(2), 134–168.

Seppälä, E. M., Nitschke, J. B., Tudorascu, D. L., Hayes, A., Goldstein, M. R., Nguyen, D. T., Perlman, D., & Davidson, R. J. (2014). Breathing-based meditation decreases posttraumatic stress disorder symptoms in U.S. military veterans: A randomized controlled longitudinal study. *Journal of Traumatic Stress, 27*(4), 397–405.

Shalev, I., Moffitt, T. E., Braithwaite, A. W., Danese, A., Fleming, N. I., Goldman-Mellor, S., Harrington, H. L. Houts, R. M., Israel, S., Poulton, R. Robertson, S. P., Sugden, K., Williams, B., & Caspi, A. (2014). Internalizing disorders and leukocyte telomere erosion: A prospective study of depression, generalized anxiety disorder and post-traumatic stress disorder. *Molecular Psychiatry, 19*(11), 1163.

Shapiro, F., & Forrest, M. S. (2001). EMDR: Eye movement desensitization and reprocessing. *New York, NY: Guilford.*

Sherin, J. E., & Nemeroff, C. B. (2011). Post-traumatic stress disorder: The neurobiological impact of psychological trauma. *Dialogues in Clinical Neuroscience, 13*(3), 263–278.

Simpson, T. L., Kaysen, D., Bowen, S., MacPherson, L. M., Chawla, N., Blume, A., Marlatt, G. A., & Larimer, M. (2007). PTSD symptoms, substance use, and vipassana meditation among incarcerated individuals. *Journal of Traumatic Stress, 20*(3), 239–249.

Singleton, M. (2010). *Yoga body: The origins of modern posture practice.* New York: Oxford University Press.

Smith, M. W., Schnurr, P. P., & Rosenheck, R. A. (2005). Employment outcomes and PTSD symptom severity. *Mental Health Services Research, 7*(2), 89–101.

Stankovic, L. (2011). Transforming trauma: a qualitative feasibility study of integrative restoration (iRest) yoga Nidra on combat-related post-traumatic stress disorder. *International Journal of Yoga Therapy, 21*(1), 23–37.

Staples, J. K., Hamilton, M. F., & Uddo, M. (2013). A yoga program for the symptoms of post-traumatic stress disorder in veterans. *Military Medicine, 178*(8), 854–860.

Steenkamp, M. M. (2016). True evidence-based care for posttraumatic stress disorder in military personnel and veterans. *JAMA Psychiatry, 73*(5), 431–432.

Steenkamp, M. M., Litz, B. T., Hoge, C. W., & Marmar, C. R. (2015). Psychotherapy for military-related PTSD: A review of randomized clinical trials. *JAMA, 314*(5), 489–500.

Streeter, C. C., Gerbarg, P. L., Saper, R. B., Ciraulo, D. A., & Brown, R. P. (2012). Effects of yoga on the autonomic nervous system, gamma-aminobutyric-acid, and allostasis in epilepsy, depression, and post-traumatic stress disorder. *Medical Hypotheses, 78*(5), 571–579.

Streeter, C. C., Whitfield, T. H., Owen, L., Rein, T., Karri, S. K., Yakhkind, A., Perlmutter, R., Prescot, A., Renshaw, P. F., Ciraulo, D. A., & Jensen, J. E. (2010). Effects of yoga versus walking on mood, anxiety, and brain GABA levels: A randomized controlled MRS study. *The Journal of Alternative and Complementary Medicine, 16*(11), 1145–1152.

Taylor, S. E., Klein, L. C., Lewis, B. P., Gruenewald, T. L., Gurung, R. A. R., & Updegraff, J. A. (2000). Biobehavioral responses to stress in females: Tend-and-befriend, not fight-or-flight. *Psychological Review, 107*(3), 411–429.

Thayer, J. F., Hansen, A. L., Saus-Rose, E., & Johnsen, B. H. (2009). Heart rate variability, prefrontal neural function, and cognitive performance: The neurovisceral integration perspective on self-regulation, adaptation, and health. *Annals of Behavioral Medicine, 37*(2), 141–153.

Thayer, J. F., & Sternberg, E. (2006). Beyond heart rate variability. *Annals of the New York Academy of Sciences, 1088*(1), 361–372.

Thordardottir, K., Gudmundsdottir, R., Zoëga, H., Valdimarsdottir, U. A., & Gudmundsdottir, B. (2014). Effects of yoga practice on stress-related symptoms in the aftermath of an earthquake: A community-based controlled trial. *Complementary Therapies in Medicine, 22*(2), 226–234.

Vaiva, G., Thomas, P., Ducrocq, F., Fontaine, M., Boss, V., Devos, P., Rascle, C., Cottencin, O., Brunet, A., Laffargue, P., & Goudemand, M. (2004). Low posttrauma GABA plasma levels as a predictive factor in the development of acute posttraumatic stress disorder. *Biological Psychiatry, 55*(3), 250–254.

van der Hart, O., Brown, P., & van der Kolk, B. A. (1989). Pierre Janet's treatment of post-traumatic stress. *Journal of Traumatic Stress, 2*(4), 379–395.

van der Kolk, B. A. (2006). Clinical implications of neuroscience research in PTSD. *Annals of the New York Academy of Sciences, 1071*(1), 277–293.

van der Kolk, B. A. (2010). *Developmental Trauma Disorder.* Chicago, IL: PESI.

van der Kolk, B. (2014). *The Body Keeps the Score: Brain, Mind, and Body in the Healing of Trauma.* New York: Viking.

van der Kolk, B. A., McFarlane, A. C., & van der Hart, O. (1996). A general approach to treatment of posttraumatic stress disorder. In B. A.

van der Kolk, A. C. McFarlane, & L. Weisaeth (Eds.), *Traumatic Stress: The Effects of Overwhelming Experience on Mind.* New York: Guilford Press.

van der Kolk, B., Pelcovitz, D., Roth, S., Mandel, F. S., McFarlane, A., & Herman, J. L. (1996). Dissociation, somatization, and affect dysregulation: The complexity of adaptation to trauma. *The American Journal of Psychiatry*, 153, 163–170.

van der Kolk, B. A., Stone, L., West, J., Rhodes, A., Emerson, D., Suvak, M., & Spinazzola, J. (2014). Original research yoga as an adjunctive treatment for posttraumatic stress disorder: A randomized controlled trial. *Journal of Clinical Psychiatry*, 75(6), e559–e565.

Washington, D. L., Yano, E. M., McGuire, J., Hines, V., Lee, M., & Gelberg, L. (2010). Risk factors for homelessness among women veterans. *Journal of Health Care for the Poor and Underserved*, 21(1), 82–91.

Wells, S. Y., Lang, A. J., Schmalzl, L., Groessl, E. J., & Strauss, J. L. (2016). Yoga as an Intervention for PTSD: A Theoretical Rationale and Review of the Literature. *Current Treatment Options in Psychiatry*, 3(1), 60–72.

West, S., King, V., Carey, T. S., Lohr, K. N., McKoy, N., Sutton, S. F., & Lux, L. (2002). Systems to rate the strength of scientific evidence. *Evidence report/technology assessment*, 47, 1–11.

West, J., Liang, B., & Spinazzola, J. (2017). Trauma Sensitive Yoga as a complementary treatment for posttraumatic stress disorder: A qualitative descriptive analysis. *International Journal of Stress Management*, 24(2), 173.

Wilson, J. P., & Zigelbaum, S. D. (1983). The Vietnam veteran on wal: The relation of post-traumatic stress disorder to criminal behavior. *Behavioral Sciences & the Law*, 1(3), 69–83.

Yackle, K., Schwarz, L. A., Kam, K., Sorokin, J. M., Huguenard, J. R., Feldman, J. L., Luo, L., & Krasnow, M. A. (2017). Breathing control center neurons that promote arousal in mice. *Science*, 355(6332), 1411–1415.

Yehuda, R., & Hoge, C. W. (2016). The meaning of evidence-based treatments for veterans with posttraumatic stress disorder. *JAMA Psychiatry*, 73(5), 433–434.

Zatzick, D. F., Marmar, C. R., Weiss, D. S., Browner, W. S., Metzler, T. J., Golding, J. M., Stewart, A., Schlenger, W. E., & Wells, K. B. (1997). Posttraumatic stress disorder and functioning and quality of life outcomes in a nationally representative sample of male Vietnam veterans. *American Journal of Psychiatry*, 154(12), 1690–1695.

Zlotnick, C., Mattia, J. I., & Zimmerman, M. (1999). Clinical correlates of self-mutilation in a sample of general psychiatric patients. *The Journal of Nervous and Mental Disease*, 187(5), 296–301.

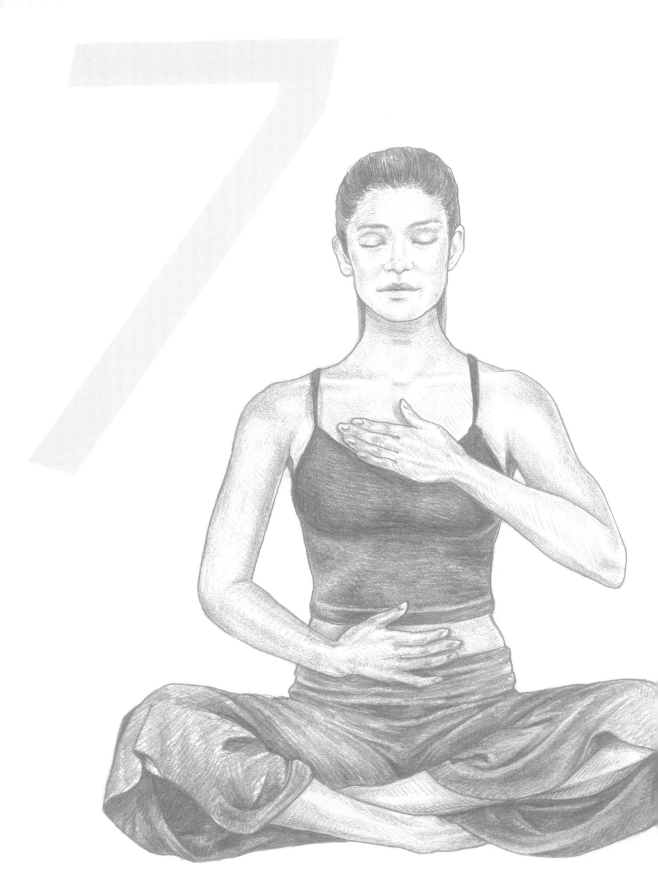

Eating Disorders

Laura Douglass and Samantha Bottrill

7

Overview

Eating disorders are devastating illnesses that dys-regulate a person's thoughts, emotions, and behaviors as they relate to food. The normal comfort of meals is gradually replaced with an obsession that centers on one or more rituals of binging, fasting, vomiting, keeping food journals, weighing, compulsive exercise, taking diuretics and/or laxatives, enemas, and calorie-counting of the smallest portions of food. Although such conditions have been documented since the 1900s, the first formal diagnosis presented to the mental health community was in 1955 (American Psychiatric Association, 2013); initially, the disorder was mischaracterized as a neurotic illness in which psychological conditions exacerbated underlying physical symptoms (Brumberg, 2000). The conception of eating disorders has changed since the 1900s, with research showing the clear genetic and sociocultural influences on the disorder (Bordo, 1992; Holland & Sicotte, 1988;). The fifth edition of the *Diagnostic and statistical manual of mental disorders* (DSM-5) includes anorexia, bulimia, binge eating (BED), pica, restrictive food intake disorder, and eating disorders not elsewhere classified (OSFED) as subsets of this complicated and life-altering condition (American Psychiatric Association, 2013). Each category is exceedingly complex, requiring a nuanced, integrative approach to wellbeing. While eating disorders impact between 7% and 10% of the total female population, the number of males, who are often silently suffering, has become a growing concern for clinicians, researchers, and loved ones alike (Birnbaum & Thompson, 2014; Sweeting et al., 2015; von Hausswolff-Juhlin, Brooks, & Larsson, 2015). Yoga may be useful for all eating disorders where emotional regulation is a concern; however, given that anorexia and bulimia are the most researched, they will be the focus of this chapter.

> Individuals suffering with anorexia become fixated on self-starvation, which leads to a host of deleterious physical problems that may include seizures, osteoporosis, and heart failure, resulting in one of the highest mortality rates of any mental illness.

In both anorexia and bulimia, individuals are beset by a negative body image and attempt to manipulate the shape of the body. Individuals suffering with anorexia become fixated on self-starvation, which leads to a host of deleterious physical problems that may include seizures, osteoporosis, and heart failure, resulting in one of the highest mortality rates of any mental illness (Hoang, Goldacre, & James, 2014). The criteria for being diagnosed with anorexia include restriction of food that leads to low bodyweight, fear of gaining weight, and a profound disturbance in the way that an individual experiences their body (American Psychiatric Association, 2013). Bulimia is characterized by binge eating followed by the use of compensatory behaviors such as vomiting, fasting, exercise, and laxatives in an attempt to avoid weight gain. The resulting destruction to their esophageal tissue, tooth enamel, and digestive system causes long-term and sometimes irreparable damage. To receive a diagnosis of bulimia, the binge eating and compensatory behaviors must both occur at least once weekly for three months (American Psychiatric Association, 2013). In addition to struggling with the basic function of feeding themselves, individuals with anorexia and bulimia are prone to self-injury, low self-esteem, crushing anxiety and incapacitating depression (Cucchi et al., 2016; Guarda, Schreyer,

Boersma, Tamashiro, & Moran, 2015; Manaf, Saravanan, & Zuhrah, 2016). The lack of nutrients and severe dehydration correlated with eating disorders engenders changes in the brain that often result in cognitive impairment. This confluence of factors makes treatment difficult, with drop-out rates as high as 58% for outpatient and inpatient care (Sly et al., 2014). This very low response rate to treatment results in a perception that those struggling with eating disorders are resistant to making changes (Aspen, Darcy, & Lock, 2014). In truth, it is challenging for those who suffer to put aside the practices they intimately know will restore some sense of balance, even if they are ultimately harmful, in favor of new, unfamiliar disciplines of the body.

Since a clear etiology for eating disorders has yet to be articulated, it is not surprising that classic psychological treatments are less effective with this population (Fennig, Brunstein Klomek, Shahar, Sarel-Michnik, & Hadas, 2015). In an attempt to clarify the risk factors associated with anorexia and bulimia, researchers point to a pattern of factors that appear to predispose individuals to suffer: genetics, an idealization of thinness, and the personality trait of perfectionism (Culbert, Racine, & Klump, 2015). A growing body of recent evidence suggests a strong correlation between trauma and eating disorder symptoms (Caslini et al., 2015; Isomaa, Backholm, & Birgegård, 2015; Lee, Zaharlick, & Akers, 2015; Monteleone et al., 2015). These are important findings as some researchers are beginning to see that the behaviors of eating disorders are a method to cope with the intense emotions that are a daily part of these individuals' lives (Polivy & Herman, 2002). Eating disorder behaviors may function as an effective method to regulate painful emotions and negative thoughts. For example, the dull, heavy sensations of hypoarousal that occur in depression may be regulated by movement such as running or vigorous yoga asana practice, while the racing thoughts that arise with anxiety are soothed through overeating.

Although the exact causes of eating disorder behavior remain disputed, what is evident is the undertow of confusion and suffering that confounds family members, therapists, psychiatrists, and nutritionists alike. Professionals are diligently searching for practices that offer the possibility of pulling individuals out of the cycle of self-destruction. Some clinicians have found hope in yoga as a mindfulness-based practice due to its capacity to produce a "…non-judgmental and accepting stance toward [the] internal experiences" of the body; clinicians hope that the awareness fostered by yoga practices will have a positive impact on the attitudes and behaviors of individuals with eating disorders (Palmeira, Trindade, & Ferreira, 2014, p. 392). While more research is still needed, existing studies suggest that the nonjudgmental acceptance of mindfulness-based practices such as yoga can teach individuals how to trust in their body's signals and thus lower their reliance on nonadaptive eating behaviors (Augustus-Horvath & Tylka, 2011; Bacon, Stern, Van Loan, & Keim, 2005; Cole & Horacek, 2010; Iannantono & Tylka, 2012).

> The tradition of yoga has a long history of working with the body as a method to bring equanimity to the mind.

Encouraged by the research and what yoga may offer their clients, psychologists and social workers in the twenty-first century began drawing on the vast literature of yoga to encourage their clients to use the body as a tool to understand their reactions to the world around them. The tradition of yoga has a long history of working with the body as a method to bring equanimity to the mind (Douglass, 2007). The fifteenth-century text, the *Hatha Yoga Pradipika*, describes working with the body as a first step in learning how to calm the mind so that the individual can experience *advaita*, or nondual consciousness (Feurstein, 2003). Yet yoga, as it is known today, is a complex transcultural tradition that is as much influenced by German gymnastic traditions as it is by ancient philosophical texts and neuroscience (Alter, 2004; Singleton, 2010). Individuals integrating yoga into the treatment of individuals with eating disorders may be inspired by philosophical texts or modern neuroscience, but their goals are essentially modest: to teach awareness of the body, and to offer practices that have the potential to free the mind from the painful habit of rumination.

Rationale and research for yoga for individuals with eating disorders

Only a small number of research trials directly support yoga as a clinical intervention for people with eating disorders and eating disorder symptoms (e.g., Cook-Cottone et al., 2008; Dale et al., 2009; Carei et al., 2010; McIver at al., 2009). Firm conclusions about yoga's effectiveness have been difficult to reach due to the wide variations in yoga interventions, clinical presentations, and the significant methodological limitations of many of the studies conducted (Balasubramaniam et al., 2013; Klein et al 2013; Neumark-Sztainer, 2013). The growing interest in yoga as an adjunctive practice for individuals with anorexia and bulimia rests, in part, on preliminary findings. These findings suggest that yoga has a potential role in treatment as one "tool in the toolbox" for individuals recovering from eating disorders (Neumark-Sztainer, 2013).

The postural and breathing practices of yoga work because the body rapidly responds to the world around us. People's deepest desires and fears are communicated through the flush of the face, the hunching of the shoulders, or a tightening of the jaw. The neuroscientist Antonio Damasio revealed that cognition happens in response to "felt sensations," which are the basic guide for our physical actions and habitual ways of being in the world (1999). Indeed, our embodied reaction to the world around us is "...the main tool we use to generate meaning, organize our experience, and shape our social identity" (Riva, 2014, p. 236).

For individuals with eating disorders, the body as a tool that maps and expresses the sense of identity becomes distorted. Sometimes, every sensation and interaction triggers repetitive negative thoughts such as "I am fat," "I am unlovable," and "I must be better." The monotony and terror of these messages persist until some effort is made to push away the unbearable discomfort and pain. A self-designed methodology emerges to regulate these felt sensations: compulsive exercising, vomiting, laxatives, binge eating, restrictive dieting, or the avoidance of food altogether. Yoga may work because it disrupts the cycle of belief and the maladaptive responses to those beliefs that have been shaped by the eating disorder. Yoga postures and breathing practices are practical tools that can foster new felt experiences of the body as relaxed, open, spacious, and at ease. During the practice of yoga, space may develop between the negative thoughts and alter the lived experience of the body as tired, stiff, and unworthy. Over time, the regular practice of yoga may enable the individual to remap their relationship with themselves.

Yoga as a form of disciplined inquiry contains a unique combination of somatic (postures and breathing practices), psychological (sense withdrawal and concentration techniques), and spiritual practices (meditation and spiritual lifestyle) that appear to be effective in bringing mental clarity to a troubled mind. Eating disorder specialist Dr. Kelly Gunderson explains that yoga has the potential to "help individuals with eating disorders self-soothe [as they]...have difficulty with feelings, anxiety, and uncertainty" (Gunderson, personal communication, October 24, 2007). Indeed, eating disorders frequently co-occur with anxiety, depression, and trauma, each of which can be exceedingly difficult to navigate for individuals who are prone to avoiding intense emotions (see Table 7.1). The practices of yoga appear to reduce the hypervigilance that so often inhibits individuals from re-envisioning new ways to relate to the sensations of

Chapter 7

Table 7.1

How yoga can help regulate symptoms associated with eating disorders

Symptom	Impact of eating disorder	How yoga helps
Emotional avoidance	Eating disorders help to distance individuals from emotions, including boredom (Crockett, Myhre, & Rokke, 2015; Evers et al., 2010)	Movement helps to regulate emotions (Shafir et al., 2016) and secure positive relationships with the body (Greenwood & Delgado, 2013)
Anxiety	Eating disorders are fueled by high levels of anxiety, including separation anxiety (Guarda et al., 2015; O'Shaughnessy & Dallos, 2009)	Research shows that yoga is effective in regulating anxiety (Javnbakht, Hejazi Kenari, & Ghasemi, 2009; Menezes et al., 2015; Subramanya & Telles, 2009; Uebelacker & Broughton, 2016)
Depression	Depression is common in individuals with eating disorders; eating disorder behavior may help to regulate depression (Michopoulos et al., 2015)	Yoga is a valuable adjunctive treatment to depression (da Silva, Ravindran, & Ravindran, 2009; Lavey et al., 2005; Pilkington, Kirkwood, Rampes, & Richardson, 2005; Streeter et al., 2007)
Trauma	Eating disorders attempt to regulate the felt sensations of trauma and/or traumatic loss (Failler, 2006; Gonçalves et al., 2016; Isomaa et al., 2015; Monteleone et al., 2015; Riva, 2014)	Yoga helps regulate the symptoms of PTSD and the addictions that help regulate the sensations of trauma (Kolk, 2014; Reddy, Dick, Gerber, & Mitchell, 2014; Spinazzola, Rhodes, Emerson, Earle, & Monroe, 2011)

the present moment. The felt sensation of relaxation (slower breathing rate, reduced tension in shoulders, jaw, and around the eyes) is linked to a psychological feeling of safety and ease that may very well enhance an individual's willingness to explore additional techniques for emotional regulation.

The ability to feel safe is a key component of an individual's capacity to regulate their emotions. Emotions have been described as the byproduct of a system that is monitoring the "discrepancy between a goal and reality" (Gross, 1998, p. 271), with positive emotions correlated with goals being achieved faster than expected, and negative emotions correlated with goals being achieved slower than expected (Gross, 1998). Individuals with eating disorders are known to experience heightened negative emotions (Lavender et al., 2015) and to have less capacity to "influence which emotions they have, when they have them, and

how they experience and express them" (Gross, 1998, p. 271). The behaviors associated with eating disorders (e.g., food avoidance, vomiting, and compulsive running) function as effective avoidance techniques (Espel et al., 2016) that give the person a sense of control over distressing emotional experiences.

Yoga teaches individuals to become aware of and accept the sensations of the present moment through a combination of slow experiential movements accompanied by verbal cues that cultivate attention to four phases of emotional regulation: (1) heart rate, breath, muscular tension, and other physiological responses; (2) identification of the internal feeling state associated with the physiology; (3) thoughts related to the emotion; and (4) behaviors related to the emotion (Füstös, J. et al, 2013). Teaching awareness is not so much discussed as it is practiced. For example, individuals who are learning to eat in the clinical setting often experience uncomfortable levels of gas that they label as fat. An effective yoga session might introduce postures that create more space in the abdomen, such as *adho mukha svanasana* (downward-facing dog) with the feet wider apart. As awareness of space in the body is created the individual may be able to relax. The class can then introduce practices that release the gas, such as *pavanmuktasana*, the wind-relieving pose. As the individual feels relief from the pressure of gas they are able to experience that the cognition "I am fat" was not as accurate as the cognition "I have gas." In addition to regulating the sensations of the present moment, the individual has learned a few tools that they can safely return to in the future that will relieve the discomfort of gas, thereby avoiding compulsive running, vomiting, or other behaviors they have used in the past.

> Individuals who are learning to eat in the clinical setting often experience uncomfortable levels of gas that they identify as fat.

Part of what individuals with eating disorders learn as they practice yoga is the ability to identify their own body sensations in the present moment (e.g., hunger, thirst, lightness, space, tension, temperature, muscular and visceral sensations). Researchers know that a high degree of interoceptive awareness has the potential to facilitate emotional regulation as it helps an individual notice the first signs of bodily sensations, thereby mobilizing a response to stimuli all the more quickly (Füstös, J. et al., 2013). Difficulty with visceral sensitivity is common in those with eating disorders (Merwin et al., 2013) and the somatic practices of yoga may teach individuals how to make clear connections between their physiological experiences, emotions, thoughts, and behaviors. While all forms of movement help to regulate emotions (Shafir, Tsachor, Welch, Watson, & Allard, 2016), the attention that yoga teachers give to assisting their students to stay present and recognize the somatic sensations, emotions and thoughts of the present moment is a crucial step in learning emotional regulation. The slow repetitive nature of yoga allows for a manipulation of the body that is at once familiar ("I can change my body for a desired mental effect") and completely new ("The practice of yoga predictably reproduces sensations of peace and ease").

In addition to the psychological benefits, yoga has the potential to mitigate some of the unpleasant physical impacts of eating disorders. The primary intervention needs to be to regain lost weight and restore normal eating patterns; however, as an adjunct, an adapted yoga practice has the potential to reverse osteoporotic bone loss (Lu, Rosner, Chang, & Fishman, 2016) and to support digestive health (Shahabi, Naliboff, & Shapiro, 2016).

Yoga's capacity to regulate the sensations of discomfort may be achieved with a strikingly small amount of consistent yoga practice. One study showed yoga was effective in reducing eating disorder symptoms in as little as one hour of twice-weekly yoga practice for eight weeks (Carei et al., 2010). In the sixteen hours of yoga practice, the yoga group (n=26) showed greater reductions in eating disorder symptoms than the control group (n=24) as measured by the global scale of the Eating Disorder Examination Interview. One participant commented that the yoga session was "the only hour in my week when I don't think about my weight" (Carei et al., 2010, p. 350). The researchers hypothesized that food preoccupation was reduced by redirecting the student's attention to the gentle yoga postures that were being taught. A more recent inpatient study hypothesized that yoga's effectiveness in reducing negative affect can be achieved in as little as 38 minutes of active standing postures, floor work, and breathing practices (Pacanowski, Diers, Crosby, & Neumark-Sztaner, 2017). The greatest impact of yoga was in lowering the negative affect prior to meal consumption (Pacanowski et al., 2017), which is significant because previous research points to the importance of improving pre-meal affect for best treatment results (Ranzenhofer et al., 2013; Steinglass et al., 2010).

Despite the limited research, the popularity of yoga as a treatment tool has continued to grow, with one study reporting that 66.7% of North American inpatient clinics have already added the practice of yoga to the therapeutic protocol of individuals with eating disorders (Frisch, Herzog, & Franko, 2006). Clinicians and researchers alike believe that exercise, binging, and fasting are an attempt to titrate the difficult sensations and emotions that people with eating disorders experience (Evers, Marijn Stok, & de Ridder, 2010; Menezes et al., 2015). Yoga can be an effective method for teaching emotion regulation (Cowdrey & Park, 2012). One of the reasons that individuals with eating disorders often find themselves in community yoga classes (Herranz Valera, Acuña Ruiz, Romero Valdespino, & Visioli, 2014) is that yoga can be a method of "self-medicating" in the hope of finding relief from stress, anxiety, and depression (Birnbaum & Thompson, 2014; Herranz Valera et al., 2014; Park, Riley, Bedesin, & Stewart, 2014). The social connection that can occur through practicing with others may be a part of that relief.

Two-thirds of clinical treatment programs in the United States include yoga as part of their treatment protocol (Frisch et al., 2006). Yoga classes that are integrated into residential and outpatient clinics usually consist of small groups of committed individuals that are guided through a combination of postures, breathing practices, deep relaxation and meditation by a trained yoga teacher (Douglass, 2009).

Recommended practices for embodied awareness

Teaching yoga to individuals who have eating disorders requires creating a space in which students begin to feel safe enough to explore the body as a trusted ally, one that imparts valuable information which can be counted on to help them respond appropriately to the present moment (Cook-Cottone & Douglass, 2017; Douglass, 2009, 2011). Focusing inward can be overwhelming for someone who has spent years denying, suppressing, or simply ignoring their physical and emotional landscape. The foundational work a yoga teacher/therapist is entrusted with necessitates establishing the classroom as a safe space to engage in unfamiliar practices and discuss problems, and one where participants are encouraged to relax and let go of some of the perceptions, thoughts, and beliefs that keep them bound. The aim for each yoga teacher/therapist is for the yoga mat to become a student's inner laboratory where they can develop new ways of understanding and regulating emotional experience; this requires the careful cultivation of a physically, psychologically, and interpersonally safe place.

> Focusing inward can be overwhelming for someone who has spent years denying, suppressing, or simply ignoring their physical and emotional landscape.

Physical considerations

From a physical perspective, students may be experiencing a range of health complications due to restricted eating, laxative misuse, excessive exercise and vomiting, all of which can lead to osteoporosis, postural hypotension, and cardiovascular complications (Casiero & Frishman, 2006). A yoga teacher/therapist should have an understanding of these conditions and be able to moderate the class taking them into consideration. They will benefit from additional training for working with eating disorders, and must ensure that students receive medical clearance before they join a yoga group or start individualized sessions. Students with eating disorders can be stuck in deeply entrenched patterns of denial and disregard with respect to their physical health, which means that yoga teachers cannot rely on self-reports from students or expect that they will arrive at classes outside of the clinical setting adequately nourished, hydrated, and able to respect their physical limits.

Psychological considerations

From a psychological perspective, an individual's sense of safety is honed through purposely cultivating emotion regulation. A good starting point for a yoga teacher/therapist is an intentional focus on grounding skills. These offer students a sense of safety and the tools and confidence to slowly reconnect with their internal world without shutting off from, or becoming overwhelmed by, their experiences. Much like with trauma work, teachers need to support students to become aware of, and work within, their therapeutic "window of tolerance" for physical and emotional experience (Ogden, Minton, & Pain, 2006). Grounding skills help to bring students back into their window of tolerance in which their nervous systems are neither hyperaroused nor hypoaroused, and offer a sense of psychological safety through presence and strength within the body. Practices may involve bringing students' attention to the connection of the feet with the ground and the felt sense of the earth beneath, or may involve simply fostering a sense of stability by drawing attention to the strength of the legs. Practices to bring students into their window of tolerance may also involve breathing techniques that involve an extended exhalation (such as *brahmari*), which can quite quickly lower sympathetic arousal, bringing a sense of calm and self-regulation.

Grounding skills provide the steady psychological base from which students can be supported to gradually develop greater interoceptive awareness; however, for many, being asked to be aware of sensations will be an abstract concept fraught with fear and self-judgment. It will be helpful for yoga teachers to offer concrete examples of what they mean by sensation— for example, numbness, tightness in the jaw, stretch when we lift the arms—while being thoughtful about using words that could trigger negative rumination about the body, for example, weight, heaviness, and spreading. It can be effective to start with grosser sensations because they are likely to be more obvious, such as the coolness of the floor, the touch of interlaced fingers, the rising of the chest on the inhalation. Then attention can be trained to move to awareness of the more subtle sensations such as tingling, pulsing, and energy moving. Certain practices such as *brahmari* breath, cat/cow, side bends, balancing poses, and supported bridge are all rich sources of sensation for most people and therefore offer an accessible way into experiencing sensation. Practices focused on interoceptive awareness that involve the body being still, such as body scans, are generally more challenging and should be short in duration, at least initially. Any invitation to attend to sensation needs to be balanced with frequent reminders that the purpose of yoga is for students to listen to what they need first and foremost; if they feel overwhelmed, they can make the choice to return to grounding skills.

As discussed earlier, interoceptive awareness provides the building blocks for greater clarity of emotional experience (Miller, 2009). When the gradual development of sensitivity to bodily signals is paired with directing a student's attention specifically to how these might relate to affective and cognitive experience, emotion regulation is enhanced. Teachers can inspire curiosity by regularly inviting students to check in with what they notice through yoga practices and how each impacts upon sensation, emotions, and thoughts. Many students experience an overwhelming rejection of what they think and feel, as well as a whole host of expectations about what they "should" or "shouldn't" be experiencing. When yoga teachers support both clarity and acceptance, they create an environment where students can welcome embodied experience (Cook-Cottone & Douglass,

2017). Many yoga teachers guide this by explicitly setting the expectation of the yoga mat as a microcosm of everyday life. For example, if students are anxious in life they are likely to meet anxiety on their mats. If individuals tend to collapse at the first sign of discomfort then they are likely to bring this pattern to *virabhadrasana,* the warrior pose. The yoga class can be an opportunity to meet themselves as they are in the given moment and to explore an alternative way of being that centers on experiencing the whole self: spiritually, physically, and emotionally. When students start to welcome the full range of their human experience from pleasure to discomfort, they open the door to developing an authentic relationship with themselves that moves them toward recovery.

People with eating disorders are often intelligent, with a tendency to want to get things right. However, the need for perfection often comes at the expense of their emotional and physical wellbeing. For example, they may force their bodies into a postural alignment that is described by the yoga teacher/therapist despite the negative thoughts and sensations that arise for them in that posture. It may not occur to these students to back away from the suggested practice. It is crucial that yoga teachers create an environment where choice is not just offered, but that choosing to adapt, adjust, and accommodate the practice is applauded as an advanced yogic practice. Teachers can model this themselves by demonstrating the simpler options of poses and taking the time to use props to support their posture. A new habit of respect for the body can then be cultivated through the combined use of language that invites a sense of gentleness with explicit instruction as to the importance of finding relative comfort in each pose.

Another challenge to teaching awareness skills is working with individuals who suffer from the habit of compulsive exercising. When someone uses exercise (often to the point of excess) to modulate the intensity

of their feelings, it can be difficult for them to practice movement as a method to explore the present moment without effort, stress, or strain. It is useful to give tangible options to students that directly support the shift from exercise to embodied awareness. This might include regularly reminding students that each pose is an opportunity to turn inward and to invite them to notice any disassociation ("spacing out") or excessive effort. A straightforward test to offer students is to say, "Could you smile if you wanted to without it feeling like a grimace, and can you take an easeful breath? If not, then this is a moment to listen to your body and back out of the pose a little." Guided self-inquiry allows the student to take the position of expert on their own body and use awareness to regulate their present moment experience, rather than using compulsive exercise to avoid feelings.

A private space without mirrors can help to de-emphasize external appearance and facilitate a focus on the felt sensations of the practice.

Yoga teachers have an important role in supporting a sense of interpersonal safety within the group context. While group classes can become another place for self-criticism, body checking, and comparison with fellow students, the teacher/therapist, or an idealized self, they can also be a place to counter the extreme loneliness of identifying so closely with the eating disorder and offer the potential of belonging to a community that is dedicated to wellbeing and recovery. A private space without mirrors can help to de-emphasize external appearance and facilitate a focus on the felt sensations of the practice. Yoga teachers might find it helpful to develop an explicit contract with students about how to reduce the likelihood that they might inadvertently trigger eating disorder thoughts or behaviors in one another. This contract might include a dress code and an agreement not to discuss eating disorder behaviors and strategies, or details of weight loss or gain (Cook-Cottone et al., 2008). Drawing students' attention to possible thoughts of competition and comparison may be useful to help them recognize and manage the habit of comparison. Yoga teachers can remove the fuel for comparison by encouraging students to return their gaze to a *drishti* (focal point) rather than looking at other students, or to reduce the power of comparison by simply and kindly labeling it as a thought, not a fact, and then directing their attention elsewhere.

Although comparison is a natural human tendency, yoga is ultimately about developing a relationship to one's own self. Developing relationships can be problematic for those who have eating disorders because the mind becomes stuck in a pattern, revolving painfully and perennially around concepts of food and weight. Turning one's attention to the present, even for a moment, reduces the extreme pain and isolation of a repetitive mind. One of the primary roles of a yoga teacher/therapist is to model a new way of relating to one's self (and to others) that is unhurried and undemanding. As the teacher/therapist's own movements begin to fill with patience and compassion, they find themselves slowing down and capable of truly being with those who are suffering. Concepts such as the "perfect" yoga sequence, the need to speak the exact right words, and striving to change students diminish, and the yoga class can become a space in which insight is gained together. Each person becomes more able to experience themselves exactly as they are, with an embodied knowledge of being good enough, exactly as they are.

Shifting the paradigm: Integrating yoga into psychological therapy

The US-based eating disorders specialist, Kelly Gunderson, stated, "I talk to my clients about how the body is a powerful tool, but what I'd like to see is a paradigm shift that imagines how I would incorporate yoga into my practice" (Gunderson, personal communication,

October 24, 2017). While the profession of psychology has yet to experience a paradigm shift that includes the body as a site of transformation, yoga is a skillset that a growing number of clinicians hope to integrate into the care they provide for their clients (Barnett & Shale, 2012; Gangadhar & Varambally, 2015; Sisk, 2007). To truly revolutionize the care those with eating disorders receive, clinicians need to develop solutions that include the body as a method to understand the social, cultural, and political implications of care for the self. The French philosopher Michel Foucault believed that repeated acts of self-care were political acts that defined how individuals were able to intimately relate to others and how to live an ethical life (Foucault, 1978). Yoga may be one method by which individuals can learn to "observ[e] and document self-limiting and self-destructive behaviors" (Heyes, 2007, p. 88) as well as the pleasures of the body.

> Through their own practice, individuals begin to acknowledge that the relationship to their body, like every relationship, requires time, communication, respect, and care.

For many clinicians, understanding the body as a site of wisdom begins with their own embodied practice of yoga. Through their own practice, individuals begin to acknowledge that the relationship to their body, like every relationship, requires time, communication, respect, and care. As clinicians begin to embody self-care through the discipline of yoga, they naturally want to share these practices with their clients. Grounding their clinical inquiry in the client's sensations in the present moment is perhaps the single most important thing clinicians can do. Clinicians can inquire, "What happens in your jaw when you speak about your partner?" or "Can you identify lightness in your spine as you speak about your college career?" The simple verbal inquiry, which may be just as effective for those with anxiety, depression, and other illnesses, begins the process of helping clients learn to be with and learn from their embodied experiences. The integration of specific yoga techniques will depend on the level of training of the clinician. Those who have training in yoga teaching or yoga therapy will be able to integrate postural work and more advanced breathing techniques. Those clinicians without such training may still be able to bring in some basic yogic breathing, body scans, and concentration techniques (assuming they have suitable clinical supervision). Alternatively, they may choose to either work alongside a yoga teacher/therapist or recommend suitable yoga classes, using psychotherapy sessions to then reflect with the client on their experience.

Stages of recovery

One of the primary challenges in integrating yoga into a private mental health practice is learning to titrate awareness practices for those who are suffering. The field of trauma uses three stages of recovery that can be valuable when adapted to recovery from eating disorders: (1) safety/stabilization, (2) acceptance, and (3) recovery/integration (Ogden et al., 2006). These stages of healing can be adapted to those with eating disorders to help clinicians match and appropriately challenge the client's understanding of embodiment, wellbeing, and self (see Table 7.2).

Safety/stabilization

In the safety and stabilization phase an individual works on keeping themselves safe by avoiding dangerous relationships, eating regularly, and avoiding cutting and other harmful activities. In this stage of recovery the emphasis is on the somatic practices of yoga. Yoga postures and breathing practices are adapted as tools that help with the emotional dysregulation that is so prevalent in the disorder. The therapist can highlight skills to calm the body, recognize and label the feeling of calm, regulate impulses, and generate an ability to self-soothe. While it is common for therapists to suggest that individuals with eating disorders attend a group yoga class, for individuals

in the safety and stabilization phase this suggestion needs to be specific about what kind of yoga would be practiced, since they are likely to be attracted to heated, athletic yoga classes that exacerbate their eating disorder (Douglass, 2009). Alternatively, the client can be referred to a yoga therapist with specific training in the use of yoga for individuals with disordered eating.

Acceptance

Once the client is able to consistently make safe choices, then they are ready to work on acceptance of the eating disorder. Clients in this stage are working on overcoming the fear of the eating disorder and are beginning to develop an appreciation for who they have become as a result of it. While group work may have been avoided or only engaged in begrudgingly before, during this stage group work helps the individual to accept their eating disorder, establish a positive identity as a survivor, and become a peer that supports their colleagues. Therapists can assist their clients to work on decreasing shame and alienation by integrating the psychological tools of yoga. Sense withdrawal and concentration techniques (e.g., studying the sense impressions and their impact on the mind, journaling, visualization, mantra, and focusing on the breath) can become important tools in helping clients develop a sense of choice and also to enhance the capacity to redirect their minds. As clients begin to experience the range of emotions that the eating disorder once held at bay, they will need a variety of techniques that are as successful as the eating disorder behavior was in retaining balance.

Recovery/integration

In the recovery and integration stage, individuals are ready to embrace a nourishing lifestyle that enables them to give back to their communities. At this stage, clients may no longer be solely practicing yoga postures and breathing practices; they may have adopted a lifestyle that is committed to health and wellbeing.

Table 7.2

How yoga provides support at each stage of recovery

Stage	Stage definition	How yoga provides support
Safety and stabilization	Learning to comprehend the effects and symptoms of an eating disorder Beginning to understand the meaning of overwhelming body sensations, intrusive emotions, and distorted cognitive schemas regarding the body Establishing bodily safety by abstaining from self-injury (e.g., laxatives, vomiting, binging, and restriction). The teacher/therapist helps clients to identify the embodied sensations that lead to self-harm	Emphasize the somatic practices of yoga as tools to regulate symptoms of the disorder Establishment of emotional stability by highlighting skills to calm the body, recognize and label the feeling of calm, regulate impulses and generate an ability to self-soothe Practices include yoga postures, body scans, yoga nidra, breath awareness, and mindful movements
Acceptance of the eating disorder	Overcoming the fear of the eating disorder and appreciation for the person you have become as a result of the eating disorder. Work on decreasing shame and alienation Normalizing a range of emotions The teacher/therapist helps the client to notice positive body sensations associated with strength, appreciation, gratitude, and beginning to connect with others	Emphasize the psychological practices of yoga as tools to work with the range of emotions and thoughts that arise Practices include sense withdrawal, alternate-nostril breathing, box breathing, and restorative yoga; and also the introduction of concentration techniques (e.g., visualization, mantra, focusing on breath, and cultivating stillness) Group yoga practices with others in recovery, and twelve-step programs
Recovery and integration	Developing a capacity for healthy attachment, and taking up personal and professional goals. Overcoming the fears of normal life. Intimacy becomes the focus of the work The teacher/therapist helps the client to notice what it feels like to truly nourish the body, and to normalize a routine of self-care The eating disorder becomes integrated into the understanding of self, but is no longer a daily focus	Emphasize the spiritual practices of yoga as tools to support and nourish one's daily activities and service to others Beginning to explore what it feels like to serve others, and to nourish the self in the same way the client nourishes others Practices include establishing a regular yoga practice outside of therapeutic settings, and participation in retreats; adapting the yoga practice for how one feels in the moment (as opposed to a prescription that is followed); volunteering to serve others; developing spiritual practices and identity in their own tradition

They may express a desire to become yoga teachers themselves as they feel they are clearly established on a path of wellbeing and yearn to share what they have learned with others; they may go on to achieve personal and professional goals unrelated to their eating disorder. As clients begin to participate in regular yoga classes and possibly attend spiritual retreats, their therapist can help them to notice what it feels like to truly nourish the body and to normalize a routine of self-care. The therapist's role becomes one that helps to solidify the relationship with the body by helping their clients to notice and articulate the positive embodied experiences such as strength, appreciation, gratitude, and the felt sensations that accompany connecting with others. The therapeutic process, at long last, focuses on helping the client to take in and truly feel their accomplishments.

Perhaps one of the most difficult challenges in integrating yoga into a clinical practice is the therapist's goal for it to have a "positive" or "healing" effect or for the client to change is some specific way. The desire for our clients to be different than they are reinforces their pattern of thinking that they need to perform or be better in order to be accepted. Psychologists who desire that their clients do yoga in order to not suffer send a message that their pain is not natural or welcome in the process of healing. While integrating yoga into clinical sessions may at times give immediate relief or increase awareness, it may also uncover tremendous pain and feelings of inadequacy. Clinicians need to be prepared to radically accept whatever arises from the practice of yoga. This acceptance recrafts the clinical space into a meeting ground on which the client's resistance to the body is explored and understood; it then becomes the client's choice to create something unexpected and new.

> A healthy relationship to the body goes a long way toward restoring connection with self and others.

Individuals with eating disorders often request prescriptions for addressing the eating disorders in the desperate hope that they will have a fix for the suffering their illness brings. It is important for mental health professionals integrating yoga into their clinical practice to bear in mind that the body heals itself; yoga merely assists the body with its natural process of healing by introducing positive habits (Satchidananda, 2011). Indeed, yoga does not so much cure illness as heal the underlying isolation from others and from their own bodies that is so common for those with eating disorders. The primary significance of yoga is as a tool that can be integrated into the therapeutic setting to help the client develop a healthy relationship with their body through establishing positive goals, introducing relaxation techniques, practicing self-acceptance, and developing positive self-talk. A healthy relationship to the body goes a long way toward restoring connection with self and

others. Like all relationships, the relationship to one's self takes time, commitment, and trust in the process.

Precautions

Viewing yoga as a supplement to therapy and nutritional counseling for individuals with eating disorders is still relatively new, and standards of care have yet to be established. When yoga classes are provided in a hospital or clinic setting the medical team is responsible for deciding a student's involvement in yoga based on health considerations. Yoga therapists are likely to have training in managing common physical issues such as osteoporosis and postural hypotension, whereas yoga teachers would likely need additional training or detailed medical guidance. The advantage of a hospital or clinic setting is that both yoga teachers and yoga therapists are able to liaise directly with a student's medical team and thus ensure that the proposed yoga practice is approved. In community-based yoga classes the lines of responsibility are less clear. Yoga therapists are qualified to conduct a comprehensive initial assessment, which can guide an individualized approach, such as deciding whether a specialized group or one-to-one sessions would be more appropriate. While yoga teachers may be aware that something is awry with their student, they may not be able to identify the symptoms of eating disorders or address student-reported challenges with osteoporosis, insomnia, and migraines. Yoga teachers are advised not to work in the community with students who currently meet eating disorder diagnostic criteria unless they gain additional training in eating disorders and related health complications. Instead, they would be better placed to deliver groups and individual sessions to those individuals who are in a much later stage of recovery and no longer engaging in food restriction and purging behaviors. Yoga teachers and yoga therapists are not medical professionals, and can be confident in knowing that it is not their role to address illness but to craft a community that is safe, nurturing, and dedicated to wellness. When yoga teachers and yoga therapists are aware of the boundaries of their discipline they can confidently refer to mental health professionals and physicians.

Despite the many benefits of yoga for self-regulation, the practice is not (nor was it traditionally intended to be) a panacea for those with eating disorders. Practicing clinicians need to be mindful of balancing the positive reports of yoga with the published case studies that link the practice of yoga to lung damage, increased pain, and the exacerbation of existing mental health problems (Campo, Shiyko, Kean, Roberts, & Pappas, 2017; Dyga & Stupak, 2015; Johnson, Tierney, & Sadighi, 2004; Lu & Lierre, 2007; Yorston, 2001). While the documented problems of yoga are in the minority, they do signal that caution is warranted until contraindications are clearly spelled out. Clinicians need to balance the positive reports with the reality that yoga can easily become another way of acting out under the guise of a healthy practice. For example, exercise addiction may lead to the compulsive practice of yoga postures as a method of detaching from and numbing psychological pain.

Clinicians and physicians must ask themselves if it is too much to add practices into the treatment of those with eating disorders. These individuals are already asked to balance the role of medication, therapy, and nutritional counseling. While group yoga classes have the potential to be safe, noncompetitive environments that encourage body acceptance and self-care, adding yoga as a method for emotion regulation means there is another thing these individuals must do in order to manage their body and establish wellness. More research is required to inform best practice, but preliminary guidance points to the importance of yoga teachers receiving additional training on adapting their practice to those with eating disorders and a shift in the culture of mainstream yoga studios to develop body-positive environments, for instance, by removing mirrors and employing teachers with a variety of body sizes (Neumark-Sztainer et al., 2011; Cook-Cottone & Douglass, 2017).

Future directions

Researchers and psychologists have found that a long-term meditation practice is correlated with increased gray matter in the brain, suggesting that meditation may lead to better memory, emotional regulation, decision making, and self-control (Schulte, 2015); that *nadi suddhi* (alternate-nostril breathing) calms the nervous system and enhances heart rate variability (Subramanian, Devaki, & Saikumar, 2016); and that yoga postures have the potential to enhance mental equanimity for a number of mental health conditions (see Table 7.1). Physicians are increasingly recommending the practice of yoga, yet no clear guidelines have been set by the American College of Physicians or the Royal College of Physicians on exactly which practices of yoga should be recommended for those diagnosed with eating disorders. For example, Duke Integrative Medicine, part of the Duke University Health System in Durham North Carolina, offers allopathic and holistic traditions as methods to support patients in their return to wellness. Their integrative yoga therapy program addresses anxiety, stress, and depression, but has yet to develop protocols for those with eating disorders. Clear guidelines for hospitals and clinics on how to integrate yoga into the healthcare system for those with eating disorders is an important next step, as individuals often turn to their physicians first for insight into the effectiveness of complementary practices such as yoga.

The use of yoga as a method to help those with eating disorders signals a shift in how those in the field of psychology think about the role of the body in mental wellness. The body is beginning to be viewed as a trusted site of wisdom that, when listened and responded to, enhances the client's ability to respond to the present moment. For those who experience the body as the primary obstacle to succeeding in life and finding happiness, it is challenging to be aware of and in the body, or *embodied*. Yet yoga is surprising. The goal of yoga, as outlined by Swami Satchidananda (2011), is to cultivate a lifestyle where the mind can be calm and allows clear seeing of one's self without any distortions. The consistent practice of yoga appears to usurp the cultural myths that with enough effort we can be thin, have endless energy, and never show signs of aging or illness. As individuals begin to accept the reality of the body, they often re-envision the authentic self. There is a shift from seeing one's self as "perfectable" to viewing one's self as "able to connect with the body," "able to connect with others," and becoming "more aware."

> The consistent practice of yoga appears to usurp the cultural myths that with enough effort we can be thin, have endless energy, and never show signs of aging or illness.

  Developing a healthy mental image of the body cannot be achieved in isolation. Wellness happens in community. The people and interactions we experience on a daily basis define the unspoken rules and regulations of relating to our bodies and ourselves. All of us (clients, clinicians, yoga teachers, and medical professionals) need to actively participate in new dialogues and practices that respect bodily diversity and the many ways individuals express powerfulness, agility, and joy through the body. It may be that some individuals have no attraction to the discipline of yoga but perhaps are attracted to mind-body centering, tai chi, powerlifting, or another somatic art that provides a similar scaffold for relating to the body and mind. Like yoga, these practices can be used for benefit or harm; individuals with eating disorders will require careful guidance no matter what somatic modality they are inspired by. In

a real sense, the paradigm shift that the discipline of yoga asks us to make is to move from the development of a strong, individualistic, well-managed ego to the development of a strong, compassionate, well-managed community. A community of wellbeing does not seek to fix the person who suffers but rather reflects their strengths while acknowledging their pain. A community of wellbeing with the body at its center naturally celebrates the strength, pleasures, and limitations of the body.

  The presence of yoga asks therapists to envisage the therapeutic landscape as a space in which the clinician and the client come together to explore embodiment. While yoga does offer powerful potential shifts in our experiences through greater self-regulation, it does not demand that we heal or become better—it merely asks us to slow down and be with what is. The philosopher Cressida Heyes asks that those of us who are concerned with the body as a site of transformation find new ways in which we can encounter ourselves (Heyes, 2007). Yoga may initially be viewed as method for self-regulation but, with time, it becomes a space in which one encounters the self and learns from the fragile, temporary strength of the body. For those with eating disorders, this exploration may only happen with the assurance and support of a therapist who can be present as they peel back the layers of suffering that have kept them from being in contact with their body, as it is, in the present moment. Changing the feeling of living in one's body takes time; the insights gained are not so much thought as they are lived.

References

Alter, J. (2004). *Yoga in Modern India*. New Jersey: Princeton University Press.

American Psychiatric Association (2013). *Diagnostic and Statistical Manual of Mental Disorders, Fifth Edition*. Washington, DC: American Psychiatric Association.

Aspen, V., Darcy, A. M., & Lock, J. (2014). Patient resistance in eating disorders. *Psychiatric Times, 31*(9), 1–4.

Augustus-Horvath, C. L., & Tylka, T. L. (2011). The acceptance model of intuitive eating: A comparison of women in emerging adulthood, early adulthood, and middle adulthood. *Journal of Counseling Psychology, 58*(1), 110–125.

Bacon, L., Stern, J. S., Van Loan, M. D., & Keim, N. L. (2005). Size acceptance and intuitive eating improve health for obese, female chronic dieters. *Journal of the American Dietetic Association, 105*(6), 929–936.

Balasubramaniam, M., Telles, S., and Doraswamy, P. M. (2013). Yoga on our minds: A systematic review of yoga for neuropsychiatric disorders. *Frontiers in Psychiatry.* 2012 3:117. Accessed from http://www.ncbi.nlm.nih.gov/pmc/articles/PMC3555015.

Barnett, J. E., & Shale, A. J. (2012). The integration of Complementary and Alternative Medicine (CAM) into the practice of psychology: A vision for the future. *Professional Psychology: Research & Practice, 43*(6), 576–585.

Birnbaum, B., & Thompson, S. H. (2014). An exploratory study of yoga practice, eating problems, depression, anxiety and desired body size among undergraduate men and women. *GAHPERD Journal, 46*(2), 16–21.

Bordo et al. (1992). *Gender/body/knowledge; feminist reconstructions of being and knowing.* New Brunswick, NJ: Rutgers University Press.

Brumberg, J. J. (2000). *Fasting Girls: The history of Anorexia Nervosa.* New York, NY: Vintage Books.

Campo, M., Shiyko, M. P., Kean, M. B., Roberts, L., & Pappas, E. (2017). Musculoskeletal pain associated with recreational yoga participation: A prospective cohort study with 1-year follow-up. *Journal of Bodywork and Movement Therapies.* Advance publication online.

Carei, T. R., Fyfe-Johnson, A. L., Breuner, C. C., & Brown, M. A. (2010). Randomized controlled clinical trial of yoga in the treatment of eating disorders. *Journal of Adolescent Health, 46*(4), 346–51.

Casiero, D., & Frishman, W.H. (2006). Cardiovascular complications of eating disorders. *Cardiology in Review, 14*(5), 227–231.

Caslini, M., Bartoli, F., Crocamo, C., Dakanalis, A., Clerici, M., & Carrà, G. (2015). Disentangling the association between child abuse and eating disorders: A systematic review and meta-analysis. *Psychosomatic Medicine.*

Cole, R. E., & Horacek, T. (2010). Effectiveness of the "My Body Knows When" intuitive-eating pilot program. *American Journal of Health Behavior, 34*(3), 286–297.

Cook-Cottone, C., Beck, M., & Kane, L. (2008). Manualized-group treatment of eating disorders: Attunement in mind, body, and relationship (AMBR). *Journal for Specialists in Group Work, 33*(1), 61–83.

Cook-Cottone, C., & Douglass, L. L. (2017). Yoga communities and eating disorders: Creating safe space for positive embodiment. *International Journal of Yoga Therapy.* Advance online publication.

Cowdrey, F. A., & Park, R. J. (2012). The role of experiential avoidance, rumination and mindfulness in eating disorders. *Eating behaviors, 13*(2), 100–105.

Crockett, A. C., Myhre, S. K., & Rokke, P. D. (2015). Boredom proneness and emotion regulation predict emotional eating. *Journal of Health Psychology, 20*(5), 670–680.

Cucchi, A., Ryan, D., Konstantakopoulos, G., Stroumpa, S., Kaçar, A. Ş., Renshaw, S., Landau, S., & Kravariti, E. (2016). Lifetime prevalence of non-suicidal self-injury in patients with eating disorders: A systematic review and meta-analysis. *Psychological Medicine, 46*(7), 1345–1358.

Culbert, K. M., Racine, S. E., & Klump, K. L. (2015). Research Review: What we have learned about the causes of eating disorders - a synthesis of sociocultural, psychological, and biological research. *Journal of Child Psychology and Psychiatry, and Allied Disciplines, 56*(11), 1141–1164.

Dale L. P., Mattison, A. M., Greening, K., Galen, G., Neace, W. P., & Matacin, M. L. (2009). Yoga workshop impacts psychological functioning and mood of women with self-reported history of eating disorders. *Eating Disorders, 17*(5), 422–434.

da Silva, T. L., Ravindran, L. N., & Ravindran, A. V. (2009). Yoga in the treatment of mood and anxiety disorders: A review. *Asian Journal of Psychiatry, 2*(1), 6–16.

Damasio, A. (1999). *The feeling of what happens.* New York: Hartcourt, Brace.

Douglass, L. (2007). How did we get here? A history of yoga in America, 1800–1970. *International Journal of Yoga Therapy,* 17: 35–42.

Douglass, L. (2009). Yoga as an intervention for eating disorders: Does it help? *Eating Disorders: The Journal of Treatment and Prevention, 17*(2), 126–139.

Douglass, L. (2011). Thinking through the body: The conceptualization of yoga as therapy for individuals with eating disorders. *Eating Disorders, 19*(1), 83–96.

Dyga, K., & Stupak, R. (2015). Meditation and psychosis: Trigger or cure? *Archives of Psychiatry & Psychotherapy, 17*(3), 48–58.

Espel, H. M., Goldstein, S. P., Manasse, S. M., & Juarascio, A. S. (2016). Experiential acceptance, motivation for recovery, and treatment outcome in eating disorders. *Eating and Weight Disorders. 21*(2), 205–210.

Evers, C., Marijn Stok, F., & de Ridder, D. T. D. (2010). Feeding your feelings: Emotion regulation strategies and emotional eating. *Personality and Social Psychology Bulletin, 36*(6), 792–804.

Failler, A. (2006). Appetizing loss: Anorexia as an experiment in living. *Eating Disorders, 14*(2), 99–107.

Fennig, S., Brunstein Klomek, A., Shahar, B., Sarel-Michnik, Z., & Hadas, A. (2015). Inpatient treatment has no impact on the core thoughts and perceptions in adolescents with anorexia nervosa. *Early Intervention in Psychiatry, 11*(3), 200–207.

Feurstein, G. (2003). *The Deeper Dimensions of Yoga.* Boston: Shambala Press.

Foucault, M. (1978). *The history of sexuality* (vol. 1). New York: Pantheon Press.

Frisch, M. J., Herzog, D. B., & Franko, D. L. (2006). Residential Treatment for Eating Disorders. *International Journal of Eating Disorders, 39,* 434–442.

Füstös, J., Gramann, K., Herbert, B. M., & Pollatos, O. (2013). On the embodiment of emotion regulation: Interoceptive awareness facilitates reappraisal. *Social Cognitive and Affective Neuroscience., 8*(8), 911–917.

Gangadhar, B. N., & Varambally, S. (2015). Integrating yoga in mental health services. *Indian Journal of Medical Research, 141*(6), 747–748.

Gonçalves, S., Machado, B., Silva, C., Crosby, R. D., Lavender, J. M., Cao, L., & Machado, P. P. (2016). The moderating role of purging behaviour in the relationship between sexual/physical abuse and nonsuicidal self-injury in eating disorder patients. *European Eating Disorders Review, 24*(2), 164–168.

Greenwood, T., & Delgado, T. (2013). A journey toward wholeness, a journey to God: Physical fitness as embodied spirituality. *Journal of Religion & Health, 52*(3), 941–954.

Gross, J. (1998). The emerging field of emotional regulation: An integrative review. *Review of General Psychology, 2*(3), 271–299.

Guarda, A. S., Schreyer, C. C., Boersma, G. J., Tamashiro, K. L., & Moran, T. H. (2015). Anorexia nervosa as a motivated behavior: Relevance of anxiety, stress, fear and learning. *Physiology & Behavior, 152*, 466–472.

Gunderson, K. (2007, October 24). Personal Interview.

Herranz Valera, J., Acuña Ruiz, P., Romero Valdespino, B., & Visioli, F. (2014). Prevalence of orthorexia nervosa among ashtanga yoga practitioners: a pilot study. *Eating & Weight Disorders, 19*(4), 469–472.

Heyes, C. (2007). *Self-Transformations: Foucault, Ethics, and Normalized Bodies.* New York: Oxford University Press.

Hoang, U., Goldacre, M., & James, A. (2014). Mortality following hospital discharge with a diagnosis of eating disorder: National record linkage study, England, 2001–2009. *The International Journal of Eating Disorders, 47*(5), 507–515.

Holland, A., & Sicotte, N. (1988). Anorexia nervosa: Evidence for a genetic basis. *Journal of Psychosomatic Research, 32*(6), 561–571.

Iannantuono, A. C., & Tylka, T. L. (2012). Interpersonal and intrapersonal links to body appreciation in college women: An exploratory model. *Body Image, 9*(2), 227–35.

Isomaa, R., Backholm, K., & Birgegård, A. (2015). Posttraumatic stress disorder in eating disorder patients: The roles of psychological distress and timing of trauma. *Psychiatry Research, 230*(2), 506–510.

Javnbakht, M., Hejazi Kenari, R., & Ghasemi, M. (2009). Effects of yoga on depression and anxiety of women. *Complementary Therapies in Clinical Practice, 15*(2), 102–104.

Johnson, D. B., Tierney, M. J., & Sadighi, P. J. (2004). Kapalabhati pranayama: Breath of fire or cause of pneumothorax? A case report. *Chest, 125*(5), 1951–1952.

Klein, J., & Cook-Cottone, C. (2013). The effects of yoga on eating disorder symptoms and correlates: A review. *International journal of Yoga Therapy, 23*, 41–50.

Kolk, B. V. D. (2014). *The Body Keeps the Score: Brain, Mind and Body in the Healing of Trauma.* New York: Penguin.

Lavender, J. M., Wonderlich, S. A., Engel, S. G., Gordon, K. H., Kay, W. H., & Mitchell J. E. (2015). Dimensions of emotion dysregulation in anorexia nervosa and bulimia nervosa: A conceptual review of the empirical literature. *Clinical Psychology Review, 40* 111–122

Lavey, R., Sherman, T., Mueser, K., Osbourne, D., Currier, M., & Wolfe, R. (2005). The effects of yoga on mood in psychiatric inpatients. *Psychiatric Rehabilitation Journal, 28*(4), 399–402.

Lu, J. S., & Lierre, J. M. (2007). Psychotic episode associated with Bikram yoga. *American Journal of Psychiatry, 164*, 1760–1761.

Lu, Y. H., Rosner, B., Chang, G., & Fishman, L. M. (2016). Twelve-minute daily yoga regime reverses osteoporotic bone loss. *Topics in Geriatric Rehabilitation, 32*(2), 81–87.

Manaf, N. A., Saravanan, C., & Zuhrah, B. (2016). The prevalence and inter-relationship of negative body image perception, depression and susceptibility to eating disorders among female medical undergraduate students. *Journal of Clinical & Diagnostic Research, 10*(3), 1–4.

McIver, S., McGartland, M., & O'Halloran, P. (2009). "Overeating is not about the food": Women describe their experience of a yoga treatment program for binge eating. *Qualitative Health Research, 19*(9), 1234–1245.

Menezes, C. B., Dalpiaz, N. R., Kiesow, L. G., Sperb, W., Hertzberg, J., & Oliveira, A. A. (2015). Yoga and emotion regulation: A review of primary psychological outcomes and their physiological correlates. *Psychology & Neuroscience, 8*(1), 82–101.

Merwin, R., Moskovich, A. A., Wagner, H. R., Ritschel, L. A., Craighead, L. W., & Zucker, N. L. (2013). Emotional regulation difficulties in anorexia nervosa: Relationship to self-perceived sensory sensitivity. *Cognition & Emotion, 27*(3), 441–452.

Michopoulos, V., Powers, A., Moore, C., Villarreal, S., Ressler, K. J., & Bradley, B. (2015). The mediating role of emotion dysregulation and depression on the relationship between childhood trauma exposure and emotional eating. *Appetite, 91*, 129–136.

Monteleone, A. M., Monteleone, P., Serino, I., Scognamiglio, P., Di Genio, M., & Maj, M. (2015). Childhood trauma and cortisol awakening response in symptomatic patients with anorexia nervosa and bulimia nervosa. *The International Journal of Eating Disorders, 48*(6), 615–621.

Neumark-Sztainer, D., Eisenberg, M. E., Wall, M., & Loth, K. A. (2011). Yoga and Pilates: Associations with body image and disordered-eating behaviors in a population-based sample of young adults. *The International Journal Of Eating Disorders, 44*(3), 276–280.

O'Shaughnessy, R., & Dallos, R. (2009). Attachment research and eating disorders: A review of the literature. *Clinical Child Psychology and Psychiatry, 14*(4), 559–574.

Ogden, P., Minton, K., & Pain, C. (2006). *Trauma and the Body: A Sensorimotor Approach to Psychotherapy.* New York: WW Norton & Company.

Pacanowski, C. R., Diers, L., Crosby, R., & Neumark-Sztaner, D. (2017). Yoga in the treatment of eating disorders within a residential program: A randomized controlled trial. *Eating Disorders, 25*(1), 37–51.

Palmeira, L., Trindade, I. A., & Ferreira, C. (2014). Can the impact of body dissatisfaction on disordered eating be weakened by one's decentering abilities? *Eating Behaviors, 15*(3), 392–396.

Park, C. L., Riley, K. E., Bedesin, E., & Stewart, V. M. (2014). Why practice yoga? Practitioners' motivations for adopting and maintaining yoga practice. *Journal of Health Psychology, 21*(6), 887–896.

Pilkington, K., Kirkwood, G., Rampes, H., & Richardson, J. (2005). Yoga for depression: The research evidence. *Journal of Affective Disorders, 89*(1–3), 13–24.

Polivy, J., & Herman, C. P. (2002). Causes of eating disorders. *Annual Review of Psychology, 53*(1), 187–213.

Ranzenhofer et al (2013 Sep). Pre-meal affective state and laboratory test meal intake in adolescent girls with loss of control eating. *Appetite.* 68:30-7. Epub 2013 Apr 18.

Reddy, S., Dick, A. M., Gerber, M. R., & Mitchell, K. (2014). The effect of a yoga intervention on alcohol and drug abuse risk in veteran and civilian women with posttraumatic stress disorder. *Journal of Alternative and Complementary Medicine, 20*(10), 750–756.

Riva, G. (2014). Out of my real body: Cognitive neuroscience meets eating disorders. *Frontiers in Human Neuroscience, 8*, 236–236.

Satchidananda, S. (2011). *To Know Your Self: The Essential Teachings of Swami Satchidananda.* Buckingham, VA: Satchidananda Ashram, Yogaville.

Schulte, B. (2015). 'Harvard neuroscientist: Meditation not only reduces stress, here's how it changes your brain.' *The Washington Post.* Accessed 9/17/2017.

Shafir, T., Tsachor, R. P., Welch, K. B., Watson, R., & Allard, E. S. (2016). Emotion regulation through movement: Unique sets of movement characteristics are associated with and enhance basic emotions. *Frontiers in Psychology*, 1–15.

Shahabi, L., Naliboff, B. D., & Shapiro, D. (2016). Self-regulation evaluation of therapeutic yoga and walking for patients with irritable bowel syndrome: A pilot study. *Psychology, Health & Medicine, 21*(2), 176–186.

Singleton, M. (2010). *Yoga Body: The Origins of Modern Posture Practice.* London: Oxford University Press.

Sisk, J. (2007). Yoga and the social worker — mantra meets mental health. *Social Work Today, 7*(2), 30.

Sly, R., Morgan, J. F., Mountford, V. A., Sawer, F., Evans, C., & Lacey, J. H. (2014). Rules of engagement: Qualitative experiences of therapeutic alliance when receiving in-patient treatment for anorexia nervosa. *Eating Disorders, 22*(3), 233–243.

Spinazzola, J., Rhodes, A. M., Emerson, D., Earle, E., & Monroe, K. (2011). Application of yoga in residential treatment of traumatized youth. *Journal of the American Psychiatric Nurses Association, 17*(6), 431–444.

Steinglass J., Albano A. M., Simpson H. B., Carpenter K., Schebendach J., & Attia E. (2012a). Fear of food as a treatment target: Exposure and response prevention for anorexia nervosa in an open series. *International Journal of Eating Disorders,*45 615–621.

Streeter, C. C., Jensen, J. E., Perlmutter, R. M., Cabral, H. J., Tian, H., Terhune, D. B., et al. (2007). Yoga asana sessions increase brain GABA levels: A pilot study. *Journal of Alternative & Complementary Medicine, 13*(4), 419–426.

Subramanya, P., & Telles, S. (2009). Effect of two yoga-based relaxation techniques on memory scores and state anxiety. *BioPsychoSocial Medicine, 3*, 8.

Subramanian, R.K., Devaki P.R., & Saikumar, P. (2016). Alternate nostril breathing at different rates and its influence on heart rate variability in non practitioners of yoga. *Journal of Clinical & Diagnostic Research, 10*(1), CM01–CM02.

Sweeting, H., Walker, L., Maclean, A., Patterson, C., RäIsänen, U., & Hunt, K. (2015). Prevalence of eating disorders in males: A review of rates reported in academic research and UK mass media. *International Journal of Men's Health, 14*(2), 86–112.

Uebelacker, L. A., & Broughton, M. K. (2016). Yoga for depression and anxiety: A review of published research and implications for healthcare providers. *Rhode Island Medical Journal (2013), 99*(3), 20–22.

von Hausswolff-Juhlin, Y., Brooks, S. J., & Larsson, M. (2015). The neurobiology of eating disorders—a clinical perspective. *Acta Psychiatrica Scandinavica, 131*(4), 244–255.

Yorston, G. A. (2001). Mania precipitated by meditation: A case report and literature review. *Mental Health, Religion & Culture, 4*(2), 209–213.

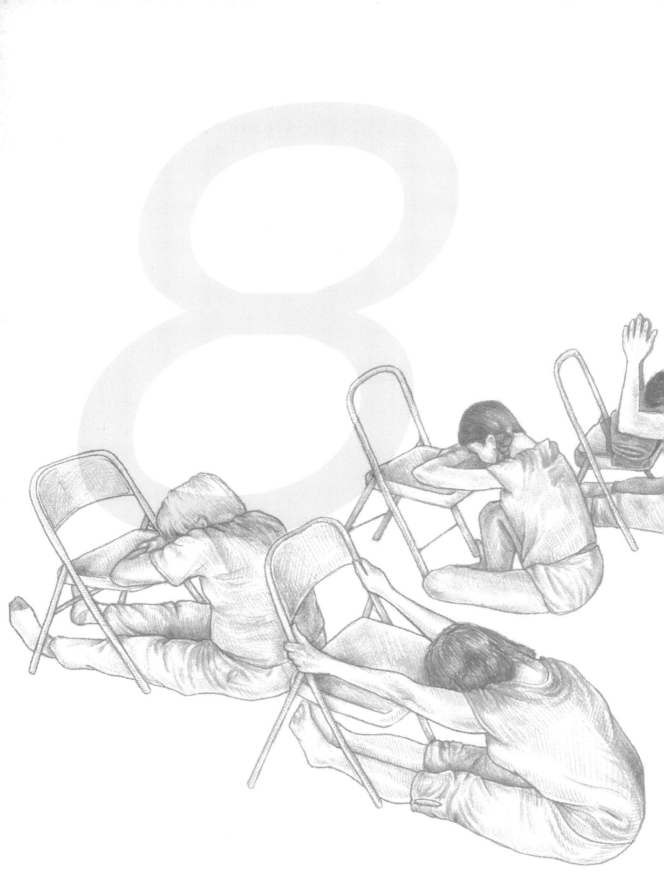

Schizophrenia

Shivarama Varambally and Elizabeth Visceglia

8

Overview

Schizophrenia, one of the most severe mental disorders, is also one of the most enigmatic illnesses that human beings suffer from. Schizophrenia is the most well-known of a group of psychiatric illnesses called *psychoses*, where the primary problems are loss of touch with reality and loss of insight into one's condition. The lifetime prevalence of psychosis is greater than 3% of the general population if all causes of psychoses are included (Perala et al., 2007). Among the psychoses, schizophrenia occurs almost universally (at a prevalence of around 0.4%) in most human populations and affects both sexes equally (Gururaj et al., 2016; Saha, Chant, Welham, & McGrath, 2005). Most patients develop the illness in the second or third decade of life (while it tends to be earlier in males), which means it affects almost all domains of their lives such as education, employment, relationships, and family life. It also can have pathoplastic effects on the personality of the individual. The current neurodevelopmental understanding of the pathogenesis of schizophrenia postulates that there is a significant genetic vulnerability, with the onset and course being linked to stress, adverse life events, and use of psychoactive substances (the "two-hit" hypothesis). Despite significant advances in understanding and treatment of psychosis, prognosis remains difficult in 40–50% of patients (Hegarty, Baldessarini, Tohen, Waternaux, & Oepen, 1994). The most recognized symptoms are delusions and hallucinations (positive symptoms), which are easily identifiable and respond well to available treatments, such as antipsychotic medications. However, the negative symptoms (amotivation, anhedonia, and emotional blunting) and cognitive deficits are also primary features of psychosis, and may precede the onset of positive symptoms by months or

years. These dimensions are more difficult to address with available treatments (Buckley & Stahl, 2007), and cause more disability. Recent research has shown that these negative and cognitive symptoms correlate better with real-life functioning and productivity of the individual. Along with neurocognitive deficits, specific deficits in social cognition have been demonstrated in these patients, which significantly influence real-world functioning and prognosis (Hofer et al., 2009; Kee, Green, Mintz, & Brekke, 2003).

> Most patients develop the illness in the second or third decade of life (while it tends to be earlier in males), which means it affects almost all domains of their lives such as education, employment, relationships, and family life.

Treatment for psychosis

The 1990s was a period when several new medications for psychosis (second-generation antipsychotics) were introduced, leading to hopes of better recovery for those patients. However, the real-life changes have been less than expected, with recovery rates remaining almost unchanged. Also, the production line of new medications appears to have stalled, leading some commentators to announce a "drug deadlock" in schizophrenia (Abbott, 2010). The other important issue apart from suboptimal efficacy of medications (particularly for negative and cognitive symptoms) is that they lead to a variety of adverse effects, ranging from extrapyramidal side effects—movement disorders such as tardive dyskinesia and akathisia, thought to be due to lack of dopamine caused by the older antipsychotics—to metabolic, cardiac, and hormonal effects with the newer medications. Hence, complementary therapies, including yoga, have emerged as important options in a multidisciplinary treatment plan. Yoga-based interventions have proven to be effective treatments in psychiatric disorders such as anxiety and depression (Rao, Varambally, & Gangadhar, 2013). However, the area of yoga as a therapy for psychosis remained uncharted territory until the early years of the twenty-first century. Possible reasons for this include apprehension about reports that meditative practices may worsen or provoke psychotic symptoms (Walsh & Roche, 1979), and also the perception that patients with psychosis may not be able to understand and follow yoga protocols. In light of these concerns, an important point to be noted about most of the research discussed in this chapter is that the components of the yoga modules were mainly yogasana and pranayama. Meditative practices have been avoided because of the concerns given, as well as the objective difficulty in verifying the actual performance of the practices.

Rationale for the use of yoga in psychosis

The term schizophrenia, which literally means "split mind," was coined by the Swiss psychiatrist Eugen Bleuler (1908); he intended it to describe the disconnection between personality, thinking, memory, and perception in a particular individual. Patients with schizophrenia show a lack of congruence between thought and affect (mood) and sometimes demonstrate clearly inappropriate emotional expressions (for example, a person with a delusional fear of being persecuted may appear unconcerned or laugh loudly during conversation). Currently, schizophrenia is understood as a neurodevelopmental disorder in which there is aberrant connectivity between different brain areas and networks, which leads to disorganization in thought processes as well as perception. People with schizophrenia also have significant disruption of self-boundaries and may find it difficult to distinguish between internal experiences and external reality. This can be reflected in the form of experiences such as hallucinations and thought-alienation phenomena where the person feels a loss of control over their body and mind and perceives these phenomena as being caused by external agencies. Recent research has shown that patients with this disorder experience a disconnect at multiple levels—neuronal networks, mental processes, and interpersonal relationships—leading to its description as a "connectopathy" (Mehta, Keshavan, & Gangadhar, 2016). Holistically viewed, a person with this disorder suffers from poor connectivity both within the self (brain/ mind) as well as externally (with family and society as a whole).

On the other hand, the term yoga is derived from the Sanskrit word *yuj* which means "to yoke together" or "to unite." The ultimate aim of yoga as enunciated by the sage Patanjali is to achieve *samatvam uchyate* (equilibrium) and merge individual consciousness with the universal. Logically, this process should be helpful in reuniting the split aspects of the individual and in reconnecting that individual to society. The body- and breath-regulation aspects of yoga should enable a person to regain a sense of control over their body, and the mindfulness aspects should similarly help with control of the mind. Further, learning yoga from a yoga teacher/therapist, particularly in a group, should foster the sense of connection and belonging. Also, yoga-based practices have been shown to improve various deficits that are seen in schizophrenia (cognitive deficits including neurocognition and social cognition, depression and anxiety symptoms) in healthy subjects as well as in patients with other psychiatric disorders. With this rationale, several studies have been done on the effects of yoga in schizophrenia and other psychoses in the last two decades, with promising results.

Studies of the use of yoga in psychosis

One of the first studies to use yoga-based practices in patients with psychosis was conducted by Nagendra, Telles, and Naveen (2000) on chronic institutionalized patients with schizophrenia. They concluded that patients were able to learn yoga and also derive some benefits in social and cognitive domains without experiencing disturbing side effects. In an early RCT, 90 patients with schizophrenia went through eight weeks of yoga practice alongside a treatment-as-usual control group (Xie, Lin, & Guo, 2006). The patients in the yoga group showed improvements in physical and psychological functioning as well as in quality of life. Another RCT using a specific yoga-based module included 61 consenting outpatients on stable medication who had moderate symptoms. They were randomized to either the yoga module or a standard set of physical exercises and were trained for one month by the same instructor. They were then advised to continue the practices at home for the next three months. The patients' symptoms were assessed using the positive and negative syndrome scale for schizophrenia (PANSS) (Kay, Fiszbein, & Opler, 1987), and social functioning was assessed using the Social and Occupational Functioning Scale (SOFS) (Saraswat, Rao, Subbakrishna, & Gangadhar, 2006). These assessments were carried out at baseline and then after four months by an independent psychiatrist. Over the four months, negative symptoms and social dysfunction reduced in both groups, with the yoga group showing greater improvement (Duraiswamy, Thirthalli, Nagendra, & Gangadhar, 2007). However, this study did not have a non-intervention control group or any measures of cognition. A subsequent RCT conducted by the same researchers (the largest published RCT of yoga for psychosis to date) included a larger number of patients (n=120) divided into three groups: yoga, physical exercise, and waitlist control (Varambally et al., 2012). This RCT used the same yoga and exercise modules and its methodology was similar to the earlier one, and assessment included the PANSS, SOFS, and a standardized tool for social cognition, the Tool for Recognition of Emotions in Neuropsychiatric Disorders (TRENDS) (Behere, Raghunandan, & Venkatasubramanian, 2008). TRENDS measures

a patient's ability to recognize facial emotions and includes standardized images of faces with different emotions as expressed by experienced actors. The sum of accurate recognitions yields the TRENDS Accuracy Score (TRACS). Improvement was operationally defined as a drop of 15 in the PANSS total score, a drop of 7 in each of the PANSS negative and positive scores, and a drop of 14 in the SOFS total score. The results of this RCT showed that significantly more patients in the yoga group improved than those in the other two groups, particularly in negative symptoms and socio-occupational functioning. Odds-ratio analyses showed that the likelihood of improvement in the yoga group in terms of negative symptoms was about five times greater than in the waitlist and the exercise groups. With regard to emotion recognition, the patients in the yoga group improved significantly in the yoga group from baseline to the second month, as well as to the end of the RCT, with no significant improvement in the other two groups (Behere et al., 2011). The NICE guidelines for management of schizophrenia (National Institute for Health and Care Excellence, 2014) cited these RCTs as good quality evidence and recommended yoga as a complementary intervention in schizophrenia.

A pilot RCT in the United States, which included eighteen institutionalized patients with schizophrenia, allocated them to either eight weeks of a yoga module, which included postures, breathing exercises, and relaxation, or a waitlist group. Once again the results showed significant improvements in positive and negative symptom scores on the PANSS, as well as on quality of life in the yoga group (Visceglia & Lewis, 2011). Another study from India evaluated a yoga module as a cognitive remediation technique in patients with schizophrenia and bipolar disorder (Bhatia et al., 2012), with results showing positive effects on several cognitive functions. The cognitive improvement was greater in subjects with schizophrenia, particularly males. An RCT using single sessions of yoga or physical exercise in patients with schizophrenia found significantly decreased state anxiety and psychological stress and increased subjective wellbeing compared with a control condition (Vancampfort et al., 2011). Another small RCT on 30 inpatients with schizophrenia found improvements in subjective wellbeing and basic living skills and reduction in disability after one month's practice of yoga (Paikkatt, Singh, Singh, & Jahan, 2012).

However, a recent single-blinded RCT that used weekly one-hour hatha yoga sessions as an adjunct to regular treatment for eight weeks found no positive changes in resilience level or stress markers. The authors commented that the duration and intensity of the yoga sessions, and the focus on patients with chronic illnesses, may explain the negative observations (Ikai et al., 2014). The majority of these RCTs included chronic patients who were stabilized on antipsychotics. In light of the fact that duration of illness is a valuable predictor of prognosis in schizophrenia, early intervention is more likely to have better effects. A recent RCT of yoga included inpatients with psychosis in the acute phase of treatment (Manjunath, Varambally, Thirthalli, Basavaraddi, & Gangadhar, 2013) using the same yoga modules as in the RCTs conducted by Varambally et al. (2012). Consenting inpatients who were deemed fit for yoga/exercise training by their treating psychiatrist (n=88) were randomized into yoga therapy (n=44) and physical exercise (*n*=44) groups. Patients were able to learn the yoga practices, and after six weeks, 60 patients remained in the RCT. Analysis showed that patients in the yoga group had significantly lower mean scores on illness severity and depression. This is an important demonstration that yoga-based interventions may be used in fairly acute phases of psychosis with some early benefits. Extending this logic and using such interventions in high-risk populations to prevent psychosis is an important and interesting future area for research.

Systematic reviews and meta-analyses looking at the effects of yoga and physical therapies in persons with schizophrenia and psychosis are now available. One such review concluded that physical interventions offered added value as part of a multidisciplinary approach (Vancampfort et al., 2012). Another review by Helgason & Sarris (2013) found positive evidence for yoga and meditative techniques in patients with psychosis. Some recent reviews have also discussed the methodological limitations in many of these RCTs conducted in psychosis. A systematic review and meta-analysis (Cramer, Lauche, Klose, Langhorst, & Dobos, 2013) found methodological limitations and a high risk of bias in most RCTs, and that only five RCTs encompassing a total of 337 patients could be included in their meta-analysis. The analysis found moderate evidence for short-term effects on quality of life compared to usual care, but no other significant effects. A subsequent publication by the same group (Cramer, Lauche, Langhorst, & Dobos, 2015) suggested that RCTs on yoga conducted in India had significantly higher odds of reaching positive conclusions as those conducted elsewhere. Possible explanations given for this were that Indian studies generally used more intense yoga programs and also more highly skilled therapists than studies conducted in western countries. A summary of controlled studies in psychosis is provided in Table 8.1.

Possible mechanisms of action of yoga in schizophrenia

Yoga-based interventions have demonstrated improvements in symptoms and cognitive measures in patients with schizophrenia. Some studies have attempted to find the mechanisms underlying these effects. A recent study assessed changes in emotion recognition and plasma levels of the hormone oxytocin, known as the "cuddling hormone" and known to be important in mother–infant bonding and also in generating feelings of wellbeing. This study

Table 8.1

Controlled studies of yoga as interventions in psychosis

Author, year	Sample	Yoga technique	Control	Duration of yoga	Results
Xie et al., 2006	Schizophrenia (n=90)	Yoga (postures, breathing techniques, meditation, relaxation)	Usual care	8 weeks	Physical and psychological functioning and quality of life improved in the yoga group
Duraiswamy et al., 2007	Schizophrenia (n=61)	Yoga module with asana and pranayama (n=31)	Physical exercise (n=30)	4 months	Patients in the yoga group had significantly better PANSS scores, functioning, and quality of life
Visceglia and Lewis, 2011	Schizophrenia (n=18)	Personalized yoga module (n=10)	Waitlist (n=8)	8 weeks; twice weekly sessions	Patients in the yoga group showed significantly greater improvements in PANSS scores and perceived quality of life
Vancampfort et al., 2011	Schizophrenia or schizoaffective disorder (n=49)	Single 30-minute yoga session (hatha yoga)	Single 20-minute session of aerobic exercise or reading	Single session	Decreased state anxiety and psychological stress, and increased subjective wellbeing in the yoga and aerobic exercise groups compared to the control group
Bhatia et al., 2012	Schizophrenia (n=88)	Yoga module with asana and pranayama (n=65)	Treatment as usual (n=23)	3 weeks	Patients in the yoga group showed greater improvement with regard to measures of attention; changes were more prominent among men
Varambally et al., 2012	Schizophrenia (n=119); RCT: 3 groups	Yoga module with asana and pranayama (n=46)	Physical exercise (n=36) Waitlist (n=37)	4 months	More patients in the yoga group improved in PANSS negative and total scores and functioning
Manjunath et al., 2013	Non-affective psychosis (n=88)	Yoga module with asana and pranayama (n=44)	Physical exercise (n=44)	6 weeks	Patients in the yoga group had CGIS, PANSS total, and HDRS

randomized consenting patients with schizophrenia to receive yoga or remain waitlisted for one month. The patients who participated obtained significant benefits in emotional recognition (TRENDS) scores following yoga, with no such benefits observed in the waitlisted patients. Plasma oxytocin levels rose significantly (nearly threefold) in the yoga group after one month of practice, while there was no change in the control group (Jayaram et al., 2013). This suggests that yoga practice is correlated with elevation of oxytocin levels, which may mediate the benefits in social cognition as well as the feeling of wellbeing that many people describe following yoga practice. This sense of wellbeing and improved ability to understand others' emotional states also improves motivation levels, especially for social interaction; this is an important negative symptom of schizophrenia, and particularly difficult to improve with medication.

> This suggests that yoga practice is correlated with elevation of oxytocin levels, which may mediate the benefits in social cognition as well as the feeling of wellbeing that many people describe following yoga.

The method of learning yoga involves conscious and mindful imitation of the yoga teacher/therapist. It requires involvement of the mirror neuron system (MNS) in the brain that was first demonstrated in monkeys, and is now understood to also be critical in learning by imitation and social cognition in humans (Rizzolatti & Craighero, 2004; Rizzolatti & Fabbri-Destro, 2008). Children with autism spectrum disorders showed improvements in imitation skills after the practice of yoga (Radhakrishna, 2010). It has been demonstrated that both mirror neuron activity (MNA) and social cognition are impaired in schizophrenia, and that there is a direct association between MNA deficits and social cognition (Mehta et al., 2014). MNA is also correlated with oxytocin levels, and oxytocin nebulization has been shown to improve gesture imitation in newborn monkeys (Simpson

et al., 2014). Nasal oxytocin has in fact been used to try and improve social cognition in patients with schizophrenia. Emerging studies are assessing MNA activity using techniques such as functional near-infrared spectroscopy (fNIRS) to examine cortical activity during action (although activity can only be detected in surface cortical areas, this is a simpler and non-invasive alternative to functional magnetic resonance imaging) and transcranial magnetic stimulation (TMS), which is another safe and non-invasive way of studying neuronal activity. Preliminary results suggest that one month of yoga practice significantly increased MNA in healthy subjects (Chhabra et al., unpublished data). Putting the above results together, we may attempt a synthetic hypothesis to explain the effects of yoga in patients with schizophrenia (see Figure 8.1). For an overview and analysis of putative mechanisms of yoga in schizophrenia, the reader would be well advised to refer to the review by Mehta et al. (2016).

To summarize, yoga as a complementary intervention in patients with schizophrenia should help patients regain a sense of control over their minds and bodies. This is particularly true for patients in the early course of illness because it may be possible to prevent or reduce the negative symptoms. These effects may occur through biological mechanisms such as elevation of plasma oxytocin levels and activation of the MNS, but yoga as a social activity can also help patients reduce some of the secondary risks associated with schizophrenia, including a sedentary lifestyle and metabolic syndrome. Furthermore, it is anticipated that these improvements in negative and cognitive aspects would have positive knock-on effects on social interaction, work performance, and quality of life, thus helping the person reintegrate into society. This reintegration, rather than merely reducing symptoms, is the ultimate aim of treatment for patients with this devastating disorder, and yoga may play a very important role in achieving this objective.

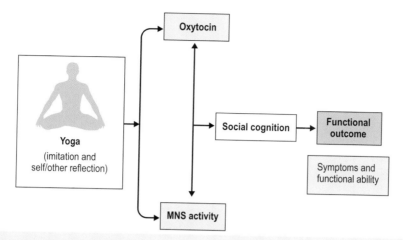

Figure 8.1

A hypothesis for the effects of yoga in schizophrenia. The impact of yoga therapy on social cognition via its engagement of neuropeptides and the mirror neuron system. Illustration by Dr. Urvakhsh Mehta. Redrawn with permission from Drs. Varambally and Mehta, NIMHANS

Yoga as a complementary intervention in patients with schizophrenia should help patients regain a sense of control over their minds and bodies.

Yogic perceptions of schizophrenia

As the concept of split mind suggests, disconnection is a defining feature of schizophrenia. This disconnection occurs on cellular/neural, personal/emotional, and social/interpersonal levels, a cascade of interdependent dysfunctions. Philosophically and practically, connection and wholeness would be the means by which to address this connectopathy. As stated in the *Brihadarankyaka Upanishad*, in yoga, "…having become calm and concentrated, one perceives the Self (Atman) within oneself" (Flood, 1996). This union is the essence of yogic practice and a much-needed addition to current approaches to schizophrenia.

In yogic perception, schizophrenia contains two spheres of imbalance in the *gunas* (qualities, or tendencies). There is an element of excess *rajasic* energy, which creates chaotic and confusing mental perceptions and hallucinations, as well as agitation and restlessness. There is also, paradoxically, an element of excess *tamasic* energy, leading to the depressive, disconnected, and apathetic aspects of this illness. The guna of balance and clarity, *sattva*, is overwhelmed by these excesses. These disparate categories of difficulties mirror the current psychiatric model of negative and positive symptoms discussed earlier.

People with schizophrenia are often highly sensitive, and in supportive circumstances this can be a strength, providing a richness of life experience. However, because of the confusion and the self-consciousness many people experience after spending years being treated as profoundly different from others and as sick, there is frequently inadequate support for many to use this sensitivity in an egosyntonic way. Furthermore, lack of sufficient energy in the grounding lower chakras leaves the excesses of the upper

Chapter 8

chakras unchecked. Once again, the psyche or energetic body is pulled apart in competing directions, rather than functioning as a unified whole. This split creates greater mental suffering.

Recommendations for practice

In the *Diagnostic and Statistical Manual of Mental Disorders, Fifth Edition* (DSM-5), a diagnosis of schizophrenia necessitates positive symptoms enduring for at least one month, and continuous signs of the disturbance presenting for at least six months; a shorter period is considered to be a brief psychotic episode or a schizophreniform disorder (American Psychiatric Association, 2013). Once an individual is diagnosed with schizophrenia, they may have frequent psychotic episodes and positive symptoms or they may never recur again. There are often ongoing negative symptoms that are typically exacerbated by antipsychotic medications. In all of these cases therapeutic yoga can be helpful. In the initial management of a psychotic episode, yoga can be part of an early intervention so that perhaps there will be less likelihood of progression to chronic schizophrenia. For those with ongoing symptoms, yoga may reduce the severity and frequency of psychotic episodes and help counteract some of the most troublesome side effects of medications, as well as improve quality of life.

> For those with ongoing symptoms, yoga may reduce the severity and frequency of psychotic episodes and help counteract some of the most troublesome side effects of medications, as well as improve quality of life.

In using therapeutic yoga for schizophrenia, it is important for the yoga teacher/therapist to be adequately trained. While this training may take a variety of forms, a thorough understanding of schizophrenia, the medications used to treat it and their side effects, and insight into the ways this illness can affect individuals are essential. People with this disorder are sensitive, and to offer yoga without this background could lead to a negative response. Some basic therapeutic principles including appropriate boundaries, transference, and countertransference, are also necessary.

Creating a safe container for group classes

The staging of the class is central, and there are important aspects to be considered when creating a safe container for students in a group class. Creating a class environment that feels safe for exploration and is supportive of each individual is the central challenge. This is accomplished by the following recommendations, starting with using a quiet, clean room where participants cannot be easily observed from outside, so that it feels private and students do not feel overly self-conscious. There should be two trained and qualified teachers present so that one of them can teach and the other one can assist anyone having difficulties. Having the flexibility of mind to meet each student where they are, rather than holding some idea of where they should be, or where they were during the last class, models this behavior for the clients themselves. Teachers and students should all be introduced to each other, and new students should be added to a group individually or by no more than two each time. Mats should be arranged in a circle so that no one's paranoia is triggered by having people behind them, and chairs should be available nearby for modifications and also to help with balance. Clients may be medicated or not, but they need to be able to follow simple instructions to participate in class. However, we recommend that those currently experiencing acute psychosis receive any necessary medication before attending class. It is best for people to follow along in their own unique way without constantly correcting them, and to encourage them by articulating that anything which feels scary or uncomfortable doesn't need to be done. For clients with enduring schizophrenia, the ability to follow instructions may be significantly compromised. There may be greater

156

neurological degeneration and the medication they are taking may influence weight and cardiovascular health, making movement and balance more challenging. It may be helpful to hold specific classes for such clients that are chair-based, while those who are physically able can participate in mat-based classes.

> There should be two trained and qualified teachers present so that one of them can teach and the other one can assist anyone having difficulties.

It's helpful to state clearly at the beginning of every class that hands-on adjustments may be offered but only after asking each person if it is acceptable to them and that it is always OK to say no. Given the sensitivity of this group, with the high levels of trauma found in their histories and their potential to misconstrue information, many yoga teachers opt not to offer physical adjustments at all, but rather cue verbal ones that rely on the student to become aware of their own body and how they are holding it. Finally, finding ways to truly enjoy the practice together is essential. Research shows that across all kinds of psychotherapy, the better the rapport between client and therapist, the more healing ensues. The same can be extrapolated to yoga therapy: the student/client and yoga teacher/therapist relationship is key.

In addition to fostering a nurturing set-up there are several other things to consider. A yoga teacher/therapist should expect a rather different experience teaching individuals with schizophrenia compared with a typical yoga class. It is important to take each class and treat each student as they are in that moment. Not having any expectations other than aware, nonjudgmental presence is essential. Perhaps more than any other mental disorder, schizophrenia is stigmatized, feared, and played upon powerfully by myriad cultural projections about madness. The willingness on the part of the yoga teacher/therapist to be fully present to their own experience, and to the experience of everyone else in the room, can create a supportive sense of spaciousness. When the mind of the teacher is uncluttered they can then attend to the moment-by-moment unfolding of the worlds inside and around them; the teacher/therapist simultaneously models this skill and creates a sense of ease for those in their presence. Learning to closely attend to personal experience, without judging or over-identifying with it, is at the heart of yoga practice.

Inviting the client(s) to be present to feel their breath, gently move their bodies, and experience whatever they feel capable of experiencing in that moment is the radical invitation of yoga. It is important to remember that a majority of people with schizophrenia do have a history of trauma, as indicated by the aforementioned two-hit theory. Although there is a genetic predisposition to schizophrenia, trauma clearly plays an important role etiologically. It has been found that children who experience severe trauma are up to three times more likely to develop schizophrenia, regardless of genetics (Bentall, Wickham, & Shevlin, 2012). As a result of the addition of trauma, it is possible for clients to experience too much all at once during yoga practice. Peter Levine's theory of *pendulation* is helpful in addressing this. In his work with Somatic Experiencing, Levine (2010) writes that "pendulation is the primal rhythm expressed as movement from constriction to expansion, but gradually opening to more and more expansion." This means that movement therapies can help clients to begin to touch the source of their suffering through breath and body awareness, and then allow them to emotionally and physically move away from this suffering when it becomes too much. As the mind and body resettle, they can move again into discomfort in an ongoing process that resembles a pendulum.

Some clients may find that certain aspects of yoga therapy trigger old traumas, so it is essential to articulate to clients that they should not feel compelled to participate in any asana or other practice that feels frightening or overwhelming. A posture such as *ananda balasana* (happy baby pose) may make students feel vulnerable because it is performed supine with the legs open; it and others like it should usually be avoided—and perhaps should never be used, at least not until a container of trust is well established. Similarly, postures such as *eka pada adho mukha svanasana* (one-legged dog pose) may also make many feel exposed. Indeed, some students may feel unexpectedly vulnerable in some poses that can't be predicted by the yoga teacher/therapist. Therefore, offering significant sensitivity to each individual is absolutely essential, and picking up on small cues can be very important. Some clients might express delusional material or regress in other ways if old traumas are triggered, and they will need particular attention and support. This matter is at the heart of the need to address every person as an individual, never overgeneralizing about what a range of people's individual experiences or needs may be. It is also vital for the yoga teacher/therapist to be well-versed in the history of each client, as well as the particulars of their illness. Coordinating care with the treatment team can be very helpful, particularly with more chronic patients.

> Offering significant sensitivity to each individual is absolutely essential, and picking up on small cues can be very important.

In the West, people with schizophrenia typically suffer from several other difficulties related to their mental illness. They are often subject to long-term institutionalization, which leads to a loss of independence as well as a loss of family or positive social supports; they are exposed to long-term treatment with medication that often worsen the negative symptoms that bother them the most while to some extent successfully suppressing the positive symptoms that are the most obvious markers of their illness; and many also experience a loss of connection with their body after years of focusing on their brain as the problem. The majority of people with schizophrenia have a history of trauma and loss, and are subject to downward socioeconomic drift. In two long-term studies of over 1200 people with schizophrenia all over the world (Leff, Sartorius, Jablensky, Korten, & Emberg, 1992; Sartorius, Gulbinat, Harrison, Laska, & Siegel, 1996), the World Health Organization found that people in developing countries have better prognoses in clinical and social outcomes than those in the United States and Western Europe. These findings were consistent and even amplified over long-term follow up. Although no one knows exactly why this is, we might hypothesize the following reasons: In developing countries people (1) tend to remain better integrated into their families and society and are less likely to be subjected to long-term hospitalization/institutionalization; (2) are less exposed to long-term treatment with antipsychotics (which have many challenging side effects for patients including, but not limited to, weight gain, movement disorders, fatigue, type 2 diabetes, dizziness, and seizures); and (3) may experience a sense of "otherworldliness" and, accordingly, are not placed on the fringes of society but are offered greater social support. Indeed, in the yogic tradition, Siva, the father of yoga, is often found covered with ash, dancing on cremation grounds with "idiots and epileptics." In this sense, the yogic tradition allows mental illness to be accepted in spiritual terms that only very rarely happens in westernized countries (Feuerstein, 1990). If a teacher/therapist tries to understand, or at least respect, the reality presented by a student in the form of a hallucination, this can be an opportunity for that student to feel listened to and thus experience healing.

> The majority of people with schizophrenia have a history of trauma and loss, and are subject to downward socioeconomic drift.

For clients with schizophrenia, therapeutic yoga can become a safe container, creating a supportive environment by focusing on the client's unique strengths, rather than simply on what is wrong with a person. This is no small task. Physicians, researchers, and yoga teachers/therapists alike believe strongly that most benefits come from a practice that integrates all categories of asana, pranayama, and appropriate kinds of meditative practice. The recent trend of focusing on certain postures to treat certain kinds of mental disorders is a reductionist and simplistic approach, unsuitable for treating complex human beings. For instance, something essential is lost when only heart-opening poses are prescribed for depressive symptoms: all the categories of asana have something to teach us. Using yoga in this prescriptive way for symptom management is an allopathic approach that diminishes part of yoga's great benefit, that is, a holistic way of viewing experience, disease, and wellbeing. Accordingly, all of these practices have a place in healing and they frequently have a synergistic effect.

Class sequencing

A very accessible and important entry point for any client, but particularly for one with schizophrenia, is the breath, and it can therefore be helpful to begin a class with attention being given to the natural breathing already present, without specific breathing techniques. The breath is something concrete that can be felt by a client by placing their hands on the belly, then later on the sides of the ribs. It is always present, and watching its rhythm and fluctuations gives each client a lesson in watching their body and thoughts without judgment but with curiosity. As the breath is part of the respiratory system, the one physiological system most of us have both conscious and unconscious control over, it becomes a doorway between these two aspects of the self. Working with the breath directly affects the nervous system and develops the client's capacity for nonjudgmental attention. Inviting an awareness of how the breathing is at that moment—observing without judging—is an excellent way to begin any therapeutic yoga practice.

For some clients, this attentiveness to the breath can be immediately relaxing; however, relaxation can feel uncomfortable and even frightening to a person whose nervous system is chronically stressed. People with schizophrenia have been found to have a low capacity for self-relaxation and a suppressed PNS (Toichi, Kubota, Murai, Kamio, & Sakihama, 1999) as well as an overactive SNS and a high baseline level of physiological arousal (Zahn, Carpenter, & McGlashan, 1981). Because of this combination, even simple breath awareness can be helpful, but it might also create new or uncomfortable feelings; here again, maintaining an awareness of each client and their unique experience is critically important, rather than simply following an idea about what should be happening. Furthermore, if at any time a client seems more upset, more engaged in delusional material, more withdrawn, agitatedly talking to themselves, not following along with the class, or exhibiting any other concerning change during breathing practices, then the yoga teacher/therapist should attend immediately to that person and make any necessary adjustments to the activity or the surroundings. This is one reason why it is recommended to always have an assistant teacher present when working with groups of people with schizophrenia, so that the class can continue even if one person needs individual attention.

Once the class has started by focusing on the awareness of the breath (and knowing that attention will wax and wane), the yoga teacher/therapist can ask the students to set an intention, or *sankalpa*, for the practice, either aloud (going around the circle) or silently. Many clients who have been subject to hospitalization have had much of their autonomy and personal authority taken from them over the years, and so by enabling them to choose some quality they would like to cultivate—for example, peace, quiet, or more energy—is empowering. These can be shared as part of a brief check-in about how each person is doing, or repeated silently.

After setting an intention, it may be helpful to ask people about any injuries or pain they are experiencing. This is not recommended in a class of people with acute psychosis, and in general too much talking is not recommended with acutely psychotic clients, but if most people are stabilized in their illness then it can be important for them to feel both invested in the class, and also that the class is committed to their wellbeing. Sometimes this question elicits delusional material and on occasion people report the same pain every time. But making it clear that the class will be moving through certain postures and stretches with the intention of relieving a particular person's suffering is quite powerful; the distressed person receives both the concern held by the class and their desire to help. At the end of the class check-in, that person almost invariably feels some relief. In individual sessions, the yoga teacher/therapist can invite the client to share an intention and then briefly discuss goals for the session as well as any injuries or limitations.

After a check-in it is very useful to do a simple grounding exercise—literally feeling the feet on the ground. For example, while standing, spending a moment feeling the feet on the ground, then inhaling to lift the toes off the floor, exhaling as the toes spread on the ground, inhaling while coming to stand on tiptoes, exhaling with feet back on the floor. A simple exercise like this is an important beginning to the practice. It is something that almost everyone can do (although standing on tiptoe can be challenging for some medicated clients due to extrapyramidal side effects) and sets the tone to attend to the experience of the body. Another warm-up option might be a modified *abhyanga*, yogic self-massage, which involves gentle but firm touching over the head, face, neck, shoulders, abdomen, back, arms, hands, legs and feet. Either cupped hands can be used to gently tap over the body or fingers can be used to massage the student's own body. Deep breathing is an important part of *abhyanga*, and clients should be prompted to notice changes in the body after self-massage.

When teaching physical practices, everything should be explained simply and clearly. The yoga teacher/therapist can demonstrate if necessary, but it is key that to convey that it is not important how the postures appear, but that the effort and mental intention are present. Simple standing postures with either breath counting or verbal reminders to breathe are vital because many people with schizophrenia have irregular breathing patterns or tend to hold their breath (Akar, Kara, Latifoglu, & Bilgiç, 2015). Modified *surya namaskar* (sun salutation), *trikonasana* (triangle pose), and balancing standing postures (remembering that balance is often impaired in schizophrenia) are excellent initial practices because they are literally grounding for the feet. The flowing rhythmic movements of *surya namaskar* are helpful in focusing attention, and should be modified as much as necessary depending on the abilities of each individual. Making the class fun and lighthearted is important, to convey the idea that feeling the body and moving it is enjoyable, and that we don't need to work too hard to do so.

> Clients should be reminded to breathe in and out through the nostrils rather than through the mouth.

When moving to the mat, *chakravakasana* (cat-cow), *dandasana* (staff pose), *balasana* (child's pose), *baddha konasana* (butterfly pose), camel, seated twists, and cobra are accessible for many. And clients typically enjoy hearing the animal names many postures are named for—for example, they can play with embodying the qualities of a lion while practicing *simhasana* (lion pose). It is important to include all categories of asana, however modified or simplified (including modified inversions like legs-up-the-wall pose), and all spinal motions: flexion, extension, rotation, and lateral flexion. Because awareness of the breath in movement is key, frequently reminding people to breathe and even counting breaths can be very helpful. Clients should be reminded to breathe in and out through the nostrils rather than through the mouth, if possible; this has many health benefits, including increased oxygen uptake, nitrous oxide production, and filtering the air before it reaches the lungs.

Working with the breath

Pranayama, which involves specific practices to focus on or change the breath rather than just observing it, can be a beneficial aspect of yoga practice, but should initially be limited in time to just a few minutes; any longer than that, and people's attention can begin to wander. Lying on the floor with the right hand on the stomach and feeling the belly fill with air with inhalation then soften with exhalation, is a great way to start. Making sure clients are using diaphragmatic breathing, rather than using the chest and accessory muscles, is important from the very beginning. Feeling the tissues of the lower back and also the sides of the ribcage expand and soften with the breath begins to cultivate a sense of the three-dimensionality of the breathing process. Feeling the movement of the breath at the nostrils while counting breaths to four is also helpful; when distracted there is a tendency to keep counting to a higher number, so this technique is extremely helpful for keeping students aware of their thoughts. If after several classes of watching the breath the client is willing, then some intentionality can be added, trying to deepen and lengthen the breath without strain.

Nadi shodhana (alternate-nostril breathing), *sama vritti* (inhalation and exhalation of equal length, aiming for five to six breaths per minute), and *dirga pranayama* are excellent for promoting balance and calm. *Nadi shodhana* can be done with the hands or mentally, depending on the capability of the students. For more practiced students without psychotic symptoms, *ujjayi* breath (a technique that produces a soft "ocean" sound by slightly constricting the glottis) is also useful. However, throughout the class, there should be repeated reminders to "breathe in" and "breathe out" to help restore a regular, deeper rhythm to the breath.

In using therapeutic yoga techniques, a long and easy exhalation is often emphasized, ideally lasting five seconds or longer. Because people with schizophrenia are often habitually shallow breathers, teaching them slowly—perhaps over weeks or even months—how to lengthen the entire breath cycle is an essential aspect of the work, because it can help rebalance the nervous system over time. In particular, slow breathing activates the PNS, which, as discussed earlier, tends to be chronically compromised in schizophrenia. The following short case report illustrates the power of breathing practices.

Chapter 8

CASE REPORT

A yoga student with schizophrenia was in Bronx State Psychiatric Hospital due to auditory hallucinations that had led him to set himself and his apartment on fire. After a year of twice-weekly yoga classes but no other significant changes in treatment, he was able to earn a higher level of privilege in the hospital and returned to making art, something he had not done in many years. His words in attributing the change were: "Now at least I remember to breathe when I am stressed out." This simple skill made a huge difference in his daily life.

Nonjudgmental attention and meditation

Throughout the course of treatment with yoga therapy there are a few objectives. One, as discussed, involves developing breath awareness and slowly deepening the breath over time. Another is to help clients more fully experience, and thus more fully inhabit, their bodies. Neurologist Antonio Damasio discusses how the "body provides a grounding reference for the mind" (1994), and yoga is profoundly useful in reestablishing this relationship between mind and body. To do so, the yoga teacher/therapist continually draws clients back to the experience of the breath and the body without judging, just observing. Repeatedly asking clients to notice and not judge—sensations, thoughts, and themselves—throughout the class is an important therapeutic technique. Finally, and closely related to this, the yoga teacher/therapist is nurturing more accurate interoceptive skills, which have been found to increase resilience to stress in all populations (Haase et al., 2016). Many people with schizophrenia have a great capacity for interoception but often the overlaid, and frequently inaccurate, cognitive interpretation of the data from the body leads to distress. For example, one yoga student with schizophrenia believed she had "fish growing in her belly," which understandably upset her. Most likely she was able to

access accurate and intense abdominal sensation, but her explanation of what she felt was possibly overlaid with the confused mental processes of schizophrenia. Helping her to simply feel the sensations of her belly without the need to judge, label or explain them, allowed her to be in touch with her body in a freer and perhaps more authentic way.

Meditation practices can be challenging for this population because long periods of silence give people an opportunity to become involved in psychotic thought processes. Guided meditation should last roughly five minutes, depending on the class. It is not recommended to have more than a minute of silence at any time, but instead to draw on yoga nidra, and the body scan in particular, as the primary meditation practice. Feeling and noticing the sensations of the body without judgment is an important skill for those struggling with schizophrenia to learn. As discussed, they often suffer with psychotic delusions about their bodies, and/or experience a deep disconnection from their embodied self because they struggle so consistently with their thoughts, but embodied practices are not a part of standard psychiatric treatment. When teaching yoga nidra it is important to limit suggested imagery; the key to working with people who have schizophrenia is using yoga for greater clarity of what is present, not adding extra layers of imagining.

> Meditation practices can be challenging for this population because long periods of silence give people an opportunity to become involved in psychotic thought processes.

Walking meditation is another excellent practice. Feeling the movement of the body, the placement of the foot as it lands and pushes off, and perhaps counting the number of steps that make up the inhalation and exhalation, is something clients can learn in class and easily continue to do outside the classroom as well. Walking meditation can also be used as part of a warm up and then repeated at the end of class to see how it feels different after doing the yogic practices. The class can try walking on tiptoes, then on the heels, then on the inside then outside edges of the feet—then return to the whole foot and notice the differences in sensation and awareness.

Precautions

In the hands of a knowledgeable yoga therapist or psychotherapist with sufficient yogic expertise, the interventions discussed are safe for most clients. Naturally, it is essential to be present to the experience of the client and to base each intervention in every moment, both on how the client feels in themselves and how they appear clinically. In addition to the considerations provided in the Recommendations for Practice section, there are general precautions for working with individuals who have schizophrenia.

- It is important to remember that, though unlikely, a person with schizophrenia could become agitated, and management of this situation is essential to safety. The room should not have objects that can be thrown and cause harm. When chairs are present they should be heavy and difficult to pick up. This will also mean that during chair postures individuals have more stability. Regarding other yoga props, depending on the group, it might be wise to exclude blocks, and straps may not be ideal. Soft pillows for sitting should be fine.

- Having an assistant in the room, well known to all the people practicing, can help relieve fear or upset should it arise.

- An unknown person can arouse suspicion, whether it be a member of staff or a new participant in the class. When anyone new is introduced, the class should be made aware of this in advance. If the new individual is a client, the yoga teacher/therapist should first hold an individual session to acclimate that person to yoga practice and then later bring them into the collective atmosphere.

- In the event that there is a problem, yoga teacher/therapists should have a well-defined strategy that is discussed with the clinic, hospital, or service offering these classes about how to deal with it. It is imperative that this is not decided alone but discussed with experts in the faculty who know the clients and the workings of the organization.

- In terms of precautions regarding practices, there are two things to avoid: overactivation of sympathetic processes and reactivation of trauma.

- Breathing should be diaphragmatic, and as slow and smooth as possible, preferably five-second inhalations, and five- to six-second exhalations or longer. Chronic mental and physiological overstimulation is part of what yogic practices aim to treat in schizophrenia, so any activating breathwork or fast movements should be used with caution (if at all). In particular, *kapalabhati* and *bhastrika* should be avoided.

- A final concern is one that is likely to be faced in teaching yoga to this population. Because most people with schizophrenia have a history of significant childhood trauma (Larkin & Read, 2008), reactivation of trauma can occur when it is least expected. To ameliorate this, the yoga teacher/therapist can foster a sense of authentic openness with the client, in addition to abiding by certain principles of trauma-sensitive practice.

The yoga teacher/therapist has a challenging job in working with this population, but the rewards are great. If the teacher/therapist is able to remain present, attentive, and flexible of mind, and to create an environment where clients feel safe and cared for, both they and their clients will experience healing, joy, and connection.

Future directions

Yoga-based interventions offer potential as a safe and effective addition to conventional therapeutic methods in the treatment of psychotic disorders, and may be an ideal complementary or adjunctive approach. Yoga also has promise for reducing the significant burden and improving the quality of life for caregivers of patients with schizophrenia. However, much work needs to be done to replicate many of the research findings, overcome inherent methodological limitations in yoga research, and demonstrate objective measures of improvement. These are essential to convince the broader medical and scientific community and to bring the benefits of yoga to a significant proportion of patients suffering from this severe mental illness. Furthermore, the spiritual aspects of yoga practice need to be explored in terms of its contribution to therapeutic effects (Varambally & Gangadhar, 2012). There could also be several other benefits from practicing yoga and meditation that the clinical scales may not tap into (and which may even be seen as adverse effects). Future research needs to find a way to overcome this limitation. The possible adverse effects of yoga practices also need to be documented and studied if yoga is to be measured in the same terms as other interventions.

References

Abbott, A. (2010). Schizophrenia: The drug deadlock. *Nature, 468*(7321), 158–159.

Akar, S. A., Kara, S., Latifoglu, F., & Bilgiç, V. (2015). Analysis of heart rate variability during auditory stimulation periods in patients with schizophrenia. *Journal of Clinical Monitoring and Computing, 29*(1), 153–162.

American Psychiatric Association (2013). *Diagnostic and Statistical Manual of Mental Disorders, Fifth Edition.* Arlington, VA: American Psychiatric Publishing.

Behere, R. V., Arasappa, R., Jagannathan, A., Varambally, S., Venkatasubramanian, G., Thirthalli, J., Subbakrishna, D. K., Nagendra, H. R, & Gangadhar, B. N. (2011). Effect of yoga therapy on facial emotion recognition deficits, symptoms and functioning in patients with schizophrenia. *Acta Psychiatrica Scandinavica, 123*(2), 147–153.

Behere, R. V., Raghunandan, V. N., & Venkatasubramanian, G. (2008). TRENDS: a Tool for recognition of emotions in neuro-psychiatric disorders. *Indian Journal of Psychological Medicine, 30,* 32–38.

Bentall, R. P., Wickham S., Shevlin M., & Varese F. (2012). Do specific early life adversities lead to specific symptoms of psychosis? *Schizophrenia Bulletin, 38*(4)734-40.

Bhatia, T., Agarwal, A., Shah, G., Wood, J., Richard, J., Gur, R. E., Gur, R. C., Nimgaonkar, V. L., Mazumdar, S., & Deshpande, S. N. (2012). Adjunctive cognitive remediation for schizophrenia using yoga: An open, non-randomized trial. *Acta Neuropsychiatrica, 24*(2), 91–100.

Bleuler, E. (1908). "Die Prognose der Dementia Praecox – Schizophreniegruppe." *Allgemeine Zeitschrift fur Psychiatrie, 65,* 434–436.

Buckley, P. F., & Stahl, S. M. (2007). Pharmacological treatment of negative symptoms of schizophrenia: Therapeutic opportunity or cul-de-sac? *Acta Psychiatrica Scandinavica, 115*(2), 93–100.

Chhabra H., Karmani S., More P., Mehta U., Varambally S., Venkatasubramanian G., & Gangadhar B. N. Effect of yoga on the mirror neuron system: A functional near infrared spectroscopy (fNIRS) study. (Manuscript under preparation for publication).

Cramer, H., Lauche, R., Klose, P., Langhorst, J., & Dobos, G. (2013). Yoga for schizophrenia: A systematic review and meta-analysis. *BMC Psychiatry, 13,* 32.

Cramer, H., Lauche, R., Langhorst, J., & Dobos, G. (2015). Are Indian yoga trials more likely to be positive than those from other countries? A systematic review of randomized controlled trials. *Contemporary Clinical Trials, 41,* 269–272.

Damasio, A. (1994). *Descartes' Error.* Penguin Books.

Duraiswamy, G., Thirthalli, J., Nagendra, H. R., & Gangadhar, B. N. (2007). Yoga therapy as an add-on treatment in the management of patients with schizophrenia--a randomized controlled trial. *Acta Psychiatrica Scandinavica, 116*(3), 226–232.

Feuerstein, G. (1990). *Holy Madness.* Hohm Press.

Flood, G. (1996). *An Introduction to Hinduism.* Cambridge University Press.

Gururaj, G., Varghese, M., Benegal, V., Rao, G. N., Pathak, K., Singh, L. K., et al. (2016). *National Mental Health Survey of India, 2015-16: Summary.* Bangalore: National Institute of Mental Health and Neurosciences.

Haase, L., Stewart, J. L., Youssef, B., May, A. C., Isakovic, S., Simmons, A. N., Johnson, D. C., Potterat, E. G., & Paulus, M. P. (2016). When the brain does not adequately feel the body: Links between low resilience and interoception. *Biological Psychology, 113,* 37–45.

Hegarty, J. D., Baldessarini, R. J., Tohen, M., Waternaux, C., & Oepen, G. (1994). One hundred years of schizophrenia: A meta-analysis of the outcome literature. *American Journal of Psychiatry, 151*(10), 1409–1416.

Helgason, C., & Sarris, J. (2013). Mind-body medicine for schizophrenia and psychotic disorders: A review of the evidence. *Clinical Schizophrenia & Related Psychoses, 7*(3), 138–148.

Hofer, A., Benecke, C., Edlinger, M., Huber, R., Kemmler, G., Rettenbacher, M. A., Schleich, G., & Wolfgang Fleischhacker W. (2009). Facial emotion recognition and its relationship to symptomatic, subjective, and functional outcomes in outpatients with chronic schizophrenia. *European Psychiatry, 24*(1), 27–32.

Ikai, S., Suzuki, T., Uchida, H., Saruta, J., Tsukinoki, K., Fujii, Y., & Mimura, M. (2014). Effects of weekly one-hour hatha yoga therapy on resilience and stress levels in patients with schizophrenia-spectrum disorders: An eight-week randomized controlled trial. *Journal of Alternative and Complementary Medicine, 20*(11), 823–830.

Jayaram, N., Varambally, S., Behere, R. V., Venkatasubramanian, G., Arasappa, R., Christopher, R., & Gangadhar, B. N. (2013). Effect of yoga therapy on plasma oxytocin and facial emotion recognition deficits in patients of schizophrenia. *Indian Journal of Psychiatry, 55*(Suppl 3), S409–S413.

Kay, S., Fiszbein, A., & Opler, R. (1987). The positive and negative syndrome scale for schizophrenia (PANSS). *Schizophrenia Bulletin, 13,* 261–276.

Kee, K. S., Green, M. F., Mintz, J., & Brekke, J. S. (2003). Is emotion processing a predictor of functional outcome in schizophrenia? *Schizophrenia Bulletin, 29*(3), 487–497.

Leff, J., Sartorius, N., Jablensky, A., Korten, A., & Emberg, G. (1992). The International Pilot Study of Schizophrenia: Five year follow up findings. *Psychological Medicine, 22*(1):131–145.

Larkin, W., & Read, J. (2008). Childhood trauma and psychosis: Evidence, pathways, and implications. *Postgraduate Medical Journal, 54*(4):287–293.

Levine, P. A. (2010). *In an Unspoken Voice: How the Body Releases Trauma and Restores Goodness.* Berkeley, CA: North Atlantic Books.

Manjunath, R. B., Varambally, S., Thirthalli, J., Basavaraddi, I. V., & Gangadhar, B. N. (2013). Efficacy of yoga as an add-on treatment for in-patients with functional psychotic disorder. *Indian Journal of Psychiatry, 55*(Suppl 3), S374–S378.

Mehta, U. M., Keshavan, M. S., & Gangadhar, B. N. (2016). Bridging the schism of schizophrenia through yoga-Review of putative mechanisms. *International Review of Psychiatry, 28*(3), 254–264.

Mehta, U. M., Thirthalli, J., Aneelraj, D., Jadhav, P., Gangadhar, B. N., & Keshavan, M. S. (2014). Mirror neuron dysfunction in schizophrenia and its functional implications: A systematic review. *Schizophrenia Research, 160*(1-3), 9–19.

Nagendra, H. R., Telles, S., & Naveen, K. V. (2000). *An integrated approach of Yoga therapy for the management of schizophrenia.* Final Report submitted to Department of Indian Systems of Medicine and Homoeopathy, Ministry of Health and Family Welfare, Government of India.

National Institute for Health and Care Excellence (2014, March). *Psychosis and schizophrenia in adults: prevention and management* (NICE Clinical Guidelines No. 178). Retrieved from: http://guidance.nice.org.uk/CG178.

Paikkatt, B., Singh, A. R., Singh, P. K., & Jahan, M. (2012). Efficacy of yoga therapy on subjective well-being and basic living skills of patients having chronic schizophrenia. *Indian Journal of Psychiatry, 21*(2), 109–114.

Perala, J., Suvisaari, J., Saarni, S. I., Kuoppasalmi, K., Isometsa, E., Pirkola, S., Partonen, T., Tuulio-Henriksson, A., Hintikka, J., Kieseppä, T., Härkänen, T., Koskinen, S., & Lönnqvist, J. (2007). Lifetime prevalence of psychotic and bipolar I disorders in a general population. *Archives of General Psychiatry, 64*(1), 19–28.

Radhakrishna, S. (2010). Application of integrated yoga therapy to increase imitation skills in children with autism spectrum disorder. *International Journal of Yoga, 3*(1), 26–30.

Rao, N. P., Varambally, S., & Gangadhar, B. N. (2013). Yoga school of thought and psychiatry: Therapeutic potential. *Indian Journal of Psychiatry, 55*(Suppl 2), S145–S149.

Rizzolatti, G., & Craighero, L. (2004). The mirror-neuron system. *Annual Review of Neuroscience, 27,* 169–192.

Rizzolatti, G., & Fabbri-Destro, M. (2008). The mirror system and its role in social cognition. *Current Opinion in Neurology, 18*(2), 179–184.

Saha, S., Chant, D., Welham, J., & McGrath, J. (2005). A systematic review of the prevalence of schizophrenia. *PLOS Medicine, 2*(5), e141.

Saraswat, N., Rao, K., Subbakrishna, D. K., & Gangadhar, B. N. (2006). The Social Occupational Functioning Scale (SOFS): A brief measure of functional status in persons with schizophrenia. *Schizophrenia Research, 81*(2-3), 301–309.

Sartorius, N., Gulbinat, W., Harrison, G., Laska, E., & Siegel, C. (1996). Long term follow up of schizophrenia in 16 countries. *Social Psychology and Psychiatric Epidemiology, 31,*249–258.

Simpson, E. A., Sclafani, V., Paukner, A., Hamel, A. F., Novak, M. A., Meyer, J. S., Suomi, S. J., & Ferrari, P. F. (2014). Inhaled oxytocin increases positive social behaviors in newborn macaques. *Proceedings of the National Academy of Sciences of the United States of America, 111*(19), 6922–6927.

Toichi, M., Kubota, Y., Murai, T., Kamio, Y., & Sakihama, M. (1997). The influence of psychotic states on the autonomic nervous system in schizophrenia. *Archives of General Psychophysiology, 2*:147–154.

Vancampfort, D., De Hert, M., Knapen, J., Wampers, M., Demunter, H., Deckx, S., Maurissen, K., & Probst, M. (2011). State anxiety, psychological stress and positive well-being responses to yoga and aerobic exercise in people with schizophrenia: A pilot study. *Disability and Rehabilitation, 33*(8), 684–689.

Vancampfort D., Vansteelandt K., Scheewe T., Probst M., Knapen J., De Herdt A., & De Hert M. (2012) Yoga in schizophrenia: A systematic review of randomised controlled trials. Acta Psychiatrica Scandinavica, 26(1):12-20.

Varambally, S., & Gangadhar, B. N. (2012). Yoga: A spiritual practice with therapeutic value in psychiatry. *Asian Journal of Psychiatry, 5*(2), 186–189.

Varambally, S., Gangadhar, B. N., Thirthalli, J., Jagannathan, A., Kumar, S., Venkatasubramanian, G., Muralidhar, D., Subbakrishna, D. K., & Nagendra, H. R. (2012). Therapeutic efficacy of add-on yogasana intervention in stabilized outpatient schizophrenia: Randomized controlled comparison with exercise and waitlist. *Indian Journal of Psychiatry, 54*(3), 227–232.

Visceglia, E., & Lewis, S. (2011). Yoga therapy as an adjunctive treatment for schizophrenia: A randomized, controlled pilot study. *Journal of Alternative and Complementary Medicine, 17*(7), 601–607.

Walsh, R., & Roche, L. (1979). Precipitation of acute psychotic episodes by intensive meditation in individuals with a history of schizophrenia. *American Journal of Psychiatry, 136*(8), 1085–1086.

Xie, J., Lin, Y.-H., & Guo, C.-R. (2006). Study on influences of yoga on quality of life of schizophrenic inpatients. *Journal of Nursing (China), 13*, 9–11.

Zahn, T. P., Carpenter, W. T., & McGlashan, T. H. (1981). Autonomic nervous system activity in acute schizophrenia: I. Method and comparison with normal controls. *Archives of General Psychiatry, 38*(3):251–258.

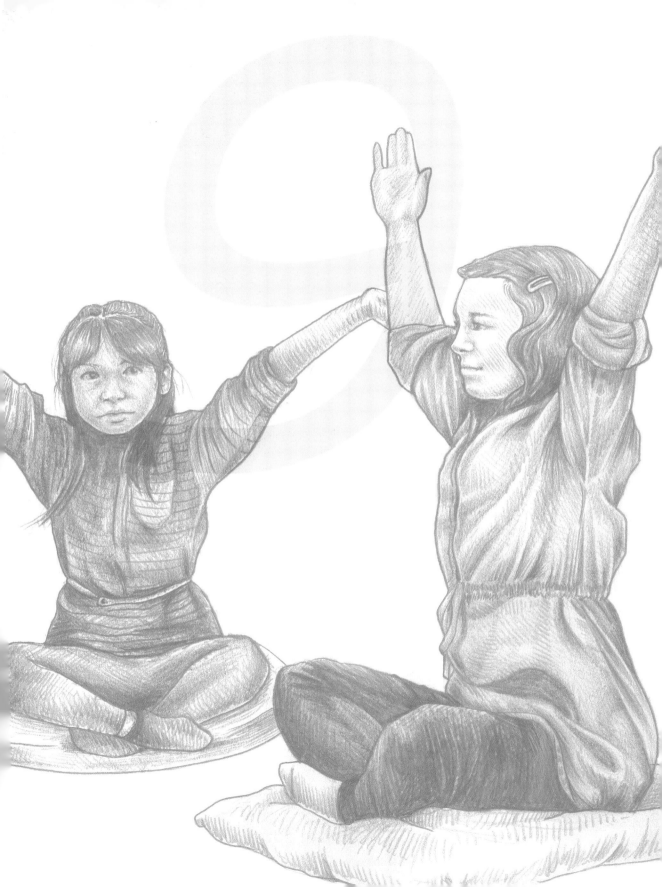

Children and Adolescents
Lisa Kaley-Isley and Michelle Fury

Overview

The mental health conditions addressed in this chapter frequently have their onset in childhood, and when they do, they often persist in some form into adulthood. Some conditions manifest symptoms very early in childhood, and therefore even from an early age a therapeutic approach is needed to compensate for (1) limitations, including communication and behavioral issues in autism spectrum disorder (ASD) and attention-deficit hyperactivity disorder (ADHD); (2) genetic predisposition, for example, anxiety (genetic risk: 33%) and depression (heritability: 40%); and (3) environmental injury, for example, from neglect, abuse, and trauma by caregivers (American Psychiatric Association, 2013). Left untreated, individual attempts to cope may result in additional co-occurring disorders and secondary consequences including eating disorders, conduct disorders, and substance abuse. The World Health Organization reports that mental health disorders such as depression and anxiety are commonly found in 28 countries canvassed, that these disorders often start in childhood or adolescence, and that the prevalence of mental health disorders seriously impairs individuals on a global scale (Kessler et al., 2009). Broderick and Metz (2009) suggest that a growing awareness of mental health issues, as well as increasing stressors on youth, has led to an increase in the diagnosis of mental health disorders.

> Yoga can be developmentally adapted to promote mental health and wellbeing in children and adolescents.

The scope of this chapter is broader than the others because in it we address the variety of disorders that first present in childhood and adolescence, rather than reviewing a single class of disorders. Some of these disorders are also covered in other chapters, so please refer to them for additional detail.

The foundations for mental health and disorders are constructed during childhood. Yoga can be developmentally adapted to promote mental health and wellbeing in children and adolescents. In this capacity, yoga serves as a protective factor intended to increase resilience and provide positive coping strategies for when conflicts, stressors, and challenges inevitably occur. As such, yoga may potentially ameliorate or prevent the future effects of disorders that begin in childhood or adolescence. Yoga can also serve a therapeutic function when development has already gone awry and symptoms of disorder are present.

Diagnostic criteria and review of the research literature

As with adults, there is a growing body of evidence to suggest that yoga is effective and beneficial for improving the mental health of youth. However, significantly fewer studies have been conducted with children and adolescents than with adults for a variety of reasons. First, children are deemed a vulnerable population and hence are subject to additional oversight regulations by internal review boards and schools. Second, children are required (where capable) to assent to participation in a study, but because they are deemed unable to give informed consent to participate, parental permission must also be obtained. Third, unless they have access to public transportation, children are unable to transport themselves to classes and appointments, so parents or other caregivers must be available, which can be problematic for working parents. Therefore, providing yoga in a setting where children are already receiving services improves the odds of participation and attendance. The majority of studies included in this review were conducted either at school, in a residential facility, or at a hospital where the child received services. The only study that offered teenagers the option to drop into yoga classes at a local yoga studio reported difficulties with ongoing participation (Hall, Ofei-Tenkorang, Machan, & Gordon, 2016).

Neurodevelopmental disorders

The *Diagnostic and Statistical Manual of Mental Disorders, Fifth Edition* (DSM-5) (American Psychiatric Association, 2013) is organized developmentally across the lifespan, listing first those conditions that arise in childhood. The first category is Neurodevelopmental Disorders, which includes ASD and ADHD. In both disorders there are high estimates of heritability, and potential pre-, peri-, and postnatal factors have been identified which can increase risk for their onset. Boys are four times more likely to develop ASD and two times more likely to develop ADHD. Developmental deficits manifest in the earliest years of life but the condition may not be formally diagnosed until the child enters school (or even later in some cases). There is a high incidence of other co-occurring learning, social-emotional, and behavioral disorders (ASD: 70%; ADHD ≤ 50%). The estimated global prevalence of ASD is 1% of the population, and for ADHD it is 5% in children and 2.5% in adults. Early intervention strategies are recommended to develop positive compensatory coping strategies that can mitigate the impact of these neurocognitive deficits.

> The estimated global prevalence of ASD is 1% of the population, and for ADHD it is 5% in children and 2.5% in adults.

Diagnostic criteria: Autism spectrum disorder

ASD is the fastest growing developmental disability tracked by the Centers for Disease Control and Prevention (CDC) according to the Autism Society (2017). About 1% of the global population meets diagnostic criteria for ASD (Centers for Disease Control and Prevention, 2014). In the United States, reported prevalence increased by 119.4% from 2000 (1 in 150) to 2010 (1 in 68) (Centers for Disease Control and Prevention, 2014). Children with ASD show behavioral symptoms of either or both limited social communication and restrictive, repetitive behavior (Mandy, Charman, & Skuse, 2012). These limitations may range from severe to barely perceptible to others. For example, an individual diagnosed with ASD may not have cognitive limitations (Nicholaidis, Kripke, & Raymaker, 2014). Communication is learned within the context of social interaction, so when impairment exists in both communication and social domains it further impairs children's acquisition of normative skills. Children with ASD may have verbal and nonverbal communication deficits, which take many forms depending upon their severity, but all of which have an effect on the communication of thoughts, feelings, and shared interaction. In addition, their repertoire of behaviors, interests, and activities are usually restricted, repetitive, and rigidly maintained. As the child ages the inability to communicate and interact socially may become increasingly distressful, leading to social isolation, attempts to self-regulate through rigid control of others, self-injurious behaviors, and aggressive or disruptive behavior. Children with ASD can learn and make developmental gains as they age, particularly with consistent, repetitive intervention and clear instructions that are geared to their needs for structure and predictability. However, children with ASD generally require greater individual support and guidance than is provided in group classrooms, putting extra demands on caregivers and schools. Yoga practices specifically tailored to children on the autism spectrum usually include the type of consistent, repetitive, and clear instructions and actions that can prove the most useful in promoting social behavior conducive to learning and the formation of more positive social relationships.

Research review: Autism spectrum disorder

A systematic review of mind-body therapies revealed three yoga interventions with ASD (Hourston & Atchely, 2017). Koenig, Buckley-Reen, and Garg (2012) evaluated a manualized yoga intervention with 25 children aged 5–12 that was incorporated into their daily morning routine using a DVD for sixteen weeks. The 20-minute integrated practices included adapted breathing techniques, yoga postures, chanting, and relaxation practices. Compared with controls, the yoga group showed a significant reduction on the Aberrant Behavior Checklist (ABC)-Total Score according to teacher reports, indicating a reduction in maladaptive and disruptive classroom behaviors.

Rosenblatt et al. (2011) evaluated eight sessions of combination interventions with 24 children aged 3–16. Each 45-minute intervention included breathing techniques, eighteen yoga postures depicted on cards, music, and dance, and yoga relaxation designed to elicit relaxation and appeal to the sensory processing sensitivites of children with ASD. The intervention was sequenced predictably, in the same order, to increase familiarity. Sensory integration and other cognitive processing issues make predictable schedules vital for children with ASD (Goldberg, 2013). Sessions were held in small groups in a hospital setting with parents participating. The yoga group achieved significant reductions on the Behavior Assessment System for Children (BASC-2) Behavioral Symptoms Index according to parent reports and a trend toward significance on the Irritability subscales of the BASC-2 and ABC, with a particularly strong response among children of latency age (5–12) indicating that negative affect decreased to a degree that was clearly apparent to parents.

Radhakrishna, Nagarathna, and Nagendra (2010) evaluated a long-term integrated approach to yoga therapy in an Indian school with six children aged 8–14. The students received five hours of weekly individual yoga instruction for 82 weeks with a parent present. The integrated intervention included breathing practices with props, postures, relaxation, and chanting, and encouraged home practice. Behavioral changes that were important to parents and teachers to promote learning and social interaction were chosen as the targets of the interventions. During the study, participants improved eye contact, ability to learn through imitation, and receptive and expressive communication; they showed greater comfort with being physically near to others, decreased self-stimulatory and self-injurious behaviors, improved alertness, slower breathing, and greater capacity for relaxation. Radhakrishna et al. asserted that "Yoga is ideally a lifetime practice, far more than an adjunctive therapy, generally discontinued after particular conditions have been corrected. Children with ASD require lifetime yoga practice. The majority require a program with repetition, structure, and continuity" (Radhakrisha et al., 2010, p. 120).

Diagnostic criteria: Attention-deficit hyperactivity disorder

The three characteristic behaviors of ADHD—inattention, hyperactivity, and impulsivity—begin early in life; the diagnostic criteria in DSM-5 (American Psychiatric Association, 2013) requires these behaviors to be evident before the age of 12 and to have persisted for at least six months at a level that is developmentally inappropriate. The behaviors must be present in two or more environments, that is, not only presenting at either home or school, and the symptoms must interfere with social, academic, or occupational functioning. Children (and adults) with ADHD may primarily demonstrate problems with inattention, or with hyperactivity and impulsivity, or they may experience all three of these. Inattention presents as a mental inability to sustain focus, which often results in disorganization and difficulties in comprehension due to a failure to take in relevant information. Hyperactivity manifests as physical restlessness, excess activity, and excessive talkativeness, making it difficult to sit still, listen, and learn. Impulsivity appears as intrusiveness, lack of self-control, failure to take into account relevant information (including potentially dangerous situations), an inability to delay gratification, and failure to modify behavior in response to potential longer-term consequences of behaviors and decisions. Impaired ability to regulate thoughts and behavior are associated with difficulties in learning, social interactions, and sense of self-efficacy that often endures into adulthood. Children with ADHD are also significantly more likely than their peers to develop conduct disorder as adolescents, antisocial personality disorder as adults, to experience substance abuse, and to be incarcerated. Early intervention through yoga practices to build cognitive and behavioral capacity for concentration, attention, and impulsive control can have a profound positive impact on the personal development of a child, and also reduce the potential negative societal impact.

Research review: Attention-deficit hyperactivity disorder

Cerrillo-Urbina et al. (2015) conducted a systematic review on the effects of physical exercise in children with ADHD that identified only one child yoga study that met their criteria. The study, by Jensen and Kenny (2004), evaluated a 20-week one-hour yoga intervention with nineteen boys aged 8–13 who were on medication to manage ADHD. The yoga intervention was administered after school at a hospital in Australia. Medication effects were reduced to thus evaluate the potential of yoga to give benefit during unmedicated periods. The controls participated in cooperative activities. The yoga intervention included breathing techniques, yoga poses (sitting and standing; supine and prone poses with flexion, extension, and lateral flexion; moving with breath, static and dynamic), progressive relaxation, and concentration with *tratak* (gazing at a word or shape with eyes open and closed). Significant improvements were achieved for both groups. The intervention led to a reduction in core ADHD symptoms, and behaviors associated with conduct disorder and mood lability. Parents' ratings on the Conners scale for the yoga group showed decreased oppositionality, emotional lability, restless/impulsivity, and total score. Both groups showed improvement on the perfectionism scale, and two DSM-IV ratings, hyperactive/impulsive and total score. The reduction on the hyperactive/impulsive scale correlated significantly with the number of yoga sessions attended such that greater reductions were achieved by boys who participated in more classes. In addition, three scale improvements correlated positively with greater amounts of home practice: (1) Test Of Variables of Attention (TOVA) response time, (2) TOVA ADHD score, and (3) emotional lability, indicating greater ability to attend and respond accurately to stimuli, and decreased mood swings, temper outbursts, and crying.

A review of ADHD and nonpharmacological treatments (Sharma, Gerbarg, & Brown, 2015) identified one additional study (Haffner, Roos, Goldstein, Parzer, & Resch, 2006) that evaluated yoga compared with exercise in nineteen children with ADHD. The study abstract reports medium-to-large improvements for the yoga group as per parents' ratings on attention and clinical scores for ADHD.

Depressive and anxiety disorders

Depressive and anxiety disorders are defined as separate disorders in the DSM-5 (American Psychiatric Association, 2013), but they frequently co-occur. In research studies evaluating yoga, measures for both conditions are often included, and the umbrella terms anxiety and depression are regularly used without a differentiation being made between them. Because extant research supports an overlap in these two diagnoses, some models of treatment, such as the transdiagnostic model, treat symptomatology rather than discrete diagnoses (Farchione et al., 2012). The presence of disorders in yoga studies is frequently defined by elevations on self, parent, or teacher report questionnaires, rather than following a formal assessment by a mental health professional. The diagnostic system used to define eligibility for special education services in US schools includes the two conditions in one single category classified as serious emotional disturbance (SED).

Females are 1.5–3 times more likely than males to develop anxiety and depression.

The DSM-5 (American Psychiatric Association, 2013) asserts that both conditions have strong genetic predispositions, with the presence of a diagnosed first-degree relative increasing the risk of a major depressive disorder by two to four times and heritability accounting for one third of the risk in generalized anxiety disorder. According to the DSM-5, females are 1.5–3 times more likely than males to develop anxiety and depression, with one exception: males are significantly more likely to meet the criteria for (the newly defined) disruptive mood dysregulation disorder, whose hallmark behavior is severe and sustained temper outbursts in children between 6 and 18 years old. Rates of first onset peak in adolescence with the onset of puberty for major depression, specific phobia, social anxiety disorder, and agoraphobia. Approximately 75% of individuals who develop social anxiety disorder will do so between the ages of 8 and 15. With some exceptions, which we will highlight, the same criteria are used in the DSM-5 to diagnose these conditions in children, adolescents, and adults.

The development of these disorders is influenced by predisposition and social/environmental factors. The primary symptoms are fear and sadness, which may be expressed as avoidance, irritability, and anger. Beginning their lives feeling unsafe and unhappy has a profound effect on children's experience of themselves and others, resulting in what are often lifelong mental health challenges. Yoga classes that provide a safe and empowering environment may be an effective antidote that these children need to develop self-efficacy and to create positive changes in their lives.

Diagnostic criteria: Depressive disorders

Children and adolescents experience depression in similar ways to adults. The only noted diagnostic difference is that children may express depression with irritability or "crankiness" rather than overt sadness. As with adults, the defining feature of major depressive disorder (MDD) is depressed mood or loss of pleasure in previously pleasurable activities. The mood needs to persist most of the day, nearly every day for at least two weeks, and must include at least four other physical, physiological, or mental-emotional symptoms from the following: (1) changes in weight and appetite (loss, gain, or in children, a failure to make developmentally expected gains); (2) sleep disruption (either excess or deficiency); (3) psychomotor disturbance (restless or slowed); (4) fatigue or loss of energy; (5) feelings of worthlessness or guilt; (6) impairment in concentration, clarity, and decision making; and (7) recurrent thoughts of death with or without suicidal ideation.

Children and adolescents may also experience persistent depressive disorder (formerly called dysthymia), although in youth, persistence for one year (rather than the two years required for adults) is sufficient to meet DSM-5 criteria. The symptoms are similar to MDD but rather than lifting they persist, and with children irritability rather than sadness may predominate. In cases of onset in childhood the course may be chronic, and the likelihood of co-occurring personality disorders and substance use disorders is increased.

The criteria for disruptive mood dysregulation disorder specify that the diagnosis is limited to children between the ages of 6 (developmental age) and 18, and the first five symptoms must be present before the age of 10. Temper outbursts must occur most days, in at least two settings, and continue for at least a year. The verbal and/or physical responses are out of proportion to the triggering event and are age-inappropriate. Children with this presentation were previously diagnosed with early-onset bipolar disorder. The DSM-5 estimates prevalence of the disorder at 2%–5% of children and adolescents, who experience the highest rates of co-occurring mental disorders than for any other condition. They are physiologically dysregulated and lack effective emotion regulation, distress tolerance, and self-soothing strategies. They present a significant behavioral challenge to parents and teachers, and multi-agent pharmacological interventions are often employed to manage them.

Diagnostic criteria: Anxiety disorders

The majority of the anxiety disorders including specific phobia, social anxiety disorder, and agoraphobia, are defined by excessive fear or anxiety in response to being in situations with a specific fear-associated stressor. In most of these disorders, the object or situation provokes fear or anxiety, it is avoided or endured fearfully, the response is disproportionate to any actual danger presented, it causes distress or impairment in functioning, and it persists for some extended period of time. The criteria specifically note that in children anxiety may be shown by "crying, tantrums, freezing, or clinging" or "failing to speak" when it would be appropriate to do so.

In separation anxiety disorder, the earliest developing anxiety disorder, the fear is about being separated from home or an attachment figure. These children worry excessively about harm coming to caregivers. They frequently refuse to go to school, to be alone, or to engage in socially appropriate activities in order to avoid separation. Their sleep is disrupted, often by nightmares. They report physical pain (sometimes referred to as "psychosomatic symptoms"), especially headaches and stomachaches, in anticipation of, and to prevent, separation. These children present a particular challenge for parents and schools. It is the most common anxiety disorder in children under 12, and it is experienced by approximately 4% of US children. The prevalence rates decrease with age, but it is estimated that 0.9%–1.9% of US adults continue to experience the disorder.

Generalized anxiety disorder differs by being a more persistent and broadly based state of excessive worry. The worry is accompanied by six potential symptoms, only one of which is required to be present in children to meet criteria for the disorder (three symptoms are required for adults): (1) restlessness, (2) fatigue, (3) difficulty concentrating, (4) irritability, (5) muscle tension, and (6) sleep disturbance. The foci of worry differ and often endure, across the lifespan. Children with this condition may be perfectionistic, overly conforming, seek excessive reassurance, and feel anxious about and dissatisfied with their performance at school and in activities.

Research review: Depressive and anxiety disorders

> The yoga group showed significantly decreased anger, fatigue, and anxiety, and significant improvements in life purpose, satisfaction, and attitude toward school.

Weaver and Darragh (2015) conducted a systematic review of yoga interventions for anxiety with children and adolescents, identifying sixteen studies that met their inclusion criteria, nearly all of which reported reductions in anxiety post intervention. Khalsa, Hickey-Schultz, Cohen, Steiner, and Cope (2012) evaluated a single semester (eleven weeks) of 30- to 40-minute yoga classes two to three times per week with 121 male and female high school students aged 15–19 years in rural Massachusetts. The students were randomized into yoga (Yoga Ed. intervention) and control groups (physical education). At the end of the semester the yoga group showed significantly decreased anger, fatigue, and anxiety, and significant improvements in life purpose, satisfaction, and attitude toward school, whereas the control group showed deterioration in functioning in these areas. Felver, Butzer, Olson, Smith, and Khalsa (2015) evaluated the acute effects of two single 35-minute Kripalu-style yoga classes and a single PE class with 47 high school students (mean age: 15.9) in rural Massachusetts. Immediately following the yoga classes participants reported significantly decreased anger, depression, and fatigue. Daly, Haden, Hagins, Papouchis, and Ramirez (2015) evaluated a sixteen-week, 40-minute thrice-weekly yoga class compared to physical education with 37 high school students aged 15–17 in New York City. The integrated intervention included a vigorous sequence of postures, breathing, relaxation, and a closing ritual designed to take the practice effects into the day. Emotion regulation significantly increased for the yoga group but decreased for the controls, and body awareness scores were significantly and positively correlated with emotion regulation change scores. Butzer et al. (2015) evaluated a ten-week, 30-minute Yoga 4 Classrooms® intervention with second and third grade boys and girls during class time with specialty trained yoga teachers in Maine. The integrated intervention included the four key elements of classical yoga: breathing, postures, relaxation and meditation. More specifically, it included singing at the beginning and end, a themed discussion on a yoga topic, primarily calming breathing practices, postures performed with shoes on while sitting at or standing by their desks, and relaxation with heads resting on the desks listening to a guided visualization. Salivary cortisol, used as a biomarker for stress, was sampled three times: after completing attention measures at the yoga class, and on the first and last days of the intervention. Second, but not third, graders showed a significant decrease in cortisol levels from the first to the last day of the intervention, but neither group showed significant decreases immediately after yoga classes.

Trauma and stressor-related disorders

Diagnostic criteria: Trauma and stressor-related disorders

To meet criteria for trauma and stressor-related disorders, the individual must experience psychological distress and disorder in response to experiencing a traumatic or stressful event. Two child-specific onset conditions are triggered specifically by inadequate caregiving in childhood. In reactive attachment disorder the neglected or deprived child becomes socially withdrawn. In contrast, in disinhibited social engagement disorder, the child has experienced neglect or repeated changes in caregivers, or has been raised in an institutional setting, and responds with indiscriminate willingness to approach and interact with unfamiliar adults.

The DSM-5 lists separate specific criteria for PTSD in children 6 years of age and younger. These children must have exposure to actual or threatened death, serious injury, or sexual violence by direct experience; they must have witnessed this, or have been told that it happened to a parent or caregiver. They must experience one or more intrusive symptoms including recurrent memories, dreams, re-experiencing, and exposure to associated cues or reminders of the event, which may be expressed in play, may not appear to be distressing, and need not be obviously connected to the traumatic event. They must demonstrate one or more symptoms that include persistent avoidance of people, places, activities, and topics that remind them of the event or demonstrate painful emotions (e.g., fear, guilt, shame, sadness, confusion), decreased pleasure in activities, social withdrawal, or reduction in positive emotional states. They must experience at least two symptoms of arousal and reactivity that worsened after the event, including angry or irritable behavior, hypervigilance, exaggerated startle response, impaired concentration, or disrupted sleep. The symptoms must last longer than a month and cause significant distress or impairment in functioning and relationships.

For children older than 6, the criteria for PTSD are primarily the same as for adults, and are very similar to the criteria for children aged 6 and younger, with similar qualifications: memories and re-experienced events may be re-enacted in repetitive play, and frightening dreams need not be obviously related to the circumstances of the traumatic event. The same caveats are cited for children with acute stress disorder, which differs from PTSD by a shorter duration of symptoms (three days to one month after the event).

Research review: Trauma and stressor-related disorders

Many experts agree that trauma treatment should include somatic interventions (Levine, 1997; Rothschild, 2000; van der Kolk, 2009). Therefore, trauma-sensitive yoga may be an ideal intervention. Beltran et al. (2016) evaluated a fourteen-week yoga-based, trauma-informed, psychoeducational group therapy intervention with ten boys aged 8–12 in an urban community mental health center. The boys were all diagnosed with ADHD and anxiety; 60% were also diagnosed with oppositional defiant disorder; and all the boys had experienced personal trauma. It should be noted that depression, anxiety, and attentional and behavioral issues are all sequelae of trauma are listed as possible symptoms of trauma in the DSM-5. The 90-minute weekly integrated intervention included breathing practices, poses, relaxation, and meditation, and was designed to strengthen six core skills: (1) safety and personal boundaries, (2) self-awareness, (3) self-soothing, (4) self-regulation, (5) competency, and (6) self-esteem. Parents' ratings showed significant improvements on interpersonal and intrapersonal strength and family involvement scales. In 2011, Spinazzola, Rhodes, Emerson, Earle,

& Monroe published a collection of case vignettes of trauma-sensitive yoga administered to traumatized youths aged 12–21 at the Trauma Center at Justice Resource Institute, and found yoga to be a viable self-regulation practice for those suffering from trauma.

Eating disorders

Diagnostic criteria: Eating disorders

Anorexia nervosa and bulimia nervosa both typically first develop in adolescence. Like anxiety and depression, they occur more frequently in females than males (10:1 ratio). Additionally, the presence of a prior anxiety disorder and first-degree relatives with anxiety or depressive disorders increases the risk of developing an eating disorder in youth. The diagnostic criteria are food- and body-based and include behaviors used inappropriately to prevent weight gain or stimulate weight loss. Individuals with anorexia are able to maintain restrictive behaviors to a degree that life-threatening weight loss may occur, and numerous physiological and cognitive impairments may result from the starvation. Individuals with bulimia episodically lose control of their desire to eat excess amounts of food and then compensate by excessive purging and exercise activities to undo the effects of their binge. Both conditions may be seen as attempts by individuals to manage intolerable emotions through their relationship with food, and thus as attempted coping strategies. The conditions tend to persist into adulthood in some form, whether as a full-blown eating disorder, body image issues, or preoccupation with food. Neurobiology, family history, and personality tendencies (such as co-occurring anxiety, depression, and/or harm avoidance), are all factors in the development of eating disorders among children and adolescents (Kargas, 2017). The current understanding is that an individual's sense of powerlessness and lack of control are key components for developing an eating disorder (Lock & le Grange, 2005; Steiner et al., 2003), especially because children and adolescents already lack control in their lives as a function of being cared for by parents and caregivers.

Research review: Eating disorders

In 2010, Carei, Fyfe-Johnson, Breuner, and Marshall evaluated an eight-week RCT with 50 girls and four boys aged 11–21 diagnosed with anorexia, bulimia, or unspecified eating disorder at Seattle Children's Hospital; participants received either standard care or standard care plus individualized, manualized yoga intervention. Measures very similar to Hall et al. (2016) were used, and assessment included a follow-up after one month. Eating disorder specific ideation decreased over time in both groups, and continued to reduce through follow-up in the yoga group, but rebounded upward in the controls. Both groups experienced decreased levels of anxiety and depression over time. Body mass index (BMI) remained stable (as intended), suggesting that the practice was gentle enough not to contribute to weight loss. Food preoccupation assessed after each class showed a steady reduction, with medium and large effect size differences from baseline to completion.

In 2016, Hall et al. evaluated a twelve-week yoga program with 20 girls aged 11–18 (no control group) with restricting eating disorders, who were all treated at an urban eating disorders clinic. The participants took up to twelve weekly classes in a local yoga studio. Classes were gentle and were not heated, to decrease the risk of weight loss. The teachers had trauma-sensitive yoga training. Classes included postures (dynamic and flow with breath), deep breathing, chanting, and seated meditation. The participants reported significantly reduced anxiety, depression, weight and shape concerns, and clinical state of anorexia.

Rationale for yoga practice

Yoga practice is the vehicle through which individuals can achieve the optimal states of being that yoga philosophy posits is the true potential of all human beings

(Rutt, 2006; Tigunait, 2014, 2017). Yoga therapy is the selection and adaptation of yoga practices and philosophy to enable and empower an individual to achieve more optimal functioning, to lessen symptoms of distress and disorder, and to improve the overall quality of their life.

Yoga offers a holistic and interdependent conceptualization of human functioning in the *panchamaya* model of the *kosha* (Kaley-Isley, 2014), and the scope of yoga therapy encompasses five domains:

1. *annamaya kosha*: the body made of food, all aspects of the physical structure of the body;

2. *pranamaya kosha*: the body made of vital energy, perceptible physiological organs and systems of the body-mind, and subtle energy systems;

3. *manomaya kosha*: the body made of thoughts, most aspects of the brain and mind;

4. *vignamaya kosha*: the body of discernment, aspects of mind characterized as deeper knowing that has qualities of truth, clarity, and wisdom referred to as intuition and inner teacher; and

5. *anandamaya kosha*: the body made of bliss, the true self that exists in a state of bliss beyond all suffering and limitation, and is veiled from awareness by the four outer sheaths.

The comprehensive scope of yoga to influence so many domains of the self is part of what makes the practices powerful and effective at creating desired changes. Most other western treatment modalities limit their scope of intervention to a single domain, such as physical therapy or surgery for the body, pharmacology to affect physiology, and talk therapies for the mind. This facilitates specialization, but misses out on the complex, multilayered reality of human existence. Through wise and skillful choices of practice elements and cultivated attitudes, the yoga teacher/therapist can promote harmony and integration of action and intention in the first three *koshas* simply by asking the student to match the pace of their breath to the pace of their movement, with sustained attention to maintain it for a set number of repetitions. By adding the instruction to "do what feels right in your body," or "choose the variation that feels best for you," the student is guided to check in with their own deeper knowing and capacity to make wise choices, thus also integrating the fourth *kosha*. When the four *koshas* of the self are working in harmony toward the same intention, rather than being in conflict with each other, there is a perceptible shift in feeling more whole and at peace. In this way, the individual experiences a taste of the fifth *kosha*: I am that joyful and free state of being.

> Through wise and skillful choices of practice elements and cultivated attitudes, the yoga teacher/therapist can promote harmony and integration of action and intention.

A second yoga conceptual model, the *gunas*, provides information about the type and direction of change needed in order to promote a beneficial effect. The *gunas* are names for qualities of energy (Frawley, 1999, Kaley-Isley, 2018) that move and change, and can therefore be influenced.

All of the mental health disorders covered in this chapter can be characterized by symptoms of excess *rajas* or *tamas*, and it can be useful for a yoga teacher/therapist to notice which qualities are out of balance in an individual or class setting. *Rajas* is accelerated movement in thought and behavior along a continuum from healthy to dysfunctional activity. *Rajas* in excess includes hyperactivity and impulsivity (ADHD); stereotyped or repetitive motor movements (ASD); mental rumination (depression); panic, agitation, restlessness, sleeplessness, and worry

(anxiety); flashbacks and re-experiencing (trauma); and excessive exercise and purging (eating disorders). *Tamas* is the opposite continuum, ranging from the healthy qualities of stability and steadiness to the symptomatic behaviors of underactivity. *Tamas* in excess includes inattention (ADHD); failure to make eye contact, initiate social interactions, imitate behaviors, and communicate verbally (ASD); diminished pleasure, hypersomnia, psychomotor retardation, and fatigue (depression); freezing (an inability to speak or act) and avoidance (anxiety and trauma); and sustained restricted eating (eating disorders). Each of the conditions includes symptoms of disorder at the two extremes, but individuals may experience symptoms predominately at one end and remain stuck there, or they may alternate between the two extremes.

Yoga practice provides the skills to move toward equilibrium between the two forces; this is *sattva*, the state of balance, integration, and harmony. The recommended direction of change toward *sattva* is by soothing, regulating, and softening the activity of *rajas* and moving from the inertia of *tamas* by stimulating, nourishing, and inspiring. Physical activity is regulated through the pace of movement in asana. The first and second *kosha* are integrated and mutually regulated through breath-focused asana and pranayama. The first three *kosha* are yoked and harmonized through mindful breath-focused asana, pranayama, guided relaxation, and meditation on an object on which the mind can become pleasantly absorbed.

> The benefit of teaching yoga to children is that development can be influenced while it is taking place.

The primary task of childhood is to develop the knowledge, skills, and abilities in all spheres that will enable children to live happy, healthy, and meaningful lives. The benefit of teaching yoga to children is that development can be influenced while it is taking place. Development occurs in nonlinear stages with critical windows of time when functions mature normally.

and it is by optimizing development as these functions unfold that yoga can play a facilitating and protective role to promote wellbeing in children and adolescents. However, in children, some circumstances and conditions already exist: a child is born into a particular family, in a particular time and place, with a certain temperament that may or may not be a good fit with their primary caregiver at a particular time, and these factors exert an ongoing influence on the child. In the earlier years development occurs at an accelerated rate, but change and the potential for growth and decline exist from the start of life, and both are influenced by changing circumstances. In the context of their environment, children must learn how to self-soothe to tolerate distress, self-regulate emotions and behavior, form relationships, make choices, and act on their intentions. Inability in one way or another to sufficiently develop these capacities underlie the mental health disorders reviewed in this chapter.

Yoga practices teach children how to consciously choose to act (move, breathe, and think), and they also heighten awareness of the immediate effect and intermediate consequences of actions undertaken, and how these improve or worsen the state of their minds and bodies. This feedback loop fosters an internal locus of control and greater self-efficacy to positively effect change in their lives.

Integration of yoga into mental healthcare

Manualized treatments are being developed, disseminated, and evaluated that will enhance the delivery of evidence-based approaches (see Table 9.1). Many involve integrating yoga with a mindfulness-based intervention, similar to how yoga was incorporated into Mindfulness-Based Stress Reduction (MBSR) (Salmon, Lush, Jablonski, & Sephton 2008). The Mindful Coping group at Children's Hospital Colorado, an outpatient therapy group for 8–12-year-olds with mood disorders, integrates yoga techniques with the Modular Approach to Therapy

for Children (MATCH), an evidence-based treatment model designed by Bruce Chorpita and John Weisz.

The pioneers of trauma-sensitive yoga at the Trauma Center at the Justice Resource Institute are evaluating the effectiveness of yoga to assist with trauma adapted for youth (Spinazzola, Rhodes, Emerson, Earle, & Monroe, 2011) using a manualized approach developed by Erica Viggiano, founder of Integrative Life Services©. Viggiano's protocol is an adolescent and pediatric trauma-focused yoga intervention that is adapted to the unique needs of youth suffering from trauma, and which empowers students to direct the yoga practice.

> Yoga is being increasingly incorporated into pediatric medical clinic services.

Yoga is being increasingly incorporated into pediatric medical clinic services. In 2016, Diorio et al. evaluated a manualized yoga intervention used in hospitals to reduce fatigue, which they planned to replicate in other hospitals. The UCLA Pediatric Pain Program (UCLA PPP) created a standardized protocol using Iyengar yoga for children suffering from rheumatoid arthritis and irritable bowel syndrome. Hainsworth et al. (2013) are using an Iyengar style of yoga in a standardized yoga sequence for youth with chronic headache. The Children's Hospital Colorado is also offering yoga practices to reduce the symptoms and frequency of headaches. The integrative headache clinic incorporated a one-hour standardized yoga practice for chronic headache in adolescents as part of a monthly specialist half-day clinic.

Recommendations for practice

There are four critical elements of clinical care for pediatric yoga therapy: (1) developmental considerations, (2) diagnostic specific interventions, (3) modality (individual, group, or family), and (4) the person delivering the intervention. The first three of these critical elements are described in the order that will

Chapter 9

Table 9.1

Adapting yoga for youth with mental health conditions

Age	Common developmental features	Contraindications	Types of poses	Other techniques
5–12 years old	• Eager to please • Like to know rules • Short attention span • Concrete thinking • Rapidly growing bodies	• Lack of structure • Long duration • Complex instructions • Excess focus on form of pose/performance	• Animal names • Challenges to gradually lengthen holds and balance • Integrate breath with sounds	• Story enacted with poses and breath • Guided visualization in rest • Cooperative games • Chanting and singing
13–18 years old	• Socially conscious of the opinions of peers • May test rules and limits • Fluctuating attention • Rapidly changing bodies • Pubertal hormonal changes to mind-body; onset of menses • Need for additional rest and sleep • Idealism • Developing self-identity and peer group	• Theme not geared to teens' interest • Positioning that creates vulnerability in mixed gender classes • Excess strain or stretch on ligaments • Risky balance poses without adequate guidance and support • Touching adjustments can feel like correction rather than support	• Younger teens are in a transitional state between adult-style asana and the playfulness of younger kids. Find the balance between both with medium length holds and a playful attitude and willingness to experiment • Older teens enjoy a class with elements similar to one for adults; and shorter class duration with mastery and challenge options	• Teen spines are already forward rounding from electronics and book bags: backbends and laterals will help counter pose • Guided yoga nidra can help teens switch off and gain much needed rest; use phones to record practice • Breathing practices they can do without attracting attention, to help calm them before tests and improve sleep at night

Diagnosis	Common diagnostic features	Suggested practice focus	Types of poses	Other techniques
ADHD	• Limited attention and concentration • Physical and mental restlessness • Impulsive action • Lack social awareness	• Gradually build capacity for sustained attention • Engage natural curiosity and enjoyment to foster positive self and social connection	• Start with doable practices to gradually build competence and confidence • Start with active poses to discharge restless energy, then transition to stillness	• Restorative yoga props and poses can increase comfort and feeling cared for to enhance capacity for rest • Teaching peers a pose creates opportunity for positive accomplishment
Anxiety	• Tendency to be shy, socially withdrawn or sensitive • Limited self-confidence and sensitive to perceived judgments • Physically and/or mentally restless • Fearful or worried	• Provide opportunities to engage or opt out • Clear rules and structure to increase feelings of safety • Breath integrated with movement to increase self-regulation and calming	• Start with more active poses and face-to-face engagement • Use repetition to build mastery and confidence • Gently challenge perceived limits by gradually increasing difficulty • Use on-the-ground poses to prepare for rest and give options to keep eyes open	• Use demonstration and verbal cues rather than touch to adjust until therapeutic relationship established • Softly sounded and balanced inhale/exhale and balanced right/left and belly breathing to regulate ANS • Mantra repetition with mudras to empower self-confidence (sahana) and to use when anxious to calm

	Characteristics			
ASD	• Rigid-like consistency • Repetitive behaviors • Limited reciprocal communication • Heightened sensory sensitivity	• Use consistency and repetition to instill safety and increase learning retention • Provide positive alternative rhythmic and repetitive behaviors	• Yoga picture cards provide method for shared communication • Limit duration to doable • Identify preferred sensory inputs and use them (chant/sing for sound, roll up in yoga mat for touch)	• Breathing with Hoberman sphere • Use verbal cues and demonstrate rather than touch to adjust • Use yoga mat to demark personal space
Depression	• Repetitive ruminative and self-critical thoughts/feelings • Physical inertia • Sadness or irritability	• Begin with gentle doable movements then increase activity • Use language cues that promote self-compassion and positive embodiment rather than accomplishment or competition • Provide experience of capacity to create desired self-change	• Start with floor-based practices to increasingly mobilize whole body and increase circulation and energy • Use contralateral body integration to engage mind-body • Coordinate breath with movement	• Balanced and full body integrated breathing • Provide alternative positive objects of mental attention in poses and rest • Restorative yoga props and poses can increase comfort and feeling cared for to enhance capacity for rest
Anxiety and depression	• Alternates between impulsive and restricted behavior • Alternates between energetic states of agitation and lethargy • Feels incapable to improve own situation (hopeless)	• Utilize an integrated practice drawing on recommendations for both conditions • Determine starting point by dominant energetic condition on the day • Build self-efficacy	• Include practices to regulate energy (if high or low adjust accordingly to balance) • Provide alternative objects of mental focus in poses and rest	• Focus on capacity to create even small desired, positive changes in feeling state and condition • Prompt awareness of subtle changes from practice and nature of conditions to change
Eating disorders	• Body dysmorphic sensitivity • Desire for weight loss • Excessive (binge, exercise) and restrictive (food intake) behaviors • Frequently co-occurring anxiety	• Find the balance between engaging attention with challenge and positive embodied sensation and excess energy discharge with desires to lose weight through excess exercise • Language and cueing that does *not* emphasis purity and lightness of being, or that provides a rationale not to eat • Encourage self-perception of subtle body signals, including appetite	• Tend to enjoy dynamic practice and poses increasing flexibility and mastery of challenging poses • Sequence and include elements to temper excess in the above and provide opportunities to feel good; not overdoing	• Yogic concepts/affirmations that promote health and wholeness and self-acceptance • Guided visualizations to make rest more accessible • Breathing practices to balance and calm hyperarousal • Alternatives to purging to feel sense of release (*kappalabhati*, lion breath). Counter pose with hold after exhale, twists, and forward bends to calm and balance to stimulate digestion
Emotional trauma	• Hyperarousal or hypoarousal of ANS • Externally hypervigilant, internally hyper-reactive • Alternately, may have blunted affect and dissociation from experiences and feelings • Associated sensory experiences can trigger memories and re-experiencing of frightening events	• Follow guidelines for a trauma sensitive yoga class: provide a safe, contained environment for practice and frequent reminders of choice during practice and invitational language in cueing and compassionate and boundarized teacher presence • Facilitate safe experiencing of physical sensations and emotions in action and stillness	• Activity level will depend on predominate energy state, similar to anxiety and depression • Integrated practice to foster balance and self-regulation, similar to anxiety and depression • Tend to prefer distraction and dynamic practice, similar to eating disorders • Mastery restores confidence	• Present moment awareness through bodily sensations and observing flow of breath can help recover from triggering events • Guided relaxation and yoga nidra help facilitate rest and sleep • Positive embodiment can rebuild sense of self-efficacy and the ability to perceive own needs and self-care

help facilitate the creation of a sequence for a single session, or a clinical treatment plan. Each of these elements take into account the individual's needs (e.g., their cognitive/developmental abilities to process instructions, as well as the symptoms to be targeted by yoga therapy), the setting in which the individual(s) receive treatment (e.g., as individuals or in a group), and the experience and scope of practice required for the yoga therapy provider to deliver the intervention.

Developmental considerations

The complexity of child development makes it challenging to ensure that yoga therapy is safe and effective. A child's developmental stage determines their physiological capabilities, perceptions of the world, and ability to process information; yet a child's developmental stage is not necessarily the same as their chronological age, for example in the case of a child who has intellectual disabilities. This chapter focuses on the developmental stages preceding and entering puberty: elementary (primary) school age (5–12 years old) and adolescence (13–18 years old). Yoga teachers/therapists working with youth need to know how to deliver yoga therapy to these different developmental stages, including how to cue instructions, sequence yoga asana and other techniques, and respond to the physical needs of growing children and adolescents.

> A child's developmental stage is not necessarily the same as their chronological age.

Elementary school-aged children (5–12 years old)

In general, children in their elementary school years are eager to please adults and are interested in the rules of games. When it comes to activities like group yoga they are typically motivated to participate and engage when asked to show what they know. An effective strategy for this age group is inviting them to take turns teaching poses from a set of yoga flashcards.

The yoga teacher/therapist may choose the poses and plan the sequence, but if the goal of the group is to work on socialization and teamwork, then the teacher/therapist may opt to have students choose the poses. When children learn to teach poses, they not only learn the poses more thoroughly, they learn to pay attention to their peers' needs. For instance, a child learns to pace instructions so that peers can follow along. However, when children are allowed to pick the sequence, the yoga teacher/therapist should choose poses for each sequence that are accessible to this age group. Children at this age are growing rapidly. Bones grow slightly ahead of muscles, so children at this age often have limited flexibility and strength. Therefore, poses should not be held for too long; for example, 3–5 counts per side for bilateral poses such as warrior poses, or 5–10 counts for unilateral poses like downward dog. Animal poses in which children can make the animal sound (such as cobra, cat or downward dog) help children to relieve stress. Balancing poses such as tree and airplane (warrior III) help teach children focus and patience. The total length of a yoga sequence including breathing and/or meditation/relaxation should not last more than 45 minutes for this age group. Breathing techniques that use body parts (such as tracing the outline of the hand) also teach focus and calming skills. Finally, to prevent injury it is important to teach children to differentiate between a healthy and a too-much stretch.

Adolescents (13–18 years old)

In contrast to elementary school-aged children, adolescents typically relate more to their peer group than to adults. It is important for a yoga teacher/therapist working with this age group to relate with their interests. For instance, a yoga teacher/therapist could mention that many professional sports teams use yoga for cross training. In addition, the therapist can ask adolescents who show enthusiasm for yoga to explain how yoga benefits them. Those who are less enthusiastic will be more open to hearing about the benefits from their peers rather than an adult. While on occasion adolescents may look and speak as if they possess adult understanding, their brains are still developing and becoming fully myelinated (especially the executive functions). Therefore, they may lack the ability to see the bigger picture, including understanding the consequences of impulsive behavior. The teacher/therapist can help them see the larger context when they don't see it by themselves, perhaps by including yoga philosophy in an age-appropriate way. Adolescents' moods can fluctuate widely as a result of pubertal hormone changes and environmental stressors. Yoga practices designed to empower adolescents can help them regulate their moods when they feel anxious, depressed, or otherwise upset.

With regard to specific yoga practices, adolescents can hold poses longer than their elementary school-age counterparts, although not for as long as adults. For instance, an adolescent can usually hold a downward-dog pose for 30 seconds to a minute. Many adolescents enjoy the flow of sun salutations, perhaps up to five repetitions. The total length of a sequence for adolescents can last up to 90 minutes, but the yoga teacher/therapist should allow for more discussion time to accommodate the shorter holdings of poses. Adolescents who are physically fit will often enjoy more challenging poses like standing balances, arm balances, and backbends. However, adolescents in the middle of a growth spurt will have decreased flexibility, which means they will need to be extra careful with regard to poses that require flexibility such as hip-openers and forward folds. Adolescents should be encouraged to use the yoga practices that help them calm, focus, and re-energize. Some adolescents prefer relaxation and/or meditation to more active poses; other adolescents prefer active, challenging practices to relaxation. For example, some adolescents who suffer from anxiety say that relaxation practices make them feel more agitated, while others claim that a practice like yoga nidra helps decrease their anxiety.

Adolescents are encouraged to find out for themselves what works best for their needs. Note that we have not seen a gender difference with their preferences.

Diagnosis-specific interventions

Autism spectrum disorders

Many children with ASD and other neurodevelopmental disorders have issues with sensory integration, and they may be either hypersensitive or hyposensitive to environmental stimuli (Rogers & Ozonoff, 2005) such as sound, sight, smell, touch and taste. Yoga in particular can be invaluable for these children. A child who is hyperaroused by visual stimuli in the environment may respond well to the visual cue of a colorful yoga mat that clearly defines their focus for practice. Another child who is hyperaroused by touch may benefit by wrapping themselves in a yoga mat while doing deep breathing exercises, which helps to create a sense of safety. Additionally, a child who is hypersensitive to kinesthetic stimuli, or who is feeling agitated or anxious, may crave deep touch pressure: allowing this child to roll up in a yoga mat at the end of class can be a great way to reward participation, and serves a therapeutic purpose. Alternatively, a child who is hypersensitive to touch will not want to be touched and may view rolling up in a yoga mat as punitive (and thus it is contraindicated for treatment).

> A useful rule when working with anxiety and/or depression is to use the yoga sequence to help the child regulate mood.

Anxiety and depression

Yoga therapy may help youth struggling with anxiety, depression, trauma, and eating disorders by helping them recognize and accept their emotions (Fury, 2015). A useful rule when working with anxiety and/or depression is to use the yoga sequence to help the child regulate mood. For instance, if a child is in a depressive state, movement may be sluggish. By starting with a seated breathing practice or small movements (such as dynamic bridge), the child begins yoga practice slowly. If this is all the child can manage, it is important to validate the effort made. If the child is able to move more energetically over the course of the session, the yoga therapist may choose some more energizing poses (such as standing poses or a sun salutation). Ending with positive affirmations or a pleasant visualization can help improve mood for a child suffering depressive symptoms. Conversely, if a child is suffering from anxious symptoms, it may be best to start with a more active practice, such as sun salutations. Over the course of the practice with an anxious child, the yoga therapist can then offer more calming practices such as forward folds and breathing techniques. Finally, the therapist should solicit the child's feedback about whether the practice is having the desired effect (e.g., regulating the child's mood).

Trauma-related disorders

The intensity of some yoga practices may be helpful in treating trauma in youth; by experiencing the intensity in yoga directly, they realize that intensity isn't always bad (as it is in traumatic events) (van der Kolk, 2009). When working with youth who have experienced trauma, a yoga therapist should either seek trauma-focused training or work closely with a mental health professional who specializes in trauma treatment, ensuring that the yoga therapist functions within their scope of practice. A yoga therapist may not know the nature of the trauma, so it is vital to attune to a child's specific needs by collaborating with them to determine which poses and techniques are beneficial. If the trauma experience was recent, it can be helpful to keep yoga movements small, and increase their size once the client indicates they are ready. Gradually increasing the time a client spends in a pose in the safe presence of the yoga therapist can help them to practice distress tolerance, a key skill in healing from trauma. Using invitational languaging for instructions allows the client to try different modifications as they choose, rather than encouraging them to push through intensity or challenge while doing a pose.

Eating disorders

Yoga provides a method to address the nonverbal, mind-body crisis of eating disorders (Fury, 2015). Klein and Cook-Cottone (2013) found that yoga practice can increase clients' body satisfaction, a key symptom in many eating disorders. Having worked with clients with eating disorders for eleven years, this author's (Michelle Fury) experience is that they love poses which stretch the fascia (connective tissue surrounding muscles and organs), including hips-openers, leg stretches, and gentle backbends. Daubenmeier (2005), as well as Klein and Cook-Cottone (2013), found that individuals with eating disorders often lose body and emotional awareness. For example, someone with anorexia nervosa must relearn how to listen to body sensations that signal hunger. Yoga retrains the individual to listen to these signals by increasing interoception (see Chapter 1, p. 2). A gentle yoga sequence that emphasizes breathing, deep relaxation, and calming strategies can increase body and emotional awareness. We recommend avoiding long holds and challenging poses that reinforce an urge to exercise, because this is often used maladaptively to manage the symptoms of disordered eating. If a client is shaking their limbs a lot while sitting or lying in *savasana*, then this could be a discreet way for them to exercise. Minimizing risk factors and negative self-talk, while increasing protective factors and experiences of competence, are critical in caring for clients with eating disorders.

Modality: Individual, peer group, and family

Individual

The purpose of individual yoga therapy is usually to target symptoms of a specific condition or behavior and, together with the child or adolescent and their parent(s) or caregiver(s), develop goals for individualized yoga practice. A yoga therapist may use whatever clinical documentation is at their disposal to create these goals. Once goals have been set then a treatment plan is created, ideally in consultation with mental or medical health professionals working with the child or adolescent. Including parents or other key family members periodically in individual yoga sessions not only helps the parents understand and see how their child is benefitting, but it can also help the entire family learn how to creatively support the child during home practice or in other areas of life. To illustrate the individual yoga therapy process, let's consider a case report.

CASE REPORT

An 8-year-old female was referred for yoga therapy to address symptoms of acute separation anxiety. Her symptoms had been intractable for four years, as evidenced by previous clinicians' notes and the family's report. This little girl threw screaming fits during which she insulted her parents and the therapist when she was asked to name emotions, to describe a fear, or to engage in usual talk therapy. Goals for treatment included identifying and labeling feelings, as well as increasing coping skills through yoga therapy. After several successful yoga therapy sessions it came to light that she had experienced a traumatic event when aged 4, when a 3-year-old friend had died, quickly followed by the death of the family dog. The treatment plan was amended to include trauma-sensitive yoga, which for this child means only attempting yoga practices that she deems safe, such as sitting quietly on her yoga mat and/or doing starfish breathing (tracing the outline of her fingers to create a regular rhythm of inhale/exhale). Her parents continue to be an integral part of all her sessions since she is now developing a repertoire of coping skills. Usually one parent attends, but on occasion the whole family (including her older sister) attends family yoga therapy, which includes partner poses that helps them to explore family dynamics.

Peer group

Group yoga therapy offers many benefits for youth. For elementary school-aged children, yoga groups offer a chance to show off skills and practice teamwork and sharing. For adolescents, the group experience can help members find a supportive social group, and can be especially useful for reluctant teens. As the group leader, the yoga therapist needs to foster a sense of safety within the group, which means establishing ground rules before introducing interventions. Whether the participants are elementary school-aged or adolescent, it is equally important to engage group members to actively establish group rules or expectations together, with the yoga therapist's guidance. This is done at the beginning of the group, or if it is a group that continues for multiple sessions, it should be done within the first session. Example of group expectations include raising hands to ask to speak, not interrupting others, using kind words, not touching without permission, and keeping safe hands (e.g., no physical aggression). Many facilities have a no-touching policy among children and teens, so it is important to know about these policies before leading groups. Individual differences exist in every group, so a yoga therapist needs to be sensitive to overgeneralizing or stereotyping, and instead listen attentively to the students' experience. Conducting check-ins and check-outs at the beginning and end of each group is a vital communication component of group yoga therapy and is one of the things that differentiates it from a non-therapeutic yoga class.

> The yoga therapist needs to foster a sense of safety within the group, which means establishing ground rules before introducing interventions.

Family

Family yoga therapy can occur with a single family or in a multifamily group setting. It takes skill to manage the group dynamics of multiple families, but the complex dynamics enable multifamily groups to provide particularly rich experiences. Setting group rules for sharing and behavior are also important in these settings. In the multifamily context, the yoga therapist and family can see the child's moods arise and be expressed in their behaviors. Partner poses and other group yoga interventions allow families to see their own behaviors and their reactions to one another. Multifamily experience provides opportunities for families to help one another and to feel supported.

Precautions

Two key questions for the yoga teacher/therapist to ask when teaching yoga to children and adolescents are: "Is it safe?" and "Is it likely to be helpful?" There are three domains of particular importance to consider: changing bodies, class composition, and adjustments.

Changing bodies

The bodies of children and adolescents are growing and transforming, and so they are naturally more malleable than adults. This malleability does not equate with meaning that they are more flexible, because the modern sedentary lifestyle has an impact on the body early in development. Many children already experience shortened hamstrings, lower and upper back pain, rounded shoulders, and protruding heads from sitting, reading, looking at computers and electronic devices, and carrying backpacks with heavy school books. Because the changes in children's and adolescent's bodies take place often unevenly in spurts, it takes time for them to adjust. They may be more vulnerable to overstretching ligaments, feel awkward or imbalanced, or in the case of pubertal changes, have mixed emotional responses to the development of secondary sex characteristics. Techniques to help youth develop curiosity and compassion for their bodies, rather than drive for performance and competition, may help engender greater awareness and positive feelings of embodiment as they develop.

Class composition

Age differences have a more pronounced impact on the structure and content of yoga classes for youth than they do for adults. In order to maintain their engagement, language cues, pacing of activities, and the duration of the class are each optimally adjusted to the ages and developmental stage of the participants. For example, the attention span of a younger child is much shorter than for a teen, so poses are held for shorter periods, and the duration of the class is often shorter as well. Younger children are more concrete in their thinking, so the cueing needs to be specific and immediately evocative. Instruction is often more about the feeling of the pose rather than the precise anatomical alignment of it. Children respond well to stories enacted in the present, and they enjoy embodying the poses with the qualities of their names, for example, becoming strong and still like a mountain, a snake hissing softly with breath, a turtle safe in his shell, or a peaceful warrior standing his ground. Young teens may still be able to enjoy this type of play, but often it feels childish to them, and so therefore groups with too large an age gap do not often mix well. A class for teens more closely resembles an adult class, but it is important to keep in mind their sensitivity to their changing bodies and in general their greater sensitivity to being corrected by adults. All of these natural tendencies may be exaggerated in children with mental health conditions. The attention span of a child with ADHD is a particular factor. A child who has experienced trauma may be more wary of touch. Additionally, there are valid advantages and disadvantages for either including mixed genders in a class or limiting a class to one gender. For example, gender mixing can either amplify or diminish competitive behaviors such as showing off, appearing tough, or being the most flexible and can either increase or decrease feelings of safety, a willingness to be curious, and the sharing of reflections. Also, in many settings the children in class know each other from other contexts, such as going to the same school or attending the same medical clinic. These outside-of-class relationships can have an inside-class effect that may be more pronounced than with adults.

Adjustments

Adolescents often have heightened body sensitivity, vulnerability, and performance concerns. They interpret suggested adjustments as evidence they are "doing it wrong," rather than as a helpful instruction. Anxious and traumatized adolescents may be particularly uncomfortable with touch and lack the empowered confidence to say so, which may mean the yoga teacher/therapist does not perform physical adjustments. Partner work can be a powerfully useful modality or a source of great discomfort that flares up anxiety. Children with ASD are often touch-sensitive, although they may respond positively to firm, clearly boundaried touch that grounds rather than corrects them. In some cultures there are prohibitions on females touching males and vice versa, and this should be respected when voiced as a preference.

Future directions

As the profession of yoga therapy develops, it is becoming evident that relevant additional training and experience are required to equip the teacher with the requisite knowledge and skills to assume the expanded role of therapist. The same principles apply for yoga teachers and therapists who wish to provide yoga to youth. In 2017, the US Yoga Alliance recommended a minimum of 95 course hours to address priority topics (Yoga Alliance, 2018); however, in reality, courses range from fourteen to 250 hours (Butzer, Ebert, Telles, & Kalsa, 2015). The vast majority of youth-specific courses prepare teachers to teach rather than to provide yoga therapy. Given the complexity of the mental health needs of children,

the evidence of yoga's potential benefits, the low cost of yoga as an intervention, and the generally positive response to yoga by youth, parents, and teachers, we anticipate that the trend will follow that of adults in offering additional specialist preparation in yoga.

We see evidence for two parallel trends in the practice of yoga with children and adolescents: (1) promotion of wellness, and (2) therapeutic intervention. The benefits of protective factors, resilience, and positive coping strategies are well established. Early exposure to yoga practices that promote these qualities through positive embodiment, and methods to self-soothe, self-regulate, and self-reflect, can increase children's resilience in facing the academic, interpersonal, and intrapsychic challenges they face during maturation (Khalsa et al., 2012). There continue to be pockets of resistance to the inclusion of yoga in schools the United States on the grounds that yoga is Hinduism, and thus violates the separation of church and state (Cook-Cottone, Lemish, & Guyker, 2017). The majority of these cases have been resolved by teachers adopting secularized language (e.g., calling meditation "time in"), not using Sanskrit or chanting mantras, and defining yoga as a method of exercise and stress reduction. Nonetheless, the current trend is expansion of yoga into more schools and we expect it to continue as a wellness modality, if not a therapeutic intervention (Butzer, Ebert et al., 2015).

The disorders covered in this chapter all frequently begin in childhood, and early intervention can change the trajectory of their development before it is deeply established. We see evidence that the therapeutic application of yoga is continuing to expand into treatment and residential facilities of various types. The pediatric research literature suggests that yoga is being more widely adopted in medical environments, and in specialty outpatient clinics in particular (Diorio et al., 2016; Ruddy et al., 2015). As the evidence base and its popular acceptance continue to grow, medical professionals are demonstrating greater willingness to evaluate the potential benefits of yoga for their patients. Healthcare professionals who are also yoga practitioners are often the driving force stimulating this change from within their organizations. The existence of manualized treatments and prerecorded classes may facilitate dissemination and adoption of yoga techniques in a wider variety of settings (Diorio et al., 2016).

> Medical professionals are demonstrating greater willingness to evaluate the potential benefits of yoga for their patients.

We would like to see yoga expand into all institutions where youth are housed, including residential treatment, juvenile justice correctional facilities, and substance abuse facilities. Youth at the high end of the service utilization continuum have profound corrective needs for positive embodiment; affect, distress, and behavior regulation; and positive social interaction where they can feel safe, relax, and be children. Harris and Fitton's Art of Yoga project for girls in the California Juvenile Justice system is an excellent example (2010).

Finally, we expect to see yoga classes and interventions being increasingly offered to a broader range of the population. For the past few decades, demographic data have revealed that yoga was primarily practiced by educated, white females. As yoga moves into mainstream and public institutions, children of all socioeconomic and ethnicity groups will have the opportunity to benefit from this ancient practice for being optimally equipped to live a happy, healthy, and meaningful life.

References

American Psychiatric Association (2013). *Diagnostic and Statistical Manual of Mental Disorders, Fifth Edition.* Arlington, VA: American Psychiatric Publishing.

Autism Society (2017, December 18). *Facts and statistics.* Retrieved from: http://www.autism-society.org/what-is/facts-and-statistics.

Beltran, M., Brown-Elhillali, A., Held, A., Ryce, P., Ofonedu, M., Hoover, D., Ensor, K., & Belcher, H. (2016). Yoga-based psychotherapy groups for boys exposed to trauma in urban settings. *Alternative Therapy Health Medicine, 22*(1), 39–46.

Broderick, P.C., & Metz, S. (2009). Learning to BREATH: A pilot trial of a mindfulness curriculum for adolescents. *Advances in School Mental Health Promotion, 2*(1), 35–36.

Butzer, B., Day, D., Potts, A., Ryan, C., Coulombe, S., Davies, B., Weidknecht, K., Ebert., M., Flynn, L, & Khalsa, S. (2015). Effects of a classroom-based yoga intervention on cortisol and behavior in second and third grade students: A pilot study. *Journal of Evidence-Based Complementary and Alternative Medicine, 20*(1), 41–49.

Butzer, B., Ebert, M., Telles, S., & Kalsa, S. (2015). School-based yoga programs in the United States: A survey. *Advances in Mind-Body Medicine, 29*(4), 18–26.

Carei, T., Fyfe-Johnson, A., Breuner, C., & Marshall, M. (2010). Randomized controlled clinical trial of yoga in the treatment of eating disorders. *Journal of Adolescent Health, 46*(4), 346–351.

Centers for Disease Control and Prevention (2014). *Autism Spectrum Disorder.* Accessed 3 May, 2018 from https://www.cdc.gov/ncbddd/autism/data.html.

Cerrillo-Urbina, A., Garcia-Hermoso, A., Sanchez-Lopez, M., Pardo-Guijarro, M., Satnos Gomez, J., & Martinez-Vizcaino, V. (2015). The effects of physical exercise in children with attention deficit hyperactivity disorder: A systematic review and meta-analysis of control trials. *Child Care Health and Development, 41*(6), 779–788.

Cook-Cottone, C., Lemish, E., & Guyker, W. (2017), Interpretive phenomenological analysis of a lawsuit contending that school-based yoga is religion: A study of school personnel. *International Journal of Yoga Therapy, 27,* 25–35.

Daly, L. A., Haden S. C., Hagins, M, Papouchis, N., & Ramirez, P. (2015). Yoga and emotion regulation in high school students: A randomized controlled trial, *Evidence-Based Complementary and Alternative Medicine.* Article publication online.

Daubenmeier, J. (2005). The relationship of yoga, body awareness, and body responsiveness to self-objectification and disordered eating. *Psychology of Women Quarterly, 29*(2), 207–219.

Diorio, C., Ekstrand, A., Hesser, T., O'Sullivan, C., Lee, M., Schechter, T., & Sung, L. (2016). Development of an individualized yoga intervention to address fatigue in hospitalized children undergoing intensive chemotherapy. *Integrative Cancer Therapies, 15*(3), 279–284.

Evans, S., Moieni, M., Sternlieg, B., Tsao, J.C.I., & Zeltzer, L. (2012) Yoga for youth: The UCLA pediatric pain program model. *Holistic Nursing Practice. 26* (5). P. 262-271.

Farchione, T.J., Fairholme, C.P., Ellard, K.K., Boisseau, C.L., Thompson-Hollands, J., Carl, J.R., Gallagher, M.W., & Barlow, D.H. (2012) Unified protocol for transdiagnostic treatment of emotional disorders: A randomized controlled trial. *Behavior Therapy.* 43 (3). p. 666-678.

Felver, J., Butzer, B., Olson, K, Smith, I, & Khalsa, S. (2015). Yoga in public school improves adolescent mood and affect. *Contemporary School Psychology*, 19(3), 184–192.

Frawley, D. (1999). *Yoga and Ayurveda: Self-healing and self-realization.* Twin Lakes: Lotus Press.

Fury, M. (2015) *Using yoga therapy to promote mental health in children and adolescents.* Edinburgh, UK: Handspring Publishing.

Goldberg, L. (2013). *Yoga Therapy for Children with Autism and Special Needs.* New York: W.W. Norton & Company.

Haffner, J., Roos, J., Goldstein, N., Parzer, P., & Resch, F. (2006). The effectiveness of body-oriented methods of therapy in the treatment of attention-deficit hyperactivity disorder (ADHD): Results of a controlled pilot study. *Z Kinder Jugendpsychiatr Psychother*, 34(1), 37–47.

Hainsworth, K., Salamon, K., Khan K., Mascarenhas, B., Davies, W., & Weisman, S. (2013). A pilot study of yoga for chronic headaches in youth: Promise amidst challenges. *Pain Management Nursing*, p. 1-9.

Hall, A., Ofei-Tenkorang, N., Machan, J., & Gordon, C. (2016). Use of yoga in outpatient eating disorder treatment: A pilot study. *Journal of Eating Disorders*, 4, 38.

Harris, A., & Fitton, M. (2010). The Art of Yoga project: A gender-responsive yoga and creative arts curriculum for girls in the California Juvenile Justice system. *International Journal of Yoga Therapy*, 20, 110–118.

Hourston S., & Atchely, R. (2017). Autism and mind-body therapies: A systematic review. *The Journal of Alternative and Complementary Medicine*, 23(5), 331–339.

Jenson, P., & Kenny D. (2004). The effects of yoga on the attention and behavior of boys with attention-deficit/hyperactivity disorder (ADHD). *Journal of Attention Disorder*, 7(4), 205–216.

Kaley-Isley, L. (2014). Adapting yoga for children and adolescents with functional disorders. In R. Anbar (Ed.), *Functional symptoms in pediatric disease* (pp. 353–371). New York, NY: Springer.

Kaley-Isley, L. (2018). Yoga therapy: Training, assessment, and practice. In S. O'Neill (Ed.), *Yoga teaching handbook: A practical guide for yoga teachers and trainees* (pp. 210–229). London, UK: Singing Dragon.

Kargas, C. (2017, 18 December). *Susceptibility to eating disorders: what does the research tell us?* Retrieved from: https://www.eatingdisorder hope.com/programs/professional-resources/susceptibility-to-eating-disorders-what-does-research-tell-us.

Kessler, R. C., Aguilar-Gaxiola, S., Alonso, J., Chatterji, S., Lee, S., Ormel, J., Ustun, T. B., & Wang, P. S. (2009). The global burden of mental disorders: An update from the WHO World Mental Health (WWMH) surveys. *Epidemiologia e Psichiatria Sociale*, 18(1), 23–33.

Khalsa, S., Hickey-Schultz, L., Cohen, D., Steiner, N., & Cope, S. (2012). Evaluation of the mental health benefits of yoga in a secondary school: A preliminary randomized control trial. *The Journal of Behavioral Health Services & Research*, 39(1), 80–89.

Klein, J., & Cook-Cottone, C. (2013). The effects of yoga on eating disorder symptoms and correlates: A review. *International Journal of Yoga Therapy*, 23(2), 41–50.

Koenig, K., Buckley-Reen, A., & Garg, S. (2012). Efficacy of the get ready to learn yoga program among children with autism spectrum disorders: A pretest-posttest control group design. *American Journal of Occupational Therapy*, 66, 538–546.

Levine, P. (1997). *Waking the Tiger—Healing Trauma.* Berkeley, CA: North Atlantic Books.

Lock, J., & le Grange, D. (2005). *Help Your Teenager Beat an Eating Disorder.* New York, NY: Guilford Press.

Mandy, W. P. L., Charman, T., & Skuse, D. H. (2012). Testing the construct validity of proposed criteria for DSM-5 Autism Spectrum Disorder. *Journal of the American Academy of Child and Adolescent Psychiatry*, 51(1), 41–50.

Nicholaidis, C., Kripke, C., & Raymaker, D. (2014) Primary care for adults on the autism spectrum. *Medical Clinics of North America*, 98 (5), 1169-1191.

Radhakrishna, S., Nagarathna, R., & Nagendra, H. (2010). Integrated approach to yoga therapy and autism spectrum disorders. *Journal of Ayurveda and Integrative Medicine*, 1(2), 120–124.

Rogers, S. J., & Ozonoff, S. (2005). Annotation: What do we know about sensory dysfunction in autism? A critical review of empirical evidence. *Journal of Child Psychology and Psychiatry*, 46(12), 1255–1268.

Rosenblatt, L, Gorantla, S., Torres. J., Yarmush, R., Rao, S., Park, E., Denninger, J., Benson, H., Fricchione, G., Bernstein, B., & Levine, J. (2011). Relaxation response-based yoga improves functioning in young children with autism: A pilot study. *The Journal of Alternative and Complementary Medicine*, 17(11), 1029–1035.

Rothschild, B. (2000). *The Body Remembers: The Psychophysiology of Trauma and Trauma treatment.* New York, NY: WW Norton & Company.

Ruddy, J., Emerson, J., McNamara, S., Genatossio, A., Breuner, C., Weber, T., & Rosenfeld, M. (2015). Yoga as a therapy for adolescents and young adults with cystic fibrosis: A pilot study. *Global Advances in Health and Medicine*, 4(6), 32–36.

Rutt, S. (2006). *An ordinary life transformed: lessons for everyone from the Bhagavad Gita.* Brookline, NH: Hobblebush Books.

Salmon, P., Lush, E., Jablonski, M., & Sephton, S. (2008). Yoga and mindfulness: Clinical aspects of an ancient mind/body practice. *Cognitive and Behavioral Practice*, 16 (1), 59-72.

Sharma, A., Gebarg, P., & Brown, R. (2015). Non-pharmacological treatments for ADHD in youth. *Adolescent Psychiatry*, 5(2), 84–95.

Spinazola, J., Rhodes, A., Emerson, D., Earle, E., & Monroe, K. (2012). Application of yoga in residential treatment of traumatized youth. *Journal of American Psychiatric Nurses Association*, 17(6), 431–444.

Steiner, H., Kwan, W., Shaffer, T. G., Walker, S., Miller, S., Sagar, A., & Lock, J. (2003). Risk and protective factors for juvenile eating disorders. *European Child & Adolescent Psychiatry*, 1(12), 38–46.

Sumar, S. (1998) *Yoga for the Special Child*. Buckingham: VA. Special Yoga Publications.

Tigunait, P. R. (2014). *The secret of the yoga sutra*. Honesdale, PA: Himalayan International Institute of Yoga Science and Philosophy of the USA.

Tigunait, P. R. (2017). *The practice of the yoga sutra*. Honesdale, PA: Himalayan International Institute of Yoga Science and Philosophy of the USA.

Weaver, L., & Darragh, A. (2015). Systematic review of yoga interventions for anxiety reduction among children and adolescents. *American Journal of Occupational Therapy*, 69(6), 1–9.

Yoga Alliance, Children's Yoga Standards, accessed 1 May 2018, from https://www.yogaalliance.org/Credentialing/Standards/ChildrensStandards.

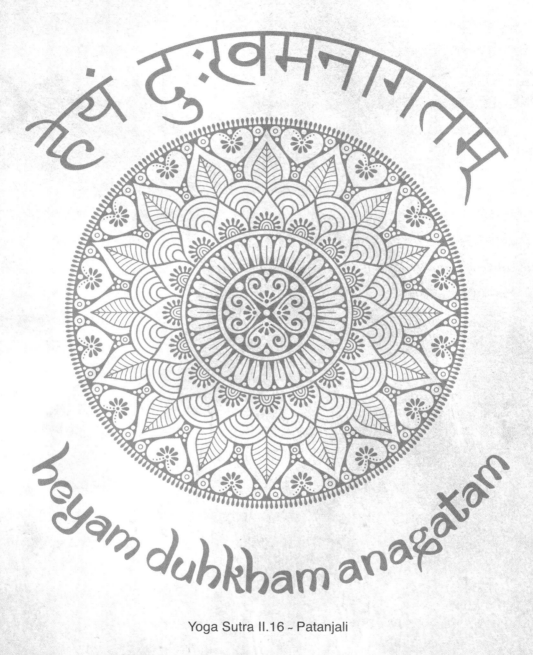

हेयं दुःखमनागतम्

heyam duhkham anagatam

Yoga Sutra II.16 ~ Patanjali

Overview

Current practice in yoga and mental healthcare

As illustrated throughout this book, research, practice, and interest in practicing yoga has grown globally in the last decade. There is evidence of this in both academic and popular literature. For example, according to a survey by the *Yoga Journal* and the Yoga Alliance in 2016, the top three reasons for practicing yoga were enjoyment of yoga itself, its impact on health, and for stress relief (Yoga Alliance, 2016). In Australia, a web-based survey of 2567 respondents found that the top reasons for practicing yoga (including asana, pranayama, meditation, and relaxation) were health and fitness, increased flexibility, and the reduction in stress and/or anxiety. Interestingly, 58.4% gave stress and anxiety reduction as a reason for starting yoga, and 79.4% cited this as a reason for continuing to practice yoga; 29% began yoga for personal development, which increased to 59% as a reason to continue practicing (Seattle Yoga News, 2018).

As many experts point out, and as this book clearly expresses, yoga has an inherent mental health benefit because, among its other effects, regular practice of yoga helps to balance the autonomic nervous system, enhance connection with self and others, and to find meaning and purpose in life. However, it is increasingly recognized that certain types of practices are beneficial for some conditions and under some circumstances for some people, and conversely some practices are contraindicated. Each chapter in this book has reviewed the current state of the research on the mental health conditions being described. This contributes greatly to a more nuanced understanding of how to specifically apply yoga in mental healthcare. Practices from yoga as a stand-alone mental health intervention and as an adjunct to psychotherapy are comprehensively described. The body of evidence presented here suggests that yoga has a place in preventing and treating mental illness and enhancing mental health and wellbeing, a notion that is being embraced across several fields of intervention including clinical psychology, mental health counseling, addiction treatment, education, and positive psychology.

Yoga and community mental health

Yoga, as a comprehensive system of mind-body practices, has evolved as a therapeutic orientation that can be applied to mental healthcare by virtue of the common factors detailed in this book. As well as being one of the main reasons that people practice yoga, mental health is one of the most frequently examined topics in yoga research. In addition, research shows that yoga's greatest efficacy is in mental health. If we also include trials that are primarily researching another condition but which also report reductions in stress, elevation in mood, and less fatigue, the corpus of trials that point to mental health benefits is even larger.

> Yoga has an inherent mental health benefit because, among its other effects, regular practice of yoga helps to balance the autonomic nervous system, enhance connection with self and others, and to find meaning and purpose in life.

In addition to reports supporting its efficacy, yoga may have a pioneering role in an alternative health model that is gaining traction in mainstream medicine due to its multifactorial approach. Often referred to as biopsychosocial, this comprehensive and holistic view of mental health sees mind and body as one functional unit that operates in a social and ecological environment. This viewpoint reduces the stigma of mental illness as a biological or personality flaw and supports psychosocial interventions. Many aspects of yoga practice and philosophy dovetail nicely with the biopsychosocial model (for example, the *kosha* model described in Chapter 1), and may support the further integration of yoga into mental healthcare as a tool to positively impact community health. Additionally, patients and clients are given tools that empower them in their mental health self-care, and multiple studies support the feasibility of yoga as an acceptable intervention. As the researcher, Sat Bir Singh Khalsa, stated: "It is acceptable, accessible, cost-effective and encourages self-reliance" (Khalsa, 2013). Furthermore, the international use of yoga in a variety of mental health conditions, along with research evidence from the last few decades to support such an application, "suggests a need to integrate yoga into mental health services" (Gangadhar & Porandla, 2015). One of the drivers for this integration into mental health services is the development of a robust research literature supporting the use of yoga.

Future directions in research

Building the evidence base

The research conducted to date has been valuable in moving the field forward, helping to document the effects of yoga for depression, eating disorders, anxiety, trauma, and other mental health conditions. However, as detailed in each chapter of this book, more research is needed to help us understand more about how and why yoga works, for whom it works, about what works in different circumstances, and, finally, how much of any one particular facet is enough. Furthermore, reviews and meta-analyses of yoga research across the field of mental health and wellbeing consistently point to the need for higher quality research.

Ensuring higher quality research

What we aim to understand is the nature of yoga and its influence in the field of mental health and wellbeing and to minimize or eradicate bias, opinion, belief, or statistical artifacts of study design (e.g., a study showing no benefits from yoga may be due to those participants only practicing yoga for 20 minutes a week or that the measuring methods adopted were poorly designed and therefore could not detect the changes that were actually taking place). Bias may occur because of researchers' own yoga practice, due to which they undertake research with an inclination toward finding positive results, and this must be addressed in future study design. Many yoga studies are underpowered (i.e., there are too few participants). Potentially positive findings may not attain statistical significance, thereby showing a lack of effect, when perhaps for that particular population yoga does indeed offer support and relief, as well as a pathway to wellbeing. Solid methodology can counter these biases and errors.

> Bias may occur because of researchers' own yoga practice, due to which they undertake research with an inclination toward finding positive results, and this must be addressed in future study design.

First, we need an accepted logic model (i.e., a framework or paradigm) detailing the key mechanisms of action and change; mediators (i.e., which mechanisms drive intervention effects); moderators (e.g., which participants will benefit the most or the least from yoga); and outcomes, as well as increased methodological rigor across studies exploring various aspects of the models of change (Da Silva, Ravindran, & Ravindran, 2009; Gard, Noggle, Park, Vago, & Wilson, 2014; Kirkwood, Rampes, Tuffrey, Richardson, & Pilkington, 2005). Furthermore, as described chapter to chapter, each area of mental health may have its own set of mechanisms that play a role in vulnerability and healing. It is not likely to be a one-size-fits-all scenario.

Second, we need a better understanding of the most effective ways to implement yoga, the role of standardization of yoga protocols, and whether specific yoga components (e.g., breath and asana) are more effective for specific concerns or if a comprehensive protocol would be best. The Essential Properties of Yoga Questionnaire (EPYQ) developed by Park et al. (2018) was designed to specifically address these questions (see p. 197).

Third, we need to know how yoga measures up against other effective mental health treatments and its use as an adjunct therapy alongside best practice protocols. The implications of this are wide-ranging, affecting reimbursement for services, access to yoga, the acceptability of yoga, and sustainability of the field. Many yoga therapists and teachers would like yoga to be a reimbursable service when utilized for those with physical and mental symptoms: this would help make yoga affordable and accessible to individuals across a wider range of socioeconomic strata. In this regard, a solid body of empirical support increases the accessibility of yoga as a valid practice for seeking and maintaining mental health and wellbeing, as well as the designing of safe and effective protocols for different mental health conditions.

Finally, sustainability of the field is enhanced by a body of empirical evidence supporting health insurance reimbursements, sustainable careers for yoga teachers and therapists, and the long-term acceptance of yoga as a valid means of access to mental health and wellbeing.

Modeling the key mechanisms of change

Researchers and theorists in the field of yoga, mental health, and wellbeing are getting closer to detailing the mechanisms that mediate some of the therapeutic benefits of yoga. The work presented here builds on years of theory and research. Rudimentary to this process is detailing the logic (or change) model. Fortunately, this is becoming standard practice, and the

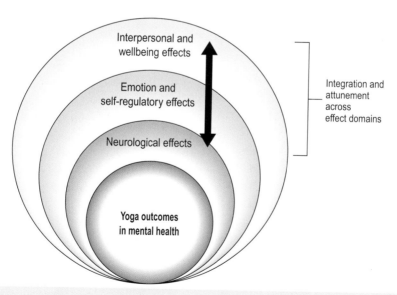

Figure 10.1

Model of change in yoga. Redrawn with permission from Catherine Cook-Cottone majority of recent research papers examining yoga for mental health and wellbeing routinely present their findings as logic (or change) models. These models of change (see Figure 10.1) are grouped into four categories: (1) neurological effects (i.e., changes at the genetic, neurotransmission, neurophysiological and neuroanatomical levels), (2) emotion and self-regulatory effects, (3) interpersonal and wellbeing effects, and (4) integration and attunement across domains of experience.

Some theorists and researchers argue for the theoretical framework to come from yoga philosophy as a way of shedding new light on the psychological mechanisms behind yoga interventions (e.g., Hendriks, de Jong, & Cramer, 2017). For example, Hendriks et al. (2017) suggest that perhaps, as stated in the Yoga Sutras of Patanjali, yoga is intended to address the fluctuations of the mind as in worrying, rumination, or mental activity. Another more complex illustration of a theoretical model that is aligned with yoga philosophy can be found in recent work by Sullivan et al. (2018), in which the yoga therapy approach is integrated with polyvagal theory (PVT); in their study, the authors explicate a framework for yoga-based practices focusing on the integration of bottom-up neurophysiological and top-down neurocognitive mechanisms. The authors propose a model of yoga therapy that converges with PVT in which the PVT is conceptualized as a neurophysiological counterpart to the yogic concept of the *gunas* (i.e., qualities of nature). They posit that the gunas provide a foundation from which behavioral, emotional, and physical attributes emerge in ways that are similar to the neural platforms detailed in PVT. This enables yoga therapy's promotion of physical, mental, and emotional wellbeing to be viewed through the PVT translational lens and to operate as a distinct practice rather than compelling yoga therapy to fit into an outside model in order to be used in clinical settings or for research.

Future directions in yoga for mental health and wellbeing will continue to explore the change model showing how and why yoga works and also how and why it works across different areas of mental health. As well-designed and well-executed research studies are conducted, the change model can be assessed, reworked, and then reassessed in the ongoing process of moving the field forward. In their meta-review of yoga programs for trauma and related mental health problems, Macy, Jones, Graham, and Roach (2015) note the complexities of conducting rigorous, randomized research on yoga. There are many factors that come into play when researchers are conducting studies in the field of yoga, mental health, and wellbeing (e.g., participant recruitment, participant dropout, diagnostic challenges, compliance with standard care during the research trial, mental health treatment trajectories, and funding).

Comparing yoga with known effective treatments

A critical area is comparing yoga interventions to already established mental health interventions (e.g., CBT) and assessing the effectiveness of (1) yoga on its own, (2) treatment as usual (TAU) on its own, and (3) yoga and TAU. In some cases, for example in clinical-level eating disorders, yoga alone may not be feasible because other forms of primary treatment are a vital component of healing, and delaying this treatment to enable it to be compared with yoga alone may place patients (in the yoga alone group) at risk. In cases like these, comparing TAU to yoga and TAU may be sufficient, as carried out by Carei, Fyfe-Johnson, Beruner, and Brown (2010) in an RCT of yoga for the treatment of eating disorders. The serum cortisol and brain-derived neurotrophic factor (BDNF) study conducted by Naveen et al. (2016) is a good example of comparing yoga, medication, and yoga with medication. Non-inferiority trials—those which show that a particular treatment works just as well as currently accepted treatments—are another interesting approach not yet widely embraced by the yoga and mental health field. Positive results may indicate good news for yoga interventions, for example, the treatment of choice may have unwanted side effects or be more costly than yoga. We can learn from study designs in the area of physical health. For example, a study by Saper et al. (2017) randomly assigned individuals with lower back pain to yoga and physical therapy (PT). The yoga group did no better than the PT group; however, instead of stating that yoga did not work because it was no better than PT, the researchers reframed the yoga comparison study as a noninferiority trial: that is, the yoga does not need to work more effectively than PT, only simply as well as PT, which it did and with a proportionally smaller drop-out rate.

The challenge of the standardized protocol

The field of mindfulness has benefited from extensive study of standardized protocols. This is most clearly illustrated by the large body of research on Mindfulness-Based Stress Reduction (MBSR) and Integrative Restoration (iRest). The MBSR research includes gold-standard meta-analyses of MBSR outcomes for wellbeing, mental health among patients with physical ailments, and effects on cancer patients (Khoury, Sharma, Rush, & Fournier, 2015). The replication of studies across research teams, countries, and areas of physical and mental health is possible because of the well-standardized methodology presented in the MBSR and iRest protocols. They are easily replicable with training available for researchers and practitioners so that the programs can be implemented with integrity. Yoga comes from a rich and diverse tradition from which many schools of yoga have evolved with varying approaches to poses, breath work, relaxation, and meditations. Some schools adhere to a strict set of practices with little variation, applying this set of practices for everyone. Other schools are very client-centered, applying specific techniques prescriptively that vary from person-to-person and session-to-session (as is common in yoga therapy). It is

for these reasons that there has been some resistance to adapting standardized protocols and standardizing client-centered protocols for research.

> Yoga comes from a rich and diverse tradition from which many schools of yoga have evolved with varying approaches to poses, breath work, relaxation, and meditations.

Effective yoga styles and components of yoga

There are two significant challenges in yoga research: the heterogeneity of yoga styles that are practiced and the huge variability in their delivery. Suggesting some commonality or common factors across yoga styles, Cramer, Lauche, Langhorst, and Dobos (2016) found that an analysis of 306 RCTs applying 52 different yoga styles indicated that the proportion of positive outcomes did not differ between yoga styles. Nevertheless, it is generally believed that the heterogeneity across styles makes comparisons across yoga studies difficult if not impossible.

The EPYQ is a recent innovation in the field of yoga research that specifically addresses the challenges of heterogeneity across yoga interventions (Groessl et al., 2015; Park et al., 2018). To develop the EPYQ the authors completed an extensive literature review, conducted focus groups with stakeholders (including a wide variety of yoga teachers and students), compiled a pool of questions and vetted those questions through cognitive interviews, reviewed and coded videos of teachers implementing yoga, and then analyzed all the data. In preliminary findings they identified fourteen factors that show up across styles and practices, including breath work, physicality, postures (active and restorative), *bandhas* (body locks), body awareness, mental and emotional awareness and release, health benefits, individual attention, social aspects, spirituality, meditation and mindfulness, yoga philosophy, and acceptance/

compassion. Yoga researchers can code their yoga interventions across these domains, enabling them to enhance the detail of the specific nature and content of the program being delivered. This is a compelling approach to documenting what has been delivered in a yoga protocol. With a better understanding of what is being emphasized in the yoga sessions and mentioned by the instructor, yoga researchers and interventionists can examine the mechanisms by which yoga improves various aspects of health. This in turn can lead to the design of yoga interventions that are better tailored to people with specific health problems and to individuals.

> Research assessing the effectiveness of yoga on mental health issues and wellness should be carefully documented, reporting specific yoga techniques used and the delivery methods.

To support this field, research assessing the effectiveness of yoga on mental health issues and wellness should be carefully documented, reporting specific yoga techniques used and the delivery methods (Büssing, Michalsen, Khalsa, Telles, & Sherman, 2012; Macy et al., 2015). This includes specific stretches and physical postures, meditation practices, and breath control exercises, as well as how much emphasis was placed on each (Macy et al., 2015). The full protocol, with a breakdown of each session including timings, along with the verbal instructions of the yoga teacher/therapist, should be detailed and accessible for those interested in understanding or replicating the study (Cook-Cottone, 2017). Any intentional philosophical or cognitive themes presented (e.g., choice, empowerment, equanimity) can be standardized, manualized, and detailed with sample teacher statements (Cook-Cottone, 2017). Researchers should report if the yoga program was delivered in an individual or a group setting, and if it was in a group setting, they should specify the size of the group (Macy et al., 2015). Details

of the setting should also be provided (e.g., room size, furniture, mirrors, and access to props).

Researchers should document the number of classes per month/days per month attended, the duration (number of minutes) of each class session, the longitudinal duration of the yoga session (i.e., days, weeks, months, years), home practice frequency and duration, the nature of the contents of each session, adherence to the yoga session, as well as measurement of any other confounding physical, especially mind/body activities and/or practices (Cook-Cottone, 2013; Macy et al., 2015; Ross, Friedmann, Bevans, & Thomas, 2012). Despite the need for guidance in this area, there are still no studies specifically addressing the dosage of yoga, including the amount of home practice (Cook-Cottone, 2013; Ross et al., 2012).

In addition to RCTs conducted within the framework of scientific methodology, another way to clarify the value of different practices would be comprehensive public health studies exploring mental health epidemiology and the role of yoga, as taught in community settings for the development and maintenance of mental health and wellbeing. Research could also be conducted that includes the participation of local stakeholders to help understand the specific needs in their communities and how to effectively meet those needs through targeted and relevant yoga programs.

> Research could also be conducted that includes the participation of local stakeholders to help understand the specific needs in their communities and how to effectively meet those needs through targeted and relevant yoga programs.

Qualities of the teacher/therapist

The qualities of the yoga teacher/therapist play a substantial role in the effectiveness of yoga interventions.

However, this area of research has yet to be studied. The key criteria to consider are the teacher/therapist's personal yoga practice and its duration, training and certification (in yoga and in mental health interventions), lineage and the fit of training and lineage with the protocol being delivered, the ability to create and maintain a therapeutic alliance, experience of working with individuals with the mental health issues being studied, their ability to take feedback, and warmth (Cook-Cottone, 2015, 2017; Macy et al., 2015). Also, the teacher/therapist's own relationship with yoga is of critical importance. Despite detailed descriptions of the MBSR protocol (i.e., "an established mindfulness meditation practice" and a "mindful movement practice"—mbpti.org), the qualities of teachers have been largely ignored in yoga literature (Cook-Cottone, 2015, 2017).

Therapeutic alliance

The therapeutic alliance refers to the relationship between those individual(s) providing the intervention and the patient(s)/participant(s) receiving the intervention. In a large, frequently cited, meta-analysis of studies in the field of psychology, Martin, Garske, and Davis (2000) found that the therapeutic alliance has a moderate, but consistent, relationship with patient outcomes. The importance of the therapeutic alliance has been established in the field of psychological intervention for mental health (Thompson & McCabe, 2012) and for physical rehabilitation (Hall, Ferreira, Maher, Latimer, & Ferreira, 2016). Despite the substantial role of the yoga teacher/therapist in the delivery of the yoga intervention, there are only infrequent mentions of the importance of the student/teacher relationship in the practical literature (Khanna & Greeson, 2013).

Unanswered questions

Despite all of the progress in the field, several questions remain to be answered in order to understand and establish the value of yoga for mental health and wellbeing (see Table 10.1). For example, does specific training lead to better outcomes, and does the yoga teacher-student alliance matter? What is the role of spirituality and how does it impact mental health and wellbeing outcomes (Weber & Pargament, 2014)? Can and should content be delivered in a secular manner to increase access? Could the introduction of yoga philosophy help construct logic models which directly address spirituality?

Potential research topics, qualitative and prospective studies

There are other research topics still to be explored, including aspects of yoga not yet addressed in the research (see Table 10.1). These include matters of methodology (e.g., randomization), the qualities of the teacher/therapist, dosage, and the therapeutic alliance.

There is a need for larger studies producing more data, with greater assessment of previous and current yoga-practicing participants. More qualitative studies—exploratory studies using interviews and observations—would reveal what individuals struggling with mental health challenges (e.g., trauma, depression, anxiety, and substance use) are seeking to gain when practicing yoga, potentially broadening current theories of change and future logic models. Prospective studies—observing the development of disease among a group of people over time—could assess risk and recovery by following cohorts of individuals as they engage in yoga practice over an extended period.

Reporting

The field of yoga research could benefit from more rigor when reporting the yoga protocols used in RCTs (see Table 10.1). This includes the diagnostic criteria used and the training of those who completed the diagnoses, effects size reporting, and collecting established

Table 10.1

Future directions for research in yoga for mental health and wellbeing

Topics to explore
• Do specific yoga teacher trainings and workshops in yoga for depression, anxiety, eating, disorders, and trauma yield more effective yoga interventions?
• The importance of the therapeutic, student/teacher alliance
• Are researchers examining what practitioners intend to achieve in yoga? More qualitative studies are necessary to ground empirical approaches into the experiences of practitioners
• The role of yoga in steadying the fluctuations in the mind (as stated in the yoga sutras) by measuring mental activities such as ruminations and worrying
• Study outcomes linked to yoga philosophy such as moksha (meaning), ananda (bliss, happiness), buddhi (wisdom), or kaivalya (detachment) (Hendriks, de Jong, & Cramer, 2017, p. 514)
• The role of spirituality and seeking spirituality in yoga outcomes in mental health and wellbeing
• Can yoga for mental health and wellbeing be simultaneously secular and spiritual?
• The influence of researchers' personal yoga practices on study outcomes
• Research into positive outcomes (i.e., more than simply the absence of mental illness) as well as negative outcomes
• Continuation of work documenting the neurophysiological effects of yoga, especially in fields where this work is critical for credibility (e.g., ADHD, depression, eating disorders)
• Commitments to replicating and extending existing research
Methodology
• Conduct a-priori sample-size calculations and power analyses to avoid under-powering studies
• Include more participants of lower socioeconomic status
• Intentionally study yoga approaches among diverse participants
• Recruit sufficient numbers of participants to study group size and different components of yoga
• Study participants' affinity for yoga as a moderator of effects
• Include comparison and active control groups
• Explore the most appropriate active control groups for mental health and wellbeing studies
• Assess previous yoga experience (and experience with other mind-body practices)
• Collaborate with yoga teachers/therapists when detailing logic models and developing study design
• Study asana (postures) on their own without including meditation or seated breathwork, to explore the unique effect of the physical practice
• Study prescriptive yoga approaches for mental health concerns (e.g., specific pranayama, mantra, and mudras for depression)
• Use designs from epidemiology (e.g., large prospective studies), education (e.g., participant action research), and program evaluation

Table 10.1 Continued

Methodology
• Compare long-term practitioners to newer practitioners across key outcomes
• Study the effects of adopting a home practice
• Empirically study yoga dosage across mental health and wellbeing issues and populations
• Integrate longitudinal studies with long-term follow-ups at three, six, and twelve months built into the study design
• Reporting requirements
• Make full and detailed protocols of yoga intervention available online
• Describe diagnostic criteria and methodology for diagnoses, including the training of those doing the diagnoses
• Measure important participant characteristics such as age, sex, and key study variables at baseline for intervention, comparison, and control groups
• Record effect sizes
• Yoga RCTs should follow accepted reporting guidelines (i.e., Consolidated Standards of Reporting Trials [www.consort-statement.org])
• Assess the influence of adherence to the intervention and treatment integrity
• Conduct and report intent-to-treat analysis
• Include safety issues (i.e., safety report), special concerns identified, dropouts due to side effects or injuries, and other adverse events
• Include any found contraindications in recommendations

guidelines for conducting clinical trials (see www. consort-statement.org).

Yoga and mental healthcare: Future directions for providers

Broader applications of yoga

The overarching theme of this book is that yoga has the potential to benefit a wide range of mental health issues. According to Khalsa (2013), even just a decade ago it would have been surprising to find yoga recommended for conditions such as schizophrenia, ADHD, and trauma; most research is focused on depression and anxiety, and yet, as demonstrated in this book, a growing body of research supports (with qualifications) the use of yoga as an adjunct therapy for such mental health concerns. There is also increasing support for the use of yoga with youth, particularly in schools and the juvenile justice system. Several authors in this book have recognized the need to conduct more research into the social aspects of yoga practice; more qualitative and long-term research on the specific mechanisms of change; and increased collaboration among mental healthcare providers, researchers, and community practitioners to find best practices in a variety of settings. A growing body of research points to broader applications of yoga, including trauma-informed yoga teaching, expanding the role of psychotherapy to include more somatic yoga practices, and increased recognition that yoga treatments for mental health often need to be tailored to individual circumstances. And, although yoga is generally considered to be safe, several authors have mentioned that there may be harmful effects as a result of inappropriate yoga practice and that adverse effects should be reported in the research literature, as well as increasing the awareness of potential harm.

Licensure, accreditation, oversight, and supervision

In most countries, yoga and yoga therapy are not state-regulated, and there is no restriction on anyone identifying themselves as a yoga teacher or yoga therapist. There are yoga associations that offer voluntary registries for yoga teachers to demonstrate that they have met minimum standards for teaching, such as the Canadian Yoga Alliance, British Wheel of Yoga, Yoga Australia, and Yoga Alliance International of India; both the US-based Yoga Alliance and the International Yoga Federation have worldwide memberships. However, there is no rigorous oversight of practitioners such as government or board regulation, little long-term supervision of yoga teachers/therapists, and few generally established ethical codes of conduct, though the International Association of Yoga Therapists (IAYT) has an ethical code as part of its individual certification (www.iayt.org/page/FinalCodeofEthics). Some yoga teachers/therapists argue that the spiritual discipline of yoga inherently includes ethical precepts, that ethical codes and state or board oversight do not guarantee ethical behavior, and that yoga teaching differs from other healing professions because it is a spiritual tradition that inherently precludes regulation. However, others believe that this position will hinder the integration of yoga into a field that requires recognizable credentials, long-term supervision before licensure, and state and board accountability in most countries.

To address such concerns, The British Wheel of Yoga has recently launched an effort to provide more oversight, and the Yoga Alliance have started using a social credentialing system to encourage accountability. The IAYT has developed an accreditation program for schools who train yoga therapists and an individual credentialing program for yoga therapists who meet the minimum standards for IAYT certification. It remains to be seen if this will lead to efforts toward state licensure in the United States. IAYT members from many other countries have accredited training programs and IAYT-certified yoga therapists.

Similarly, there are currently no regulations covering the ability of licensed mental health professionals seeking to incorporate yoga into their clinical practice, although discussions concerning this are ongoing.

Following are some suggestions for providers who offer yoga as a stand-alone mental health practice, as an adjunct practice, or in a clinical setting.

Competencies for yoga teachers/therapists working in mental healthcare

Some yoga teachers/therapists work through specifically integrating into mainstream healthcare systems. As suggested by the body of work presented on this text, this may be the next logical step. However, the form of the process across treatment areas (e.g., depression, eating disorders, anxiety, PTSD) may vary substantially based on the state of research and practice. According to Moonaz, Jeter, and Schmaltzl (2017), research literacy in yoga therapists is lacking and yet it is essential if they desire to collaborate with and integrate into healthcare settings. This is equally true for yoga teachers/therapists who wish to specialize in mental healthcare. Substantial psychological research from the last decade provides teachers/therapists with many studies on mental health treatments to refer to, as well as the continued increase in yoga research to draw from.

For some of the more severe mental health issues such as PTSD, complex trauma, eating disorders, and schizophrenia, researchers and experts agree that yoga should be an adjunct to support psychological treatments. For example, as previously noted, in the field of eating disorders there have been no comparative studies examining yoga on its own without mental health treatment (compared with several studies of yoga as an adjunct intervention). In this case, due to the high mortality rates among those with eating disorders, it would not be ethical to suggest that yoga on its own is a sufficient treatment approach for an individual with an active eating disorder, without them engaging in traditional eating disorder treatment. Accordingly, those in the field of yoga who would like to be involved in the treatment of those with clinical mental illness are advised to appreciate the importance of working within an integrative team. Furthermore, to promote safety, those using yoga with individuals who have acute mental health disorders should keep up to date with the latest research, both in the use of yoga and the mental health disorder being treated. To have an evidence-informed practice, which includes the incorporation of best practices, yoga teachers/therapists need to be able to incorporate research knowledge into their teaching and therapy. As Moonaz et al. (2017) point out, evidence-informed practice incorporates not only research evidence but also "expert opinion … and client values." This means that yoga professionals will still be able to use traditional teachings and their own professional experience, along with the client's collaborative input, to deliver appropriate yoga practices to their clients.

> To promote safety, those using yoga with individuals who have acute mental health disorders should keep up to date with the latest research, both in the use of yoga and the mental health disorder being treated.

Along with the need to understand the research for integration and collaboration with mental health professionals, the increase of yoga's popularity has brought with it an increasing variety of yoga offerings within mainstream society. In addition, a reliance on evidence-based practices among medical and mental health professionals has brought yoga techniques into the clinical domain. As the body of research grows, mental health professionals are delivering these techniques to their clients. Well-informed yoga professionals can offer an important service to the public by understanding and communicating what has, and what has not, been supported by the research literature regarding yoga's efficacy.

Independent yoga teachers/therapists

Some yoga therapists specializing in mental health work as professionals in their own field, rather than integrating into mental healthcare systems. In this case more than a basic knowledge of psychological, psychotherapeutic, and other conditions is necessary, including trauma, psychosis, and personality disorders, as well as the common factors in therapeutic change.

Many clients and students will have pre-existing diagnoses from their mental health or primary care clinicians. Not only will knowledge of these diagnoses inform the yoga therapist as to how those symptoms might impact on yoga protocols in both group and individual settings, but it will also help them use a common language when collaborating with mental health providers, especially in cases of acute or severe disorders. There are many ways that yoga teachers/therapists can educate themselves, from independent study, to shadowing healthcare providers and mental health professionals, to attending formal training.

Ethical considerations

To ensure that ethical boundaries are maintained, a yoga therapist independently working in mental health needs to know and operate within their scope of practice and training, establish a network of referrals with mental health providers, and have a clear understanding of when to refer to those providers. Other considerations include quality control measures such as establishing regular supervision or mentorship, meeting with peers to discuss treatment plans, understanding the rules governing client confidentiality and when these must be broken (e.g. when mandatory reporting is required in the area where they operate), and keeping a list of local emergency and mental health services in the community such as suicide hotlines, readily available for clients.

Mental health clinicians incorporating yoga into clinical practice

Current research shows that yoga appears in general to be a safe intervention (Cramer et al., 2015). Therefore, a variety of simple practices may be used with safety by qualified mental health providers, such as simple breath practices to regulate the nervous system. However, as has been repeatedly emphasized throughout this book, many experts consider it vitally important to match the treatment with the client/student, especially where mental health stability may be an issue of concern. This calls for more training in, for example, some pranayama practices that can powerfully affect the CNS and are contraindicated for certain individuals.

A yoga teacher/therapist often assesses individuals using different criteria to those a mental health professional may use. For example, many yoga teachers/therapists use the *kosha* model (see Chapter 1). A mental health provider will need to be aware of how the different yoga tools can affect each *kosha*, and it may be beneficial for them to be trained in this model before incorporating anything beyond the simplest yoga techniques into clinical practice. Similarly, we recommend caution when incorporating yoga asana into clinical settings without undertaking the appropriate training beforehand.

Therefore, the future of yoga therapy for mental health providers will ideally include training in specialized programs where they can learn skills such as pranayama, meditation, and yoga asana, which can then be incorporated into clinical practice. In addition, we would hope to see more yoga therapy/techniques included in training programs in psychology, psychotherapy and counseling, and medical education. Currently, yoga is incorporated into a few university curricula, for example, at Boston University School of Medicine and in counseling programs at the University of Buffalo, SUNY.

A clinician may also collaborate with a yoga therapist for instruction and to consult about when to refer a client to the yoga therapist. Networking with yoga teachers and therapists to find who has expertise in mental health is good practice.

Although qualified mental health professionals will be familiar with interpreting research, for providers who wish to incorporate yoga into clinical settings in order to offer best practices, they need to remain informed about current yoga research across the areas of mental health.

Practicing new tools

We recommend in particular that anyone—whether a yoga teacher/therapist or a mental health provider—using yoga tools in mental healthcare have an ongoing regular yoga practice and always practice new tools before teaching them to patients.

Referrals and outreach

There is currently a lack of formal procedures for yoga teachers/therapists and mental health providers to refer clients to each other. Perhaps in the future it will be possible for a psychiatrist or psychologist to write a prescription for yoga. One way forward may be the model of social prescribing that has been introduced into the NHS in the UK, whereby physicians can refer patients to group programs that teach and cultivate health-promoting behaviors, supporting the notion of social connection as beneficial to both mental and physical health.

One way forward may be the model of social prescribing that has been introduced into the NHS in the UK, whereby physicians can refer patients to group programs that teach and cultivate health-promoting behaviors.

Both yoga teachers/therapists and mental health providers establish a collaboration by reaching out to each other in local networks. Yoga teachers/therapists can increase their visibility and public knowledge of the specific mental health benefits of yoga by speaking at community centers, educational institutions, at conferences and workshops, and so on. This underscores the importance of research literacy for yoga teachers/therapists, as well as an ability to use medical and psychological language in a way that is appropriate and relevant for the audience they wish to reach. A clear sense of the physiological and psychological mechanisms that underpin yoga's efficacy, as well as having a collection of case studies to report, will serve to scaffold this work.

Another option for incorporating yoga into clinical settings is the treatment team approach. In this situation the yoga teacher/therapist meets with mental healthcare providers and they work collaboratively on treatment plans for specific clients/patients.

Yoga and the wider society

The majority of yoga research has included predominantly white, educated, relatively well-off women, which makes it difficult to apply findings and best practices to the wider society. We must be careful not to impose research findings onto other socioeconomic, ethnic, or marginalized groups. Although research in these underserved areas is sparse, it is increasing. There is a growing trend in the yoga community to reach out and overcome the barriers blocking the access to yoga for these populations.

Conclusion

There has been a global awakening to yoga's value for mental health, driven by the rising incidence of mental health problems, the research literature on yoga's benefits, a need to stem rising healthcare costs in many countries, and the grassroots adoption of yoga for mental health by consumers. As the body of research continues to develop, it will help to inform practice. Research will enhance our understanding of how and why yoga works and the best methods for applying yoga for specific issues and concerns. Despite yoga's ancient heritage, recent research demonstrates that it is a novel and innovative intervention for many current-day issues that rely on surgical, pharmaceutical, or talking remedies. As observed throughout this book, yoga outcomes are often comparable to those from standard treatments but with fewer negative side effects, and yoga also offers additional outcomes such as improved balance, strength, and cognitive and physical flexibility.

Yoga as a comprehensive system for mind and body both stands alone as a treatment tool for promoting mental health and also as a powerful adjunct to clinical psychotherapy.

Yoga as a comprehensive system for mind and body both stands alone as a treatment tool for promoting mental health and also as a powerful adjunct to clinical psychotherapy. Perhaps, however, the most important contribution of yoga to mental healthcare will be in the realm of prevention, by reducing the risk factors for a variety of mental health disorders across modern society. As Sat Bir Singh Khalsa states: "It is clearly more cost-effective and efficacious to prevent mental health diseases, than to treat them once they have manifested as clinically significant conditions" (Khalsa, 2013). Indeed, we can refer back to Patanjali's Yoga Sutras for advice on this topic: *Heyam duhkham anagatam* (YS 11.16) states that we can "prevent the suffering that is yet to come" (Holcombe, 2012) through the practice of yoga.

Yoga's ancient wisdom ultimately points to a way of alleviating mental and emotional suffering at the most fundamental level. Embodiment of yoga principles and lifestyle, with regular and individualized practices, create a foundation for a population healthier in body and mind.

References

Büssing, A., Michalsen, A., Khalsa, S. B. S., Telles, S., & Sherman, K. J. (2012). Effects of yoga on mental and physical health: A short summary of reviews. *Evidence-Based Complementary and Alternative Medicine.* Article publication online.

Carei, T. R., Fyfe-Johnson, A. L., Breuner, C. C., & Brown, M. A. (2010). Randomized controlled clinical trial of yoga in the treatment of eating disorders. *Journal of Adolescent Health, 46,* 346–351.

Cook-Cottone, C. P. (2013). Dosage as a critical variable in yoga therapy research. *International Journal of Yoga Therapy, 23,* 11–12.

Cook-Cottone, C. P. (2015). *Mindfulness and Yoga for Self-Regulation: A Primer for Mental Health Professionals.* New York, NY: Springer Publishing Company.

Cook-Cottone, C. P. (2017). *Mindfulness and Yoga in Schools: A Guide for Teachers and Practitioners.* New York, NY: Springer Publishing Company.

Cramer, H., Lauche, R., Langhorst, J., & Dobos, G. (2016). Is one yoga style better than another? A systematic review of associations of yoga style and conclusions in randomized yoga trials. *Complementary Therapies in Medicine, 25,* 178–187.

Cramer, H., Ward, L., Saper, R., Fishbein, D., Dobos, G., & Lauche, R. (2015). The safety of yoga: A systematic review and meta-analysis of randomized controlled trials. *American Journal of Epidemiology, 182*(4), 281–293.

Da Silva, T. L., Ravindran, L. N., & Ravindran, A. V. (2009). Yoga in the treatment of mood and anxiety disorders: A review. *Asian Journal of Psychiatry, 2,* 6–16.

Gard, T., Noggle, J. J., Park, C. L., Vago, D. R., & Wilson, A. (2014). Potential self-regulatory mechanisms of yoga for psychological health. *Frontiers in Human Neuroscience, 8,* 770.

Gangadhar, B., & Porandla, K. (2015). Yoga and mental health services. *Indian Journal of Psychiatry, 57*(4), 338.

Groessl, E. J., Chopra, D., & Mills, P. J. (2015). An overview of yoga research for health and well-being. *Journal of Yoga & Physical Therapy, 5,* 1.

Groessl, E. J., Maiya, M., Elwy, A. R., Riley, K. E., Sarkin, A. J., Eisen, S. V., Braun, T., Gutierrez, I., Kidane, L., & Park, C. L. (2015). The

Essential Properties of Yoga Questionnaire: Development and methods. *International Journal of Yoga Therapy, 25,* 51–59.

Hall, A. M., Ferreira, P. H., Maher, C. G., Latimer, J., & Ferreira, M. L. (2016). The influence of the therapist-patient relationship on treatment outcome in physical rehabilitation: A systematic review. *Physical Therapy, 90,* 1099–1110.

Hendriks, T., de Jong, J., & Cramer, H. (2017). The effects of yoga on positive mental health among healthy adults: A systematic review and meta-analysis. *The Journal of Alternative and Complementary Medicine, 23,* 505–517.

Holcombe, K. (2012). Life happens: The yoga sutras' take on suffering. Retrieved November 2017 from https://www.yogajournal.com/yoga-101/life-happens

Khalsa, S. B. S. (2013). Yoga for psychiatry and mental health: An ancient practice with modern relevance. *Indian Journal of Psychiatry, 55* (Suppl 3), S334–S336.

Khanna, S., & Greeson, J. M. (2013). A narrative review of yoga and mindfulness as complementary therapies for addiction. *Complementary therapies in medicine, 21,* 244–252.

Khoury, B., Sharma, M., Rush, S. E., & Fournier, C. (2015). Mindfulness-based stress reduction for healthy individuals: A meta-analysis. *Journal of Psychosomatic Research, 78,* 519–528.

Kirkwood, G., Rampes, H., Tuffrey, V., Richardson, J., & Pilkington, K. (2005). Yoga for anxiety: A systematic review of the research evidence. *British Journal of Sports Medicine, 39,* 884–891.

Klatte, R., Pabst, S., Beelmann, A., & Rosendahl, J. (2016). The efficacy of body-oriented yoga in mental disorders: A systematic review and meta-analysis. *Deutsches Ärzteblatt International, 113,* 195.

Lauche, R., Langhorst, J., Lee, M. S., Dobos, G., & Cramer, H. (2016). A systematic review and meta-analysis on the effects of yoga on weight-related outcomes. *Preventive Medicine, 87,* 213–232.

Macy, R. J., Jones, E., Graham, L. M., & Roach, L. (2015). Yoga for trauma and related mental health problems: A meta-review with clinical and service recommendations. *Trauma, Violence & Abuse.* Advance publication online.

Martin, D. J., Garske, J. P., & Davis, M. K. (2000). Relation of the therapeutic alliance with outcome and other variables: A meta-analytic review. *Journal of Consulting and Clinical Psychology, 68,* 438–450.

Moonaz, S., Jeter P., & Schmalzl, L. (2017). The importance of research literacy for yoga therapists. *International Journal of Yoga Therapy, 27*(1), 131-133.

Naveen, G. H., Varambally, S., Thirthalli, J., Rao, M., Christopher, R., & Gangadhar, B. N. (2016). Serum cortisol and BDNF in patients with major depression—effect of yoga. *International Review of Psychiatry, 28,* 273–278.

Park, C., Rani Elwy, A., Maiya, M., Sarkin, A. J., Riley, K. E., Eisen, S. V., Gutierrez, I., Finkelstein-Fox, L., Casteel, D., Braun, T., & Groessl, E. J. (2018). The Essential Properties of Yoga Questionnaire (EPYQ): Psychometric properties. *International Journal of Yoga Therapy.* Advance publication online.

Ross, A., Friedmann, E., Bevans, M., & Thomas, S. (2012). Frequency of yoga practice predicts health: Results of a national survey of yoga practice. *Evidence-based Complementary and Alternative Medicine*. Article publication online.

Saper, R. B., Lemaster, C., Delitto, A., Sherman, K. J., Herman, P. M., Sadikova, E., Stevans, J., Keosaian, J. E., Cerrada, C. J, Femia, A. L., Roseen, E. J., Gardiner, P., Barnett, K. G, Faulkner, C., & Weinberg, J. (2017). Yoga, physical therapy, or education for chronic low back pain: A randomized noninferiority trial. *Annals of Internal Medicine, 167*, 85–94.

Seattle Yoga News (2018). *Yoga in America 2016*. Retrieved from https://seattleyoganews.com/yoga-in-america-2016-statistics/.

Sullivan, M. B., Erb, M., Schmalzl, L., Moonaz, S., Noggle Taylor, J., & Porges, S. W. (2018). Yoga therapy and polyvagal theory: The convergence of traditional wisdom and contemporary neuroscience for self-regulation and resilience. *Frontiers in Human Neuroscience, 12,* 67.

Thompson, L., & McCabe, R. (2012). The effect of clinician-patient alliance and communication on treatment adherence in mental health care: A systematic review. *BMC Psychiatry, 12,* 87.

Weber, S. R., & Pargament, K. I. (2014). The role of religion and spirituality in mental health. *Current Opinion in Psychiatry, 27,* 358–363.

Yoga Alliance (2016, January 13). 2016 Yoga in America study conducted by Yoga Journal and Yoga Alliance reveals growth and benefits of the practice. [Press Release] Retrieved from https://www.yogaalliance.org/Contact_Us/Media_Inquiries/2016_Yoga_in_America_Study_Conducted_by_Yoga_Journal_and_Yoga_Alliance_Reveals_Growth_and_Benefits_of_the_Practice.

INDEX